CAMBRIDGE LIBRARY COLLECTION

Books of enduring scholarly value

History of Medicine

It is sobering to realise that as recently as the year in which On the Origin of Species was published, learned opinion was that diseases such as typhus and cholera were spread by a 'miasma', and suggestions that doctors should wash their hands before examining patients were greeted with mockery by the profession. The Cambridge Library Collection reissues milestone publications in the history of Western medicine as well as studies of other medical traditions. Its coverage ranges from Galen on anatomical procedures to Florence Nightingale's common-sense advice to nurses, and includes early research into genetics and mental health, colonial reports on tropical diseases, documents on public health and military medicine, and publications on spa culture and medicinal plants.

Manual of Lunacy

A controversial psychiatrist, Lyttleton Stewart Forbes Winslow (1844–1913) grew up around the lunatic asylums run by his father, Forbes B. Winslow, who was a specialist in the treatment of mental illness, establishing also medical grounds for the plea of insanity in criminal defence. Lyttleton spent much of his own medical career attempting to show the courts that crime and alcoholism were linked to mental illness, though he later gained notoriety for his amateur detective work: he claimed to know the identity of Jack the Ripper. Published in 1874, this book examines, often through case descriptions, the legal framework within which the mentally ill were managed, and comparisons are made with the status quo elsewhere in the world. It is an enlightening but often disturbing insight into the institutional treatment of mental illness in the late nineteenth century.

T0188079

Cambridge University Press has long been a pioneer in the reissuing of out-of-print titles from its own backlist, producing digital reprints of books that are still sought after by scholars and students but could not be reprinted economically using traditional technology. The Cambridge Library Collection extends this activity to a wider range of books which are still of importance to researchers and professionals, either for the source material they contain, or as landmarks in the history of their academic discipline.

Drawing from the world-renowned collections in the Cambridge University Library and other partner libraries, and guided by the advice of experts in each subject area, Cambridge University Press is using state-of-the-art scanning machines in its own Printing House to capture the content of each book selected for inclusion. The files are processed to give a consistently clear, crisp image, and the books finished to the high quality standard for which the Press is recognised around the world. The latest print-on-demand technology ensures that the books will remain available indefinitely, and that orders for single or multiple copies can quickly be supplied.

The Cambridge Library Collection brings back to life books of enduring scholarly value (including out-of-copyright works originally issued by other publishers) across a wide range of disciplines in the humanities and social sciences and in science and technology.

Manual of Lunacy

*A Handbook Relating to the Legal Care
and Treatment of the Insane in the Public
and Private Asylums of Great Britain, Ireland,
United States of America, and the Continent*

Lyttleton S. Winslow

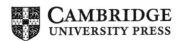

CAMBRIDGE
UNIVERSITY PRESS

CAMBRIDGE
UNIVERSITY PRESS

University Printing House, Cambridge, CB2 8BS, United Kingdom

Published in the United States of America by Cambridge University Press, New York

Cambridge University Press is part of the University of Cambridge.
It furthers the University's mission by disseminating knowledge in the pursuit of
education, learning and research at the highest international levels of excellence.

www.cambridge.org
Information on this title: www.cambridge.org/9781108063494

© in this compilation Cambridge University Press 2014

This edition first published 1874
This digitally printed version 2014

ISBN 978-1-108-06349-4 Paperback

A HANDBOOK

RELATING TO THE

LEGAL CARE AND TREATMENT OF THE INSANE.

MANUAL OF LUNACY:

A HANDBOOK

RELATING TO THE

LEGAL CARE AND TREATMENT OF THE INSANE

IN THE PUBLIC AND PRIVATE
ASYLUMS OF GREAT BRITAIN, IRELAND, UNITED STATES OF
AMERICA, AND THE CONTINENT.

BY

LYTTLETON S. WINSLOW, M.B. & M.L. Cantab.,
M.R.C.P. Lònd., D.C.L. Oxon.

WITH A PREFACE
BY
FORBES WINSLOW, M.D., D.C.L. Oxon.
ETC. ETC.

LONDON:
SMITH, ELDER, & CO., 15 WATERLOO PLACE.
1874.

TO

HER MAJESTY'S

COMMISSIONERS IN LUNACY

𝕿𝖍𝖎𝖘 𝖂𝖔𝖗𝖐 𝖎𝖘 𝕽𝖊𝖘𝖕𝖊𝖈𝖙𝖋𝖚𝖑𝖑𝖞 𝕯𝖊𝖉𝖎𝖈𝖆𝖙𝖊𝖉

BY THEIR OBEDIENT SERVANT

THE AUTHOR.

communicated with the most distinguished continental *alienists*, as well as with the lunacy officials of Scotland and Ireland, and they have kindly placed at his disposal much valuable information relative to the laws regulating the confinement of the insane in their respective countries, which has been embodied in these pages.

He hopes that this volume will fill a gap existing in medico-psychological literature. No medical practitioner having access to it can for the future plead ignorance of the law as an excuse for its violation, as he will find here clearly specified everything that he is required to know in regard to the legal confinement of persons (paupers as well as others) alleged to be of unsound mind, not only in licensed, but unlicensed, houses as "single patients."

The author has also drawn attention to the documents the physician is required to arrange and sign, in conformity with the provisions of the Lunacy Acts, previously to, and after, placing a patient under restraint. Instructions are also given for drawing up the official records necessary to be kept by the resident medical or non-resident medical officer of an asylum, and suggestions are made as to the mode of signing the medical certificates, order, and statement, authorising the use of restraint, and of filling up the reports it is obligatory for the medical officer to make for the inspection of those appointed by the government to visit asylums, and to report as to their condition.

But, what is of more importance to the busy prac-

titioner (who, in moments of difficulty, may have
no authoritative work at hand to consult, and no
experienced legal friend on the spot to whom he may
apply for information), he will find pointed out in
this volume the rocks and dangerous quicksands to
be avoided; in other words, he can easily ascertain
what he may, and may not, do in reference to the
confinement and detention of persons alleged to be
mentally unsound, and fit subjects for surveillance.

The "pains and penalties" to which he makes
himself liable for any infraction of the lunacy laws
are here distinctly detailed, so that he who runs
may read and understand his responsible duties
when called upon to assist in temporarily curtailing
the liberty of a person on the plea of his being mis-
chievously insane, and consequently unfit to be at
large, govern himself, or to manage his own affairs.

The reader will also find in this manual valuable
statistical facts relating to the insane in this and
other countries, with an account of the principal
asylums, public and private, the names of the proprietors, resident and consulting medical officers, and
information with regard to the scale of charges for
the maintenance of the patients, as well as instructions for obtaining ready admission for these afflicted
persons, should it be necessary to place them under
"care and treatment" in asylums specially or-
ganised for their reception.

The author has analysed the Acts of Parliament
that refer to Commissions of Lunacy and Chancery
patients, and briefly indicated the course to be

pursued should it be necessary to petition the Lord Chancellor to issue a writ *De Lunatico Inquirendo,* in order to enable the Court to protect and administer the property of insane persons.

In the final chapter are delineated the characteristic symptoms of the various phases of insanity, which the physician has to describe when certifying to a person's mental derangement prior to his being placed under restraint, with a short explanation of the nosological terms representative of particular types of insanity which he will be required to define, when giving evidence in a court of law as to the existence of the unsoundness of mind of persons accused of crime, or alleged to be deficient in testamentary capacity.

I wish to add two or three words in conclusion. I offer no apology for saying, what the diffidence of the author would obviously preclude him from stating, that he has brought to the composition of this work a considerable amount of knowledge acquired from a careful study of the literature of insanity, as well as valuable practical experience regarding the laws regulating asylums and the confinement of insane persons, from his having resided for several years in my establishment at Hammersmith, and taken an active part in its management.

FORBES WINSLOW, M.D.

CAVENDISH SQUARE:
October 1873.

CONTENTS.

CHAPTER VIII.

COMMISSIONS IN LUNACY AND CHANCERY LUNATICS.

CHAPTER IX.

ST. LUKE'S AND BETHLEHEM HOSPITALS FOR LUNATICS.

CHAPTER X.

LIABILITIES INCURRED BY THOSE CONCERNED IN THE CONFINEMENT OF PERSONS ALLEGED TO BE INSANE.

CHAPTER XV.

LUNACY IN GERMANY.

CHAPTER XVI.

LUNACY IN UNITED STATES OF AMERICA.

CHAPTER XVII.

LUNACY IN RUSSIA.

CHAPTER XVIII.

RECENT LUNACY STATISTICS AND INSTRUCTIONS.

CHAPTER XIX.

DEFINITIONS AND EXPLANATIONS OF TERMS.

APPENDICES.

LUNACY ACT, 1845, 8 AND 9 VICT. C. 100.

Appointment of Commissioners in Lunacy—Particulars relative to the Commissioners in Lunacy—Secretary to Commissioners—Appointment of Clerks—Oath taken by Commissioners—Jurisdiction of Commissioners—Licences—Special Meetings of Commissioners —Visitor of Asylums beyond the Jurisdiction of the Commissioners in Lunacy—No Commissioner, Visitor, or Secretary to act as such if interested within one Year in a Licensed House—Alteration of Asylum—Notice to be given to the Commissioners—Licences granted by Justices—Renewal of Licence, what to contain—Licence to be made out in a given Form—Charge for Licence—Annual Accounts made out by Secretary of Commissioners and Clerk of the Peace—Provision when the Person licensed is dead or incapacitated—Provision when Licensed House is rendered unfit by Fire or otherwise—Revocation of Licence—Hospitals containing Lunatics to have Printed Regulations and Medical Attendant—Licence required for two, or more than two, Patients—Book of Admissions—Notice of Admission of Patient sent to the Commissioners—Notice of Escape sent to Commissioners—Statement of Death sent to Commissioners—Ill-treatment of Lunatics—Residence of Medical Officers in Licensed Houses—Medical Visitation Book in Licensed Houses—Case Book—Visitation of Licensed Houses by the Commissioners—Licensed Houses beyond the Jurisdiction of the Commissioners inspected by Visitors—Commissioners at Visitation to examine House and all Lunatics therein confined—Enquiries made by Commissioners at their Visitation—Official Books placed before Commissioners—Visitor's Book—Patient's Book—Copy of Official Entries transmitted to Board—Doubtful Cases to be mentioned in Patients' Book — Visiting Commissioners' Report to Commissioners in Lunacy of Houses not within the immediate Jurisdiction of the latter—Power of Commissioners to make Rules—Visitation of Asylums by Night—Who may authorise the Discharge of a Patient from an Asylum—Dis-

II. LUNACY ACT, 1853, 16 & 17 Vict. c. 96.

III. LUNACY ACTS AMENDMENT ACT, 1862, 25 & 26 Vict. c. 111.

The Author will be obliged to any of his readers if they will have the kindness to point out any errors into which he may have fallen in preparing this volume for the press, or to forward him any important information relative to the subject matter of this work, which, if used, he will be happy to acknowledge and embody in subsequent editions.

SUSSEX HOUSE, HAMMERSMITH, W.:
November 1873.

MANUAL OF LUNACY.

CHAPTER I.

HISTORY OF LUNACY LEGISLATION.

I PROPOSE in this chapter briefly to sketch the progress made in lunacy legislation from the earliest period in which we have any record of statutory enactments for the protection of the insane.

The recognition of insanity by the ancients is clearly established. Our Classical writers, who lived many years before Christ, frequently allude to the subject. *Recognition of madness by the ancients.*

Repeated reference is made in the Bible to persons mentally afflicted.

The madness of Saul may be mentioned as one of the first instances of mental disease that we possess. David was supposed to have subdued by music his attacks of maniacal fury. *The madness of Saul, one of the first allusions to insanity.*

David, who reigned from 1055 to 1015 B.C., feigned madness, and in the first book of Samuel (chap. xxi.) we find this simulation alluded to as follows :—" Then said Achish unto his servants, Lo, ye see the man is mad: wherefore then have ye brought him to me? Have I need of madmen, that ye have brought this *fellow* to play the madman in my presence? Shall this fellow come into my house?" *David's feigned madness mentioned in the Bible 1055 B.C.*

Notwithstanding the constant allusions to madness

B

among the ancients, we do not meet with any account in the writings of that period of hospitals appropriated to the insane, or of any legislative enactments for their protection.

The first institution for the insane was established in the East. In the year 491 one existed at Jerusalem.

In the twelfth century, Benjamin of Tudela mentions there was a large edifice at Bagdad, called "*Dal Almeraphtan*" or "House of Grace." In this building all persons of unsound mind were received in summer, and kept confined in chains until they recovered.

This establishment was visited by the magistrates every month, whose duty was to examine the state of the patients, and to discharge those who had recovered.

In the same century, the Emperor Alexius founded hospitals for the insane. Asylums were common among the Moors. About thirty years ago there was at Fez, the holy city of the empire of Morocco, a *Muriston*, or Asylum, in which the poor patients were chained, and treated as cruelly as lunatics were in the *Timarahane* at Constantinople during the sixteenth century.

Under the feudal system in this country, when lands were held under military tenure, subject to military services, when the vassal was rendered incapable of performing such duties, the lord seized upon his rents and profits; this custom applied to all idiots and infants.

The lawless and violent practices of the ancient barons made it reasonable to suppose, that in consequence of the spoliation and waste that constantly occurred in the property of lunatics, the Legislature was induced to place them under the immediate protection of the Crown; but the exact period at which this change was effected is unknown, and we do not even know by what statute the King first acquired this jurisdiction. It appears to have had no existence in the time of John, as no allusion to any prerogative of this nature can be found in Magna Charta; and Bracton, who wrote in the reign of Henry III., does not mention it.

We are informed by Fleta that certain persons called *Tutores* used to have the custody of the lands *idiotarum et stultorum*, and he states that in consequence of an abuse of their trust, a statute was made in the reign of Edward I., 1272, by which " the custody of the persons and the inheritances *idiotarum et stultorum*, being such *a nativitate*, was given to the King, with a reservation to the lord of all his lawful claims for awards, relief, and the like." This statute is not in print, but in the subsequent reign the Act " *De Prærogativa Regis* " was passed, the ninth chapter of which enacts that " the King shall have the custody of the lands of natural fools, taking the profits of them without waste or destruction, and shall find them with necessaries, of whose fee soever the lands be so holden ; and, after the death of such idiots, he shall render it to the right heirs ; so that such idiots shall not alien, nor their heir be disinherited." *(margin: The person and property of the lunatics formerly in the hands of "Tutores.")*

Also, " the King shall provide, when any that beforetime hath had his wit and memory happen to fail of his wit, as there are many *per lucida intervalla*, that their lands and tenements shall be safely kept without waste and destruction, and that they and their household shall be maintained comfortably with the profits of the same ; and the residue shall be kept for their use, to be delivered unto them when they come to be of right mind."

By this it appears, that the duty of protecting all mentally afflicted devolved originally upon the King in his capacity as *parens-patriæ*. *(margin: The King originally considered to be the protector of lunatics)*

We perceive by this brief sketch that the object of the Legislature was to protect the person and property of lunatics, little if any attention being given to their medical or moral treatment. We have abundant evidence, that before asylums were founded, lunatics were *(margin: Lunatics subjected to cruelties in the olden time.)*

treated with great cruelty. They were frequently cast into prison, and their delusions, from a misconception of their nature, punished with death.

Anecdote showing the inhuman feeling entertained towards lunatics in 1660.

The prejudice against, or rather the inhuman feeling entertained towards persons mentally afflicted, is curiously illustrated by an anecdote mentioned in the History of the Royal Society :—

In 1660, when experiments were being made in the "transfusion of blood," an account was received by the Society of two experiments made in Paris before the Academy of Sciences, on a youth and on an adult, whose veins were opened and injected with the blood of lambs.

The experiment having succeeded so well, the Royal Society became anxious to perform it in England. Sir George Ent suggested, that it would be advisable to perform this operation upon some mad person at Bethlehem. This proposal having met with the approbation of the Society, Dr. Allen, the medical officer at Bethlehem, was called upon to produce a lunatic for the experiment; he, however, positively refused to grant their request. In Paris, the operation was attempted by M. Denis, but the lunatic during the process died in his arms. Many lunatics in the olden time were burnt for witchcraft, others were confined in dens fit only for wild beasts.

Insanity in the reign of Elizabeth.

During the reign of Elizabeth, we read of the insanity of Arthington, Coppenger, and Hacket. Arthington was under the delusion that Coppenger was a prophet of mercy, and that Hacket was king of Europe : these two were to go before him and separate the sheep from the goats. Arthington was hanged, drawn, and quartered.

We read of another lunatic named Venner, who was under the delusion that all human governments were about to cease, and in consequence of this belief, he proclaimed our Saviour king in the public streets. He was followed by a rabble, who were attacked by the militia. Venner was executed in January, 1660, protesting his belief that Cromwell and Charles II. were Christ's usurpers.*

"Many of these poor creatures had more need to be relieved than chastised; more mete were a preacher to admonish them than a jailer to keep them, and a physician more necessary to helpe them than an executioner or tormentor to hang and burn them." †

The oldest hospital in Europe for the insane is Bethlehem.

In 1247 Simon Fitz-Mary, one of the Sheriffs of London, in consequence of the superstition then existing, was desirous of founding a religious house.

1247. Bethlehem founded as a priory.

By a deed of gift which is still extant, he appropriated all his lands situated in the parish of St Botolph, the spot known as Old Bethlehem, for the foundation of a priory.

The prior, brethren, canons, and sisters, for whose maintenance he provided, were distinguished by a star upon their mantle, and were directed to receive and entertain the Bishop of St. Mary of Bethlehem, the canons, brothers, and messengers of such order, as often as they came to England.

We read nothing more of Bethlehem until 1547, in which year Henry VIII., in abolishing monasteries, seized upon it and presented it to the City of London, with all its revenues, as a residence for lunatics. This was the first asylum established in England; and Lord Ashley, in 1845, previously to introducing into the House of Commons a bill for the protection and care of lunatics, said "that the whole history of the world, until the era of the Reformation, does not afford an instance of a single receptacle assigned to the pro-

1547. Henry VIII. presents Bethlehem to the City of London, to be used as a hospital for the insane; the first institution established in Europe.

* "Biographical History of England," 1784.
† "Discovery of Witchcraft," Scot, 1665.

tection and care of these unhappy sufferers, whose malady was looked upon as hardly within the reach or hope of medical aid.

If dangerous, they were incarcerated in the common prison; if of a certain rank in society, they were shut up in their houses, under the care of appropriate guardians: chains, whips, darkness, and solitude were the approved and only remedies."

At that time Bethlehem was situated in a dark and confined neighbourhood, and was quite inadequate for the purpose for which it was intended. In consequence of either the gradual increase of insanity, or from more attention being paid to this disease, it became necessary to build a new and larger hospital for the reception of lunatics.

In 1644, during the reign of Charles I., it was proposed to enlarge the old building, but the close and confined situation would not allow of the hospital being rendered more commodious. In the reign of Charles II.,

1675. Bethlehem rebuilt at cost of 17,000l., the design taken from Tuileries.

April 1675, in consequence of the meagre accommodation for lunatics, the Lord Mayor, Aldermen, and Common Council of the City allotted to the Governors a large piece of ground, situated near London Wall, on the south side of the lower quarter of Moorfields.

The erection of the new building was completed by July of the following year, at a cost of 17,000l. The hospital afforded accommodation for one hundred and fifty patients.

The design of the hospital was taken from the Tuileries in Paris.

Old rules in Bethlehem for the guidance of attendants.

Rules were framed for the guidance of those who were interested in the welfare and management of the patients confined therein; one of the rules was :—" That no keeper or servant should beat or ill-treat a lunatic, without he considered it absolutely necessary for the better governing of the lunatic."

In 1734, during the reign of George II., two additional wings, capable of receiving one hundred patients incurable of each sex, were added.*

In consequence of the insufficient accommodation for lunatics in 1751, St. Luke's Hospital was founded by voluntary contributions, and Manchester, York, and other large cities built hospitals for the confinement of the insane.

1751.
St. Luke's Hospital built.

The first legislative enactment for the protection of lunatics was made in 1744. The "Vagrant Act" contained a section dealing with persons "furiously mad, or so far mentally disordered as to be dangerous if left at large." By this section two justices of the peace were authorised to issue a warrant for the arrest of any lunatic, who was to be locked up in a secure place, and if it was found necessary, he was to be chained and confined in his own parish, and if in possession of any property, it was to be expended for his maintenance. This clause did not afford any real protection for the insane.

1744.
First legislative enactment passed for the management of the insane.

In 1763 a Committee was appointed by the House of Commons to enquire into the condition of the insane. This Committee confined its investigations to two cardinal points.

1763.
Committee appointed by Parliament to enquire into condition of lunatics.

1st. The manner of admitting patients into houses kept for the reception of lunatics.

2nd. The treatment of them during their confinement.

The chief witnesses who were called were persons who had been surreptitiously enticed away from their homes by relatives under false pretences and placed in asylums.

The evidence of the witnesses examined before this

---

* In 1814 the hospital was pulled down, and the patients transferred to a new building in St. George's Fields, which was enlarged in 1838.

Committee proved, beyond all doubt, that there were many persons illegally confined under the plea of insanity.

The treatment to which they were subjected was harsh in the extreme. They were excluded from all intercourse with the outward world, and many of them were cruelly chained.

Evidence given before Committee. Two keepers of a notorious madhouse stated " that during the six years they had resided in the asylum they had never admitted a single patient of unsound mind into the house, and that the patients received were drunkards and sane people placed there by their friends and treated like lunatics." No medical man visited the asylum, and the inmates received no medical treatment.

Such, then, was the deplorable condition of the insane in 1763, before any legislative measures were proposed by Parliament for the alteration of the law relating to the confinement of persons alleged to be insane.

Resolution adopted by Committee. The Committee of the House of Commons, after examining several witnesses, proposed and adopted the following resolution : " That it is the opinion of this Committee that the present state of madhouses requires the interposition of the Legislature."

1774. First Lunacy Act. The subject of the then existing condition of lunacy having been brought conspicuously before the House of Commons, a discussion arose in the House, but which failed to lead to any immediate results until 1774, in which year was passed the first Act for the regulation of madhouses.

1773. Mr. Townshend introduces the Bill. On February 1, 1773, Mr. Townshend moved the first reading of the bill for the " better regulation of madhouses." He drew the special attention of Parliament to the abuses then existing in these institutions. He said "that the facts which had come to his immediate knowledge were such as would awaken the compassion of the most callous heart," showing that these unhappy creatures were subjected to barbarous treatment which could not be equalled in any other European State.

This motion was seconded by Mr. Mackworth, who stated that " he had written evidence of such character as to shock the most hardened heart. The scenes of distress lie hid in obscure corners, but if gentlemen were once to see them, I am convinced they would not rest a day until a bill for their relief was passed, and for my part I solemnly protest that I will neither mind time nor trouble, but employ every hour until some relief may be obtained."

On February 11, Mr. Townshend moved that the report which was made by the Committee, upon February 22, 1763, appointed to enquire into the state of the private madhouses in this kingdom, might be read.

Leave being given to bring in the bill, Mr. Townshend, in moving the second reading on April 22, 1773, informed the House that he had framed the bill with a view of remedying two evils :—

1st. The incarceration of sane persons in asylums ;
2nd. The barbarous treatment of those admitted.

He told the House that asylums were under no regulations, receiving who and what they pleased ; that the inmates were subjected to no inspection, and received no remedial treatment of any sort ; and that within seven miles of London eighteen of these madhouses could be found in which sane persons were undoubtedly confined.

In his bill he proposed :—

1st. That no person should be received into these institutions without having been first examined by persons nominated by the College of Physicians.

2nd. That the College of Physicians should appoint inspectors to examine into asylums, and personally inspect the persons confined, once or twice annually.

3rd. That the proprietor of an asylum should be

Purport of Mr. Townshend's Bill.

compelled to take out a licence from the said College of Physicians.

The chief object of this bill was to prevent any one being illegally confined as a person of unsound mind, and to protect the interests of those properly placed under restraint.

The bill was then read a second time, and became law on November 20 of that year.

Chief sections in Act.

It prohibited any person taking care of or receiving more than one lunatic into his house, without a licence.

It enacted that five Fellows of the College of Physicians, elected by the President and Members, should be appointed to act as Commissioners, and authorised to visit asylums and grant licences. No person was to act in this capacity for three consecutive years.

An oath was taken by each of these Commissioners not to reveal to the proprietor of the asylum the date of their proposed visit.

The Commissioners met annually on the third Wednesday in October, for the purpose of granting licences.

These licences were made out under the seal of three of the Commissioners, and a specified charge, according to the number of patients, was made.

By this Act, the Commissioners were to examine into the condition of the licensed houses once a year.

It was enacted that the Act of 1774 should continue in force for the term of five years. At the expiration of this time it was deemed advisable to have it renewed for a further period of seven years, the Act becoming perpetual in the 29th year of the reign of George III., 1789.

1813.
Mr. Rose's
Lunacy Act
rejected.

Nothing important in lunacy legislation occurred until 1813. During this year a bill was brought before Parliament for the better regulation of asylums, but in consequence of the opposition the bill received from the House, Mr. Rose, who had proposed the bill, withdrew it.

1814.
Attention of

The attention of the House of Commons was again

drawn to the condition of the insane on April 5, 1814, by Mr. Rose, who narrated to the House some most aggravated cases of persons in these establishments who were of sound mind.

He mentioned the case of a lady who had been placed in an asylum by her husband, who, upon being asked whether he considered his wife mad, replied, "Oh, no! but I consider the place a kind of Bridewell." *

Mr. Rose informed the House that, notwithstanding the other Lunacy Acts which had been passed, it was even then the custom to admit patients without previously enquiring into their state of mind. He drew their attention to the extraordinary fact, that ten years had elapsed before the resolution passed by the Committee in 1763 had been adopted, and that the Act passed in 1774 was found to be quite inadequate to prevent the evil then existing.

After describing to the House the condition of one of these asylums, in which the patients were confined in cells on the ground-floor, nine feet long, the ground wet, and the only furniture consisting of a box which contained straw to be used as a bed, he moved for leave to bring in his bill for the better regulation of private asylums ; the chief purport of his bill being to the effect, that the magistrates in the different counties should periodically visit the private madhouses within their respective counties and report on the subject.

This bill passed the House of Commons, but was ultimately rejected by the House of Lords. The rejection led to a motion being passed for the appointment of

* Edward VI. founded a hospital in the vicinity of St. Bride's well, one of the holy wells of London, situated near St. Bride's Church in Fleet Street. This hospital was afterwards converted into a receptacle for disorderly people. The name of "Bridewell" is constantly given to houses of correction situated in different parts of the country, in consequence of the hospital having been the first institution used for that purpose.

a Committee of the House of Commons to enquire into the management of lunatic asylums in the United Kingdom. The Committee, notwithstanding they were appointed in 1814, did not commence the examination of witnesses until a year afterwards.

1815.
Report of
Committee
brought con-
spicuously
before
House of
Commons.
Conclusions
arrived at
from con-
sideration of
report.

The report of this Committee was brought up before the House by Mr. Rose on July 11, 1815, and contained some most startling and heartrending details. The chief conclusions arrived at were :—

1st. The indisputable necessity for legislative interference.

2nd. That the treatment of lunatics was worse than the treatment of prisoners in gaols.

3rd. That the authorities who were deputed to take care of these unhappy creatures were quite incompetent to do so, in consequence of which, barbarous treatment was frequently resorted to.

4th. The Committee had reason to believe that many lunatics would ultimately recover if the legislative measures were sufficiently stringent, so as to guarantee their proper surveillance and treatment. To further this end, and as proof of this last statement, the report contained an account of a poor insane woman, who, having for some time been chained to the floor in a parish workhouse, disturbed all the other inmates by her cries, and who, on being removed to a proper place of confinement, was by judicious treatment cured in the space of five months.

1815.
Report
ordered to
be printed.
1816.
Committee
of House
again sit.

The report of the Committee having been read before the House, it was ordered to be printed.

This Committee again sat in 1816, and it was found necessary to make a more searching enquiry into the condition of the insane. Most painful disclosures were revealed, and the Committee decided that immediate legislative interference was requisite.

In consequence of this decision of the Committee,

legislative measures were from time to time introduced, but they were all rejected by the House, and it was not till 1828 that any bill was passed relating to the care of the insane.

1828. Lunacy Act of Mr. Gordon passes both Lords and Commons.

It is not proposed to give any abstract of the various bills brought before Parliament between 1816 and 1828, as they were all rejected.

In 1828 Mr. R. Gordon brought in his bill to amend the law for the regulation of lunatic asylums. He called the attention of the House to the report issued by the Committee which had sat during the previous session. The result of the enquiry was such as to fully justify him in bringing in his bill. He drew the attention of Members to the fact that, under the existing defective state of the law, there was nothing to interfere with the incarceration in an asylum of any person possessing a large income, by any one of his friends, relatives, or acquaintances, who from interested motives desired to place him in confinement as a lunatic. He said that the only provision of the law against the illegal confinement of an individual under the plea of insanity was that the keeper of a lunatic asylum could not receive any one as a lunatic without a certificate signed by a physician, surgeon, or apothecary; and he drew the especial attention of the House to the derivation of the term "apothecary," "a seller of drugs," so that any dealer in drugs had the privilege granted to him of signing a certificate and so sending one of his fellow-creatures to an asylum; and not only the apothecary, but the boy in the shop, who was his apprentice, could do the same as soon as his indentures were terminated. Thus the poor ignorant apothecary, possessing no diploma, and, perhaps, never having entered a hospital, might send to an asylum a person perhaps labouring under the delirium of fever, mistaking it for the delirium of insanity.

1828. Mr. Gordon introduces his bill.

Mr. Gordon told the House that it was the business of the Legislature to prevent, as far as possible, the illegal confinement of persons, and all the witnesses examined before the Committee had agreed that some new enactments were necessary to regulate the mode of granting certificates. Passing on to consider the deficiencies in the existing law, he stated to the House that the only regulation in the law for the protection of lunatics had been violated, in consequence of the five Commissioners appointed by the College of Physicians having neglected their duties to visit asylums and patients annually, and report the results of such visits to the College. In conclusion, he told the House "that in Holland, France, Italy, and even in Spain, there were establishments existing for the reception of lunatics, which, to those of this country who had visited them, were the subject of envy and admiration."

1828.
Lord Ashley
seconds the
bill.

The motion was seconded by Lord Ashley, and leave was given to bring in the bill. The chief difference existing between this Act and the one passed in 1774, had special reference to the granting of medical certificates. It was herein ordered that every certificate for a patient's admission was to be signed by two medical men, who had to separately visit and examine the patient, and to state that he was a fit person to be confined in an asylum. The medical men who signed the certificate must have no interest in the asylum, or be connected with it in any way.

1828.
Chief clauses
in Act.

The Act enabled the Commissioners (fifteen in number, and appointed by Government) to revoke or refuse any licence they might think proper.

The person who signed the order for the patient's admission was obliged to visit the patient at least once every six months, and if prevented from doing so, he was to delegate some one to visit in his place.

The Commissioners had power, if they thought

proper, to order the liberation of any person from the asylum.

Every asylum was to be visited at least four times a year by three of the Commissioners.

Notice of discharge or death of a patient was to be given to the Commissioners within three days from the time of such discharge or death.

Notice of the patient's admission had to be sent to the Commissioners within seven days from the date of such admission.

All asylums containing more than one hundred patients were required to have a resident medical officer; if containing a less number of patients, it was requisite for a medical man to visit the asylum three times during the week.

No single patient could be placed under care or treatment without first obtaining two medical certificates and an order, except in the case of a relative, and any person keeping an asylum without a licence was liable to an action for misdemeanour.

We thus see, that before the passing of this Act in 1828, there was no power to punish any infraction of the law, or to refuse, or revoke a licence.

The medical certificate was signed in a very loose way, and one only required, and this frequently signed by an uneducated person, or by the superintendent of the asylum—who was not prohibited from signing in his medical capacity—and under whose care the patient was to be confined.

Licensed houses were only required to be visited once a year, and the proprietor had no power to discharge any person who might have recovered, and no plans of houses were requisite previously to the licence being granted.

No return of single patients was made, and no medical visitation necessary.

1833.
Amendment
Act, chief
alterations.

This Act was amended in 1833 ; the chief alterations were the appointment of Commissioners by the Lord Chancellor, with a much wider jurisdiction, called the "Metropolitan Commissioners," who were to hold quarterly meetings for the purpose of granting licences.

1845.
Lord Ash-
ley's Lunacy
Act, the Act
now in force.

Nothing important occurred in lunacy legislation until 1845, in which year Lord Ashley brought in his celebrated Lunacy Act. This bill was introduced in consequence of an elaborate report presented to the Lord Chancellor by the Commissioners in Lunacy in 1844, giving the result of their enquiries as to the condition of the insane in England and Wales.

This report plainly pointed out the evils then existing in consequence of an insufficient accommodation for pauper lunatics, and directed attention to the evil practices and injurious treatment of patients confined in licensed houses. The report concluded by recommending various suggestions, twenty-five in number, for the amendment of the law.

Lord Ashley, towards the close of the year 1844, brought this report before Parliament, and, in order to show the condition of lunacy even as late as 1844, I will quote the last few lines from the speech of Lord Ashley in introducing his bill.

Lord Ash-
ley's speech
in intro-
ducing his
bill.

"The House possesses the means of applying a real and a speedy remedy. These unhappy persons are outcasts from all the social and domestic affections of private life—nay more, from all its cares and duties, and have no refuge but in the law. You can prevent by the agency you shall appoint, as you have in many instances prevented, the recurrence of frightful cruelties ; you can soothe the days of the incurable, and restore many sufferers to health and usefulness ; for we must not run away with the notion that even the hopelessly mad are dead to all capacity of intellectual or moral exertion. Quite the reverse, their feelings too are painfully active.

I have seen them writhe under supposed contempt, while a word of kindness and respect would kindle their whole countenance into an expression of joy. Their condition appeals to our highest sympathies,

' Majestic in ruin.'

For though there may be in the order of a merciful Providence some compensating dispensation which abates within the horrors manifested without, we must judge alone by what we see; and I trust, therefore, that I shall stand excused, though I have consumed so much of your valuable time, when you call to mind that the motion is made on behalf of the most helpless, if not the most afflicted portion of the human race."

Lord Ashley succeeded in passing his bill in 1845. It contained 114 sections.

The principal Act now in force, with slight amendments in those of 1853 and 1862, is that introduced by Lord Ashley in 1845.

1853-1862.
Amendment
Act.

It is a cause for congratulation that we now have so perfect a law for the protection of lunatics. I speak with some knowledge of this subject, as I have carefully watched its working, in all its details, for some years. Any infringement of it meets with the immediate attention of the Commissioners, who do all in their power to enforce its rigorous fulfilment. A debt of gratitude is due to these gentlemen, who spare neither time nor trouble in promoting the interests of the insane.

The general impression appears to have been, that if the Commissioners appointed under the Act of 1828 had faithfully discharged their duty there would not have been any justification for the merited rebuke which Lord Ashley administered to them when introducing his bill. I have carefully avoided entering into minute details concerning the barbarous treatment to which lunatics were formerly subjected. Had I been desirous of revealing

c

startling and well-authenticated facts, I should have had but little difficulty in awakening a thrill of horror in many an apathetic heart by the narration of the in-human treatment and unnecessary cruelty to which lunatics were exposed before the Legislature took up their cause.

Comparison between the treatment of lunatics previous to and at the time of Lunacy Act 1845.

The insane are no longer treated like wild beasts. Our asylums no longer resemble the Spanish Inquisition, or the hold of a slave ship; the inmates of these institutions are not now exposed to the painful cut of the whip, or chained like felons to the floor of some pestilential dungeon, uncared for, forgotten, there left to drag their miserable life away until death put an end to their frightful sufferings; and, while there, exhibited to the eager inspection of those desiring to satisfy their morbid curiosity.

Gratitude and immortal honour must be given to those who exposed and laid bare these frightful atrocities.

CHAPTER II.

PRESENT STATE OF LUNACY IN ENGLAND AND WALES.

THE Annual Report of the Commissioners in Lunacy is always looked forward to with interest by all engaged in the special study of mental disease, inasmuch as it places before us an official and authentic account of the existing state of lunacy and lunatic asylums throughout England and Wales, and records the history of their progressive improvement under the suggestions which the Commissioners from time to time find it expedient to make.

The last report of the Commissioners in Lunacy, July 1872, presents a variety of very interesting and valuable information on the present state and statistics of insanity throughout England and Wales, and contains much matter for reflection, both in a moral and social aspect. It is shown in the report that on January 1, 1872, there were 58,640 insane persons in England and Wales. This number includes both pauper and private patients. On January 1 of the previous year, the number recorded was 56,755, a difference of 1,885 between the two years.

Besides the number of persons of unsound mind returned on January 1, 1872, there are 170 lunatics found so by inquisition, and residing in charge of their Committees elsewhere than in asylums, hospitals, and licensed houses.

Commissioners' Report, 1872.

58,640 insane persons on Jan. 1, 1872, in England and Wales, being an increase of 1,885 on the previous year.

The table below shows the classification and distribution of the patients.

	Private			Pauper			Total		
	M.	F.	T.	M.	F.	T.	M.	F.	T.
In County and Borough Asylums	138	167	305	13,495	15,841	29,336	13,633	16,008	29,641
In Registered Hospitals	1,104	998	2,102	197	179	376	1,301	1,177	2,478
In Licensed Houses	1,602	1,477	3,079	379	715	1,094	1,981	2,192	4,173
In Naval and Military Hospitals, and Royal India Asylum	380	15	395	—	—	—	380	15	395
In State Criminal Asylum	290	51	341	116	32	148	406	83	489
Private Single Patients	168	252	420	—	—	—	168	252	420
In Workhouses	—	—	—	5,878	7,730	13,608	5,878	7,730	13,608
Out-door Paupers	—	—	—	3,071	4,365	7,436	3,071	4,365	7,436
Total	3,682	2,960	6,642	23,136	28,862	51,998	26,818	31,822	58,640

Probability of Recovery.

Out of the 29,641 patients confined in county and borough asylums, 2,635 only are deemed curable. Out of the 2,478 patients confined in registered hospitals the number deemed curable is 413.

Of 4,173 cases confined in metropolitan and provincial licensed houses the number returned as curable is 527.

All patients maintained in the various State asylums are included among those returned as belonging to the private class, not being chargeable to parishes, unions, counties, or boroughs, with the exception of the 148 pauper patients who are confined in Broadmoor Criminal Asylum.

No reliable statistics of insanity were published until

1844, and upon referring to the statistical table of the Commissioners published in that year, we find that the number of persons of unsound mind was 20,611. First reliable statistics of insanity published in 1844.

On January 1, 1861, out of a population of 20,119,314 there were 38,058 insane persons, making a ratio of 1·91 in every 1,000 of the population, and on January 1, 1871, out of a population of 22,704,108 there were 56,755 insane people, making the ratio of 2·49 in every 1,000 of the population. We see by this that the population, between the years 1861 and 1871, has increased to the extent of 1,415,206, but there are 18,697 more lunatics residing in England and Wales in the year 1871 than in the year 1861, and the ratio per thousand to the population is double, proving a decided increase of insanity beyond that of the increase of the population. I give a table showing the number of patients admitted, discharged, or died, between the years 1859 and 1870. Insanity on the increase.

From this it is seen that the number of patients admitted into asylums every year is greatly in excess of the number who are discharged. So long as this is the case, the number of insane persons on the Commissioners' register must gradually and progressively increase.

Statistical table of admissions, discharges, and deaths between the years 1859 and 1870.*

Years	Admissions	Discharged Recovered	Discharged not Recovered	Deaths	Total Discharges and Deaths	Accumulation
1859	9,310	3,270	2,850	2,332	8,452	858
1860	9,512	2,954	2,671	2,757	8,382	1,130
1861	9,329	3,182	2,110	2,657	7,949	1,380
1862	9,078	3,342	1,963	2,637	7,942	1,036
1863	8,914	3,150	1,958	2,747	7,855	1,059
1864	9,473	3,256	1,950	3,174	8,380	1,093
1865	10,424	3,290	2,515	3,161	8,966	1,458
1866	10,051	3,439	2,229	3,337	9,005	1,046
1867	10,631	3,581	2,327	3,377	9,285	1,346
1868	11,213	3,707	2,617	3,367	9,691	1,532
1869	11,194	3,801	2,304	3,825	9,930	1,264
1870	11,620	3,968	2,853	3,805	10,626	1,994
Totals .	120,749	40,940	28,347	37,176	106,463	15,186

Institutions for the insane in England and Wales, 180.

There are at present existing in England and Wales 180 asylums, hospitals, and licensed houses for the reception of persons of unsound mind, and all subject to statutory and other visitation by the Commissioners. Of this number 54 are county and borough asylums, 16 registered hospitals, 4 State asylums, 41 metropolitan licensed houses, 65 provincial licensed houses.

New county asylums opened during the year 1871.

During 1871 three large county asylums were opened—at Hereford for the county and city of Hereford, Beverley for the East Riding of Yorkshire ; and one at Macclesfield for the county of Chester.

Extra accommodation for patients required in Middlesex and Surrey.

The Commissioners, in their report, draw attention to the fact that extra accommodation for lunatics is required in Middlesex. It was decided at the Court of Quarter Sessions, held in November 1871, to appoint a committee of eighteen justices to negotiate for the purchase of land, and procure plans and estimate of cost for the erection of a third county asylum in Middlesex.

* Dr. Maudsley's Paper on Statistics of Insanity, "British Medical Journal," January 20, 1872.

Additional accommodation for lunatics is also required in Surrey to prevent the overcrowding of asylums, as is at present the case.

The reports made by the Commissioners upon the occasion of their statutory visits to the county asylums of England and Wales, now 54 in number, were on the whole very favourable.

Various alterations and additions have been made in the county and borough asylums.

The weekly cost per head of patients confined in county and borough asylums averaged 9s. 8¼d. In the previous year the average cost per head was 9s. 5½d., whereas in 1858 the average weekly cost for pauper lunatics, including maintenance and clothing, was at the rate of 6s. 8d. per head.

Average weekly cost for patients confined in county asylums is 9s. 8¼d. per patient.

The Commissioners during 1871 visited 219 workhouses, and in all 9,738 patients, showing an increase of 2,043 upon the number seen the previous year; the reports were generally favourable.

The number of metropolitan private licensed houses amounts to 41; the number of provincial licensed houses to 66.

Private asylums.*

Most of these establishments possess every accommodation and convenience which comfort and even luxury can require, and in these institutions the patients are treated kindly and judiciously. These remarks apply not only to houses which are situated in the metropolitan district, but also to the provincial ones, and it is satisfactory to be able to quote as follows from the last Commissioners' report, in their remarks upon the metropolitan licensed houses: — " Happily there has not been any occurrence in any of the houses requiring special interference or censure of the Board."

* A list of metropolitan and provincial asylums will be found at the end of the chapter relating to the admission of "private patients" into asylums.

Registered Hospitals, and State, Naval, and Military Asylums.

County	Hospital	Medical Superintendent	Private — Patients remaining on January 1, 1872			Pauper — Patients remaining on January 1, 1872			Total Lunatics on Jan. 1, 1872
			M.	F.	Total.	M.	F.	Total.	
Devon	Wonford House, Exeter	Dr. T. Lyle	37	39	76	—	1	1	77
Gloucester	Barnwood House, Gloucester	Dr. A. J. Wood	38	39	77	—	—	—	77
Lancaster	Liverpool Lunatic Hospital	J. Stockwell (Surgeon)	21	19	40	—	—	—	40
	Manchester Royal Lunatic Hospital, Cheadle	G. W. Mould (Surgeon)	64	76	140	—	—	—	140
„	Royal Albert Asylum for Idiots, Lancaster	Dr. G. E. Shuttleworth	67	—	67	7	—	7	74
Lincoln	Lincoln Lunatic Hospital	F. D. Walsh (Surgeon)	37	35	72	—	—	—	72
Middlesex	St. Luke's Hospital, Old Street	Dr. Eager (Surgeon)	44	88	132	—	—	—	132
Norfolk	Bethel Hospital, Norwich	C. M. Gibson (Surgeon)	25	48	73	4	2	6	79
Northampton	Northampton General Lunatic Hospital	J. Bayley (Surgeon)	57	54	111	162	151	313	424
Notts	Nottingham Lunatic Asylum, The Coppice, Nottingham	Dr. W. B. Tate	31	32	63	—	—	—	63
Oxford	Warneford Asylum, Headington Hill, near Oxford	Thomas Allen (Surgn.)	29	28	57	—	—	—	57
Stafford	Charitable Institution for the Insane, Coton Hill, near Stafford	Dr. J. D. Hewson	68	66	134	—	—	—	134
Surrey	Bethlehem Hospital, Lambeth Rd.	Dr. W. R. Williams	94	151	245	—	—	—	245
„	Asylum for Idiots, Earlswood, near Reigate	Dr. G. W. Grabham	360	179	539	—	—	—	539
York	York Lunatic Hospital, Bootham	Dr. F. Needham	80	57	137	24	25	49	186
„	The Retreat, York	Dr. J. Kitching	52	87	139	—	—	—	139
	Total		1,104	998	2,102	197	179	376	2,478
Berks	State Criminal Asylum, Broadmoor	Dr. W. Orange	290	51	341	116	32	148	489
Hants	Netley Abbey, Southampton	Dr. T. Blatherwick	72	—	72	—	—	—	72
Middlesex	Royal India Lunatic Asylum	Dr. T. M. Christie	103	15	118	—	—	—	118
Norfolk	Royal Naval Hospital, Yarmouth	{ Dr. W. Macleod (Deputy Inspector Gen.) }	205	—	205	—	—	—	205
	Total		670	66	736	116	32	148	884

The three following very interesting Tables are taken from the Commissioners' Report 1872:—

TABLE I.—*Showing the Number and Distribution of all Lunatics, Idiots, and Persons of Unsound Mind, on the 1st January in each of the Years 1859-72, inclusive.*

On 1st January	In County and Borough Asylums		In Registered Hospitals		In Metropolitan Licensed Houses		In Provincial Licensed Houses		In Naval and Military Hospitals and Royal India Asylum	In Workhouses	Residing with Relatives or Others		Total		In Broadmoor Criminal Asylum		Grand Total	Annual Increase
	Private	Pauper	Private	Pauper	Private	Pauper	Private	Pauper	Private	Pauper	Private	Pauper	Private	Pauper	Private	Pauper		
1859	227	15,617	1,639	216	1,287	1,264	1,541	924	164	7,963	122	5,798	4,980	31,782			36,762	—
1860	227	17,209	1,616	233	1,342	602	1,606	750	157	8,219	117	5,980	5,065	32,993			38,058	1,296
1861	212	18,380	1,739	258	1,380	573	1,638	512	174	8,543	123	6,115	5,266	34,381			39,647	1,589
1862	267	19,387	1,752	262	1,437	695	1,656	605	162	8,603	146	6,167	5,420	35,709			41,129	1,482
1863	259	20,314	1,797	306	1,448	826	1,705	552	145	9,208	153	6,405	5,507	37,611			43,118	1,989
1864	231	21,800	1,780	348	1,479	843	1,685	448	176	9,710	159	6,541	5,510	39,190		95	44,795	1,677
1865	208	22,077	1,815	363	1,485	870	1,669	453	176	9,756	212	6,557	5,565	40,076		309	45,950	1,155
1866	229	23,414	1,835	380	1,635	897	1,027	304	176	9,973	227	6,580	5,679	41,548		421	47,648	1,698
1867	216	24,374	1,844	374	1,680	914	1,650	336	190	10,307	223	6,638	5,703	42,943		440	49,086	1,438
1868	219	25,461	1,869	412	1,555	991	1,599	499	182	10,684	274	6,829	5,698	44,876		426	51,000	1,914
1869	225	26,642	1,939	413	1,662	1,020	1,461	653	209	11,181	324	6,987	5,820	46,896	404	57	53,177	2,177
1870	259	27,721	1,969	400	1,666	1,034	1,478	726	198	11,258	356	7,086	5,926	48,325	354	108	54,713	1,536
1871	287	28,692	2,045	345	1,543	978	1,489	678	354	12,161	392	7,331	6,110	50,185	344	116	56,755	2,042
1872	305	29,336	2,102	376	1,573	683	1,506	411	395	13,608	420	7,486	6,301	51,850	341	148	58,640	1,885

TABLE II.—*The Ratio per 1,000 of the Total Number of Lunatics, Idiots, and Persons of Unsound Mind, to the Population, in each year from 1859–1872, both inclusive.*

YEAR	Population	Total Number of Lunatics, Idiots, &c., on January 1	Ratio per 1,000 to the Population
1859	19,686,701	36,762	1·86
1860	19,902,713	38,058	1·91
1861	20,119,314	39,647	1·97
1862	20,336,467	41,129	2·02
1863	20,554,137	43,118	2·09
1864	20,772,308	44,795	2·15
1865	20,990,946	45,950	2·18
1866	21,210,020	47,648	2·24
1867	21,429,508	49,086	2·29
1868	21,649,377	51,000	2·35
1869	21,869,607	53.177	2·43
1870	22,090,163	54,713	2·47
1871	22,704,108	56,755	2·49
1872	23,074,600	58,640	2·54

In the above Table the population for each year has been taken from the Annual Report of. the Registrar-General, and is applicable to the middle of the year.

TABLE III.—*Showing in juxtaposition the Proportion of Deaths to the Daily Average Number Resident, and to the Total Number under Treatment, for each Year.*

YEAR	Aggregate of Asylums, Hospitals, &c.		County and Borough Asylums		Registered Hospitals		Metropolitan Licensed Houses		Provincial Licensed Houses	
	Number of Deaths to 100 of the Daily Average Number Resident	Number of Deaths to 100 of the Total Number under Treatment	Number of Deaths to 100 of the Daily Average Number Resident	Number of Deaths to 100 of the Total Number under Treatment	Number of Deaths to 100 of the Daily Average Number Resident	Number of Deaths to 100 of the Total Number under Treatment	Number of Deaths to 100 of the Daily Average Number Resident	Number of Deaths to 100 of the Total Number under Treatment	Number of Deaths to 100 of the Daily Average Number Resident	Number of Deaths to 100 of the Total Number under Treatment
1859	9·90	7·22	10·25	7·76	6·53	4·61	12·41	7·82	7·60	5·36
1860	11·28	8·26	12·16	9·12	6·45	4·57	11·04	7·76	8·56	5·92
1861	10·33	7·74	11·03	8·52	7·38	5·26	10·60	7·32	6·78	5·03
1862	9·77	7·44	10·16	7·95	7·61	5·56	11·08	7·84	7·11	5·09
1863	9·81	7·54	10·42	8·18	7·93	5·93	8·54	6·36	7·41	5·43
1864	10·88	8·35	11·73	9·20	6·89	5·00	10·91	7·95	7·17	5·33
1865	10·42	7·89	10·95	8·46	7·99	5·96	11·31	8·16	7·95	5·31
1866	10·59	8·11	10·76	8·48	7·97	5·84	13·67	9·18	9·72	6·86
1867	10·29	7·90	10·66	8·38	8·57	6·33	11·75	8·26	8·08	5·71
1868	9·78	7·53	10·15	7·99	7·52	5·62	9·73	7·33	9·97	6·90
1869	10·72	8·28	11·16	8·76	9·12	6·61	9·69	7·36	10·64	7·49
1870	10·29	7·94	10·81	8·48	7·33	5·36	9·48	6·97	10·19	7·54
1871	10·23	7·66	10·71	8·09	7·47	5·57	9·97	6·98	9·76	6·98
Averages .	10·33	7·83	10·84	8·41	7·59	5·55	10·78	7·63	8·53	6·07

CHAPTER III.

EPITOME OF THE LUNACY ACT.

On the Law relating to Private Patients.

THE following is an epitome of the first part of the Lunacy Act, relating to the Masters and Commissioners in Lunacy and the granting of licences.

In the succeeding chapter I propose to refer to that part of the Act principally relating to the management of asylums.

Lunacy Act 1845.   The Lunacy Act 1845 repeals 2 and 3 William IV. c. 22 ; 1 and 2 Vict. c. 73 ; 5 Vict. c. 4 ; 5 and 6 Vict. c. 87.

Masters in Lunacy.

Masters in Lunacy.   The Masters in Lunacy are two in number. They act as judges in all proceedings under the writ "*de lunatico inquirendo.*" The present Masters are—Francis Barlow, Esq., and Samuel Warren, Esq., F.R.S., D.C.L. Oxon. The salary is 2,000*l.* per annum exclusive of travelling expenses.

Oath taken by a Master in Lunacy.   Before acting officially, an oath is required to be taken.

Masters in Lunacy appointed by Lord Chancellor.   The Masters are appointed by the Lord Chancellor, and they must be barristers of ten years' standing, or serjeants-at-law.

Commissioners in Lunacy.

Commissioners in Lunacy.   Six gentlemen are appointed to act as visiting Commissioners in Lunacy ; of this number, three are medical men and three are barristers. The three Medical Commissioners are—James Wilkes, Esq., F.R.C.S.; John D. Cleaton, Esq., M.R.C.S.; and Robert Nairne, Esq., M.D.

The three Legal Commissioners are—William George Campbell, Esq.; Charles Palmer Phillips, Esq.; and the Hon. Greville Howard.

The unpaid and non-visiting Commissioners are—the Right Honourable the Earl of Shaftesbury (chairman); Francis Barlow, Esq.; Hon. Dudley F. Fortescue, M.P.; B. W. Proctor, Esq.; and John Forster, Esq.

The Secretary is Charles Spencer Perceval, Esq. The office, 19 Whitehall Place, London, S.W.

It is their duty to grant licences, visit and regulate asylums, report to the Lord Chancellor as to the condition of the same, and conduct and manage everything connected with certified lunatics in England and Wales.

A report once a year is issued by the Board of Commissioners, in which a vast amount of carefully drawn-up statistics and useful information relating to lunacy is published. *Report of Commissioners.*

This report is ordered to be printed by the House of Commons, and is directed to the Lord Chancellor.

The salary of a Commissioner in Lunacy is 1,500*l.* per annum, and no person can act as a Commissioner, Secretary, or Clerk to the Commissioners, if at that time, or within a year preceding, he is or has been interested directly of indirectly in any house licensed for the reception of lunatics, or derives profit from such reception. *Salary of Commissioners.*

The Commissioners are prohibited from holding any other office, or practising in their respective professions.

Before any one can act as Commissioner, he must have been a physician, surgeon, or barrister of at least five years' standing.

The Commissioners have a common seal, which is attached to all licences, orders, and instruments. *Seal of Commissioners.*

Chairman of Commissioners. The office of Chairman to the Board of Commissioners is a permanent one; and no physician or barrister can act as such. No remuneration is attached to it.

Salary of Secretary. The Secretary's salary is 800*l.* per annum.

Limits of Commissioners' jurisdiction. The limits of the immediate jurisdiction of the Commissioners comprise the following places:—

The city of London, the city of Westminster, the county of Middlesex, the borough of Southwark.

The following places in the county of Surrey:—

Barnes, Camberwell (St. Giles), Dulwich, Battersea, Clapham (Christ Church), Graveney, Bermondsey (St. Mary Magdalene), Kennington, Brixton, Deptford (St. Paul's), Kew Green, Lambeth (St. Mary), Mortlake, Merton, Newington (St. Mary), Mitcham, Norwood, Peckham, Roehampton, Stockwell, Putney, Rotherhithe (St. Mary), Streatham, Wandsworth, Tooting, Wimbledon, Walworth.

The following places in the county of Kent:—

Blackheath, Greenwich, Charlton, Lee, Woolwich, Deptford, Lewisham.

The following places in the county of Essex:—

East Ham, Leytonstone, Plaistow, West Ham, Leyton, Low Leyton, Walthamstow, Southend.

And every other place (if any) within the distance of seven miles from any part of the cities of London and Westminster, or borough of Southwark.

Licensed houses beyond immediate jurisdiction of Commissioners. All houses not within the " immediate jurisdiction " of the Commissioners are visited by persons nominated at the Michaelmas Quarter Sessions in each year. The licences for these houses are granted by the Justices at the Quarter Sessions. These visitors are appointed in every county or borough.

The visitors consist of three or more justices, who act gratuitously, and one (or more) surgeon, physician, or apothecary, who receives remuneration.

Incapacity of a visitor from acting. If any of the visitors die, or from any cause become unable to officiate, it is lawful for the justices of the county or borough to appoint a visitor to fill up the vacancy, the appointment being made at the Quarter Sessions.

A list of visitors of licensed houses not within the immediate jurisdiction of the Commissioners is published by the Clerk of the Peace, and a copy sent to the Commissioners in Lunacy.

The appointment of Clerk to the Visitors is made at the Quarter Sessions.
Clerk to Visitors.

The visitors and the clerk take an oath of fidelity and secrecy, and must not be interested in any licensed house.

Two of the visitors, one being a medical man, are required to visit four times during the year all asylums beyond the immediate jurisdiction of the Commissioners. And by the amended Act 1862, in addition to these visits, the asylum must be visited by one or more of the visitors twice during the year.
Visitation of asylums beyond the immediate jurisdiction of Commissioners.

The official books required for the visitors' reports, are, "the Visitors' Book," "the Patients' Book," and "the Medical Visitation Book." A copy of these entries must be sent to the Commissioners and Clerk of the Visitors within three days from their visitation, and be placed before the justices when the yearly licence is granted.

In addition to being officially visited, as stated above, all houses not within the "immediate jurisdiction" of the Commissioners in Lunacy are supervised by two of the Commissioners (one being a barrister, and the other a medical man) twice every year.
Commissioners' supervision of asylums beyond their immediate jurisdiction.

The Commissioners in Lunacy make entries in the official books. A copy of these entries is sent within three days after such visitation to the Commissioners and to the Clerk of the Visitors.

Visitation of Commissioners.

The Commissioners visit all licensed houses within their immediate jurisdiction six times a year.

Four of these visits are made conjointly by a medical and legal Commissioner, and two single visits are made by a legal Commissioner.

Enquiries made by the Commissioners at the time of their Visitation.

1st. Number of patients then in the house.

2ndly. Number of patients admitted since their last visit.

3rd. Number of patients discharged or died since their last visit.

4th. Particulars relating to carriage drives and walks of the patients.

5th. Number of patients attending Divine Worship.

6th. Particulars relating to the occupations and amusements of the patients.

7th. Number of patients then under medical treatment.

8th. Particulars relating to restraint and seclusion made since last visit.

9th. Particulars relating to the visitation of the patients by their friends.

Night Visitation.

Two or more of the Commissioners may visit any licensed house or hospital, at any hour of the night they think proper.

Single Patients in Unlicensed Houses.

No one deriving profit from the care or charge of a person of unsound mind can receive a patient into his house without the necessary " order " and " medical certificates," as required in the case of patients confined in asylums.

This does not apply to persons found lunatic by inquisition, to whom reference is made in the chapter on Chancery Lunatics.

Two or more Patients.

In the case of two or more persons of unsound mind being received into a house with a view to profit, a special licence from the Commissioners is necessary.

Licence required for more than one patient.

Property of Lunatics.

The Commissioners have to report to the Lord Chancellor if the property of the lunatic is not duly protected or administered.

Commissioners enquire into the property of patients not duly protected.

Visitation of Gaols and Workhouses.

Two or more of the Commissioners are empowered to visit all workhouses and gaols in which any lunatic, or alleged lunatic is confined, and to ascertain if all the provisions of the law have been carried out, and make other enquiries they may think proper as to their management, &c.

Dangerous Lunatics.

No lunatic, if certified to be dangerous, can be removed from any house or hospital, without first obtaining the consent of the Commissioners and visitors.

Discharge of dangerous lunatics prohibited, except by consent of Commissioners.

Discharge of Patients can be ordered by Commissioners.

The Commissioners have power to discharge any patient confined in an asylum or licensed house, if after two visits they consider him to have been improperly detained. Seven days must intervene between these visits. This does not refer to Chancery lunatics or persons confined by order of the Secretary of State.

Commissioners can order the discharge of patients.

D

Licences.

The Commissioners meet at their office, 19 Whitehall Place, S.W., on the first Wednesday in the months of February, May, July, and November, to receive applications for licences; but they are also empowered to receive and determine such application at any special meeting summoned for the purpose.*

Form of Application for Licence.

Application must be made by the person or persons applying for the licence, fourteen days previous to the meeting of the Commissioners.

An application for the renewal of the licence must have attached to it a statement of the number and names of the patients, male and female, at that time resident in the asylum.

If the application refers to a house that has not been previously licensed, it must be accompanied by a plan of the house drawn upon a scale of not less than one-eighth of an inch to a foot, number and size of the rooms, quantity of land attached, &c. The number of patients for which the licence is required must also be stated, and whether it is proposed to use the house for male or female patients, together or separately.

The Commissioners in their thirteenth Report, dated March 31, 1859, state clearly what course they pursue in dealing with applications for licences.

I quote from their report:—

" In reference to our practice of granting licences, it is not necessary to enumerate the instances in which we have considered it our duty to refuse them. The Legislature has given us a discretion on the subject; and the question to be considered by us on receiving such ap-

* *Vide* Schedule A, 8 and 9 Vict. c. 100, and Schedule A, 25 and 26 Vict. c. 111.

plications, appears to be whether or not an additional
house is required for the accommodation of insane
persons, and also whether the qualifications of the
persons applying are such as (under other circumstances) would induce us to grant the licence.

In some districts the number of houses licensed is
already too numerous.

Should it seem advisable to grant a new licence, it
is our custom to propose the following questions :— *Questions asked by the Commissioners before granting a new licence.*

1. State your age, and whether you are married or
single, and whether you propose to reside on the premises to be licensed.

2. If married, is it proposed that your wife (or
husband) should reside in the house to be licensed, and
take any, and if any, what part in the charge and management of the patients ?   Have you any children, and
if so, of what age and sex respectively, and is it proposed that they, or any of them should be resident in
the licensed house ?

3. Are you a medical man ?   If so, state where you
received your professional and general education, what
degree you have received, or examination you have
passed, and where and for how long you have been engaged in the practice of your profession.   If not a
medical man, state what your profession or occupation
has been.   Also state the name and address of the person
who is to act as the medical visitor and attendant of the
patients.

4. State the nature and amount of your education,
training, and experience with reference to the care and
treatment of the insane, and when, and where, and under
what circumstances obtained.

5. Produce testimonials or other satisfactory evidence as to your skill and experience as a medical practitioner, and as a person fit to be entrusted with the

charge of the insane; and also as to your possession of
the necessary pecuniary means for enabling you to carry
on and maintain the establishment in a comfortable state.

6. What is the nature and extent of the interest
which you possess in the house and premises proposed
to be licensed? Have any other persons, and who, by
name and description, any and what interest in the house
and premises jointly with yourself or otherwise, or in the
profits to be derived from the establishment?

7. What class, and number of patients, and of
which sex do you propose to receive into the house, and
paying what weekly or other rate of board?'

Licences
granted for
new houses.

Should the foregoing be satisfactorily answered, an
inspection of the premises is undertaken, and a report
made by one or more Commissioners as to their general
capabilities for the number and class of patients for
which a licence is desired.

The Board subsequently considers the question, and,
if satisfied, grants the licence, subject, if necessary, to
such stipulations as the case may require.

On granting licences for new houses, or promoting
changes in houses already existing, we endeavour to
secure for the inmates free intercourse within doors, and
a ready access to the open air.

These advantages being often curtailed when patients
of both sexes are placed in dwellings of an ordinary size,
standing in limited grounds or gardens, we have generally required that the proprietor of such houses should
admit only one sex.

The result of the progressive change thus effected,
by means of the foregoing requisitions and stipulations,
will be made evident by stating that out of the 40
metropolitan houses, only 17 are now licensed for the
admission of both sexes; and in order that the most
competent parties only should be allowed to act as superintendents of the insane, we have had it under serious

consideration whether it might not be expedient, as a
general rule, to grant new licences only to medical
men."

In their fourteenth Report, the Commissioners make
the following additional remarks :—

"For a statement of our practice in granting licences
for the first time, we take leave to refer your Lordship
to our last report (p. 58), and more especially to the
questions, of which a copy will there be found, required
to be answered by applicants.

Practice of
Commis-
sioners in
granting a
licence for
first time, as
stated in
14th Report,
1860.

The subject generally of licences for the reception
of lunatics, and their grant, renewal, and transfer, has
continued during the past year to engage our serious
attention, and the importance of the considerations involved induces us, upon this occasion, shortly to re-
iterate the principles by which we are guided in dealing
with applications.

As respects the metropolitan district, we have prac-
tically come to the resolution not to add to the number
of licensed houses, unless for special reasons applicable
to the particular case. In the event of a medical man
or other person of high character and qualifications, and
possessing adequate pecuniary resources, applying for a
licence to receive private patients in a suitable house, we
should be disposed to make an exception, but should in
that case, generally, if not invariably, limit the licence
to patients of one sex.

The licensed houses within our immediate jurisdiction, judging from the actual number of patients
resident therein, appear fully to meet, not merely the
requirements of the special locality (which would be
comparatively unimportant, inasmuch as private patients
are, for the most part, sent to asylums not in the neighbourhood of their homes), but in general the wants of
the community.

We have also to observe, that in consequence of the

now rapid withdrawal of the pauper patients from the five large metropolitan houses at present licensed to receive that class of the insane, extensive provisions will shortly be made for the accommodation of patients of the middle and poorer classes, for whom it is hoped that ultimately adequate means of care and treatment will be afforded in public hospitals.''

An absolute discretion is vested in the Commissioners to grant or withhold the licence applied for, as they think fit.

Duration of Licence.

Licence available for thirteen months.

A licence is granted for a period of thirteen calendar months.

Cost of Licence.

Ten shillings paid for every patient in licence.

The sum of 10s. is paid for every private patient for which the asylum is licensed.

Residence of Licensed Person in the Asylum.

A licence granted for the first time to any applicant, after the passing of the Lunacy Act 1845, requires the person to whom it is granted to reside on the premises.*

Licence when granted to two or more persons.

If the licence is granted to two or more persons, then one or all of them are required to reside in the asylum. This refers to houses licensed for the first time after the Act of 1845 came into force, and not to houses licensed prior to that time.

Asylums licensed before passing the Act of 1845.

An asylum which was licensed before the Act of 1845 may have a medical superintendent residing in it, who need not be licensed, but he must be approved of by the Commissioners in Lunacy.

* 16 and 17 Vict. c. 96, s. 2.

Residence of Medical Officer in Asylums.

It is compulsory for every hospital for the insane to have a resident medical superintendent. Residence of medical officer in asylums.

Every asylum licensed for less than one hundred or more than fifty patients, is required by Act of Parliament to be visited daily by a medical man, provided there is no resident medical officer. If it contain more than 50 patients and less than 100.

Every asylum licensed for less than fifty patients (provided such asylum is not kept by, or have a resident medical officer) must be visited twice during the week by a physician, surgeon, or apothecary. The Commissioners have power to increase the number of medical visitations, according to their discretion. If it contain less than 50.

If the house is licensed for less than eleven patients the Commissioners have power to lessen the number of medical visits. Asylum licensed for less than 11 patients.

Licences may include more than one House.

The Justices or Commissioners, as the case may be, have power to include in one licence any buildings detached from the principal house, if described in the notice and plan required to be sent to the office when application is made for a licence. This is only done when these buildings are not separated from the house by land not the property of the person applying for the licence. More than one house can be included in one licence.

Death or Incapacity of the Person licensed.

If the person to whom a licence is originally granted die, or from any cause becomes incapacitated from acting, the licence may be transferred by consent of the Commissioners to any other person. If two persons are conjointly licensed, and one of them dies or becomes incapacitated, the licence is still valid with respect to the other person licensed. Licence can be transferred on death or incapacity of licensee.

Refusal to renew Licence.

Lord Chancellor has power at the request of Commissioners to refuse or revoke any licence.

The Lord Chancellor may, at the request of the Commissioners in Lunacy, recall or refuse to grant a renewal of the licence, and any person keeping such house after the expiration of two clear months from the revoking of such licence is guilty of a misdemeanour. Before the Commissioners revoke the licence, notice is given to the proprietor of the asylum, and the fact is published in the " London Gazette."

CHAPTER IV.

ON THE MANAGEMENT OF ASYLUMS AND LICENSED HOUSES.

ON the admission of a patient into an asylum, it is the duty of the medical superintendent to carefully examine the order, statement, and medical certificates, with the view of ascertaining their legal accuracy. No patient can be received into an asylum and detained there if, *[Duties of medical officer on the admission of patients into an asylum.]*

1st. The order be signed by a person who has not seen the patient within a month from the time of certifying. *[Illegal grounds for detaining patient.]*

2ndly. The "date of examination" of the patient stated in the certificate be longer than seven days prior to the patient's admission. Facts stated in the certificates must have been observed on the day of the examination of the patient.

3rdly. The medical certificates are signed by the persons who are prohibited by Act of Parliament from signing.*

Omissions and mistakes are frequently made in the order, statement, and medical certificates, but these inaccuracies do not necessarily render them invalid. After being forwarded to the Commissioners, they are returned by them for alteration, fourteen days being allowed to the proprietor of the asylum to obtain the required amendments. *[Mistakes made in the medical certificates.]*

* *Vide* 16 and 17 Vict. c. 96, s. 12.

Admission Book.

Admission
Book.

The name, &c., of the patient must be entered in the Admission Book* within two days from the patient's reception into the asylum.

Case Book.

Case Book.

The medical officer is required by Act of Parliament to keep a Case Book.

The Commissioners in Lunacy, in their annual report dated March 20, 1863, issued the following regulations respecting this :—

Case Book.—Revised Order (8 and 9 Vict. c. 100, s. 60).

Directions
for making
entries in the
Case Book.

"The Commissioners in Lunacy, by virtue of the power vested in them by the Act of Parliament passed in the session holden in the 8th and 9th years of the reign of her present Majesty, intituled ' An Act for the Regulation of the Care and Treatment of Lunatics,' do hereby order and direct—

That the medical Case Book, by the said Act directed to be kept in every licensed house and hospital, shall be kept in the form hereinafter mentioned, viz. :—

1st. A statement of the name, age, sex, and previous occupation of the patient, and whether married, single, or widowed.

2ndly. An accurate description of the external appearance of the patient upon admission ; habit of body and temperament ; appearance of eyes, expression of countenance, and any peculiarity in form of head ; of the physical state of the vascular and respiratory organs and of the abdominal viscera, and their respective functions ; of the state of the pulse, tongue, skin, &c.

3rdly. A description of the phenomena of mental

* Schedule E, 8 and 9 Vict. c. 100.

disorder; the manner and period of the attack, with a minute account of the symptoms, and the changes produced in the patient's temper or disposition; specifying whether the malady displays itself by any and what illusions, or irrational conduct or morbid or dangerous habits or propensities; whether it has occasioned any failure of memory or understanding, or is connected with epilepsy, or ordinary paralysis, or symptoms of general paralysis, such as tremulous movements of the tongue, defect of articulation, or weakness or unsteadiness of gait.

4thly. Every particular which can be obtained respecting the previous history of the patient; what are believed to have been the predisposing and exciting causes of the attack, what the previous habits, active or sedentary, temperate or otherwise; whether the patient has experienced any former attacks, and if so at what periods; whether any relatives have been subject to insanity, and whether the present attack has been preceded by any premonitory symptoms, such as restlessness, unusual elevation or depression of spirits, or any remarkable deviation from ordinary habits and conduct, and whether the patient has undergone any and what previous treatment, or been subjected to personal restraint.

5thly. During the first month after admission entries to be made at least once in every week, and oftener where the nature of the case requires it. Afterwards in recent or curable cases, entries to be made at least once in every month, and in chronic cases subject to little variation, once in every three months.

An accurate record must be kept of the medicines administered, and other remedies employed, and all injuries and accidents should be stated.

That the several particulars hereinbefore required to be recorded, to be set forth in a manner so clear and distinct, as to admit of being easily referred to, and extracted whenever the Commissioners shall so require. And that the present order be in substitution for that of the 9th of January, 1846, and that a copy thereof be inserted at the commencement of the Case Book.

Dated this 20th day of March, One thousand eight hundred and sixty-three.

Office of Commissioners in Lunacy,
No. 19, Whitehall Place."

Copy of Medical Certificates and Order.

A copy of these documents, according to the amended Acts, must be sent to the Commissioners within twenty-four hours from the patient's admission. The copy of the certificates must be a fac-simile of the original, containing all erasures and alterations.

Statement of Mental and Bodily Health.

The patient must be examined by the medical attendant after two clear days and before the expiration of seven clear days from the date of admission.

This statement must be sent to the Commissioners in Lunacy by the proprietor or superintendent.*

Discharge of Patients.

Notice of the discharge of a patient must be given to the Commissioners within two days from the discharge, and must state whether the patient has been discharged as " recovered," " relieved," or as " not improved." †

The medical attendant is also required to make an entry of the patient's discharge in the Discharge Book.‡

* A copy of this statement will be found in Schedule C at the end of the Lunacy Act 1853 (16 and 17 Vict. c. 96), printed at the end of the book.

† 8 and 9 Vict. c. 100, Schedule E 2.

‡ 8 and 9 Vict. c. 100, Schedule E 1.

This is required to be done within two clear days from the discharge.

Death of Patients.

Notice of death must be forwarded,

1st. To the Commissioners in Lunacy, within two clear days from the time of the death. Notice of death.

2nd. To the coroner of the district.*

3rd. To the person to whom notice of death has to be sent, whose name is mentioned in the statement of admission.

4th. To the parish registrar of deaths.

A copy of the notice to the Commissioners must be entered in the Case Book.†

Medical Journal.

The Medical Journal‡ must be filled up and signed every week. It must contain the number and names of the patients who have been under medical treatment during the week, and also the nature of their bodily ailment, the number of patients in the house, the patients who have been restrained, or secluded, since the last week's entry, and the reason for this restraint or seclusion; the names of those patients who have died, or who have received any injury during the week. Medical Journal, what it is to contain.

Books to be placed before the Commissioners at the Time of their Visit.

The following six books have to be placed before the Commissioners in Lunacy at the time of their visitation: Official books to be placed before Commissioners at time of their visit.

1st. Medical Journal.

* 25 and 26 Vict. c. 111, s. 44.

† A form of the notice of death will be found at the end of the book.

‡ Schedule D, 16 and 17 Vict. c. 96.

2nd. Book of Admission.

3rd. Book of Discharges.

4th. Case Book.

5th. Visitors' Book. In this the Act of Parliament is printed in full, and here the Commissioners write their report and particulars of their visit.

6th. Patients' Book.

Patients' book.

In this book special remarks relating to individual cases are made by the Commissioners.

All recent medical certificates have also to be placed before the Commissioners.

Commissioners' Entries in Official Books.

Commissioners' entries in official books of the asylum.

A copy of the entries made in the Visitors' and Patients' Book must be sent to the Commissioners within three days from their visitation, written on foolscap paper. A blank margin of about two inches had better be made on the left-hand side of the copy, and a margin of about half an inch on the right, leaving room for any remarks to be made by the Commissioners in Lunacy at their office.

Escape of Patients.

Escape of patients, notice to be sent to Commissioners within two clear days.

If a patient escapes from a licensed or private house, notice of the fact must be sent to the Commissioners in Lunacy. If the patient has escaped from a house not within their immediate jurisdiction, the notice is then to be sent to the visitors. In each case, the notice must be sent within two clear days, and must contain the name of the patient, his condition of mind at the time of the escape, and the circumstances connected with it. Notice of recapture must be sent to the Commissioners or visitors, as the case may be, within two days from such recapture. A patient who has escaped can be recaptured within *fourteen* days, upon the original order and medical certificates; if this time has elapsed, the medical certificates and order become invalid.

Patient can be recaptured within fourteen days.

Notice of escape and recapture may be sent at the same time.

Transfer of Patients from one House to another after the Expiration of Licence.

If any licensed house is pulled down, or occupied under the provisions of any Act of Parliament, or by fire, tempest, or any other accident is rendered unfit for the accommodation of lunatics, or if the proprietor of a licensed house desires to remove his patients from one house to another, the Commissioners have power to grant to such person whose house has been rendered unfit for occupation, and who shall desire to transfer his patients, a licence for such time as the Commissioners think proper. Seven clear days' notice must be given to the Commissioners of the proposed change, together with plans, statement, and description of the new house to which it is proposed to transfer the patients. (This does not, of course, apply to cases of fire and tempest.) Notice is also required to be sent to the persons who signed the "order," or to the person who made the last payment.

A patient can be transferred from one house to another after expiration of licence.

Transfer of a Patient from one Asylum to another.

If it be deemed desirable to remove a patient from one asylum to another, application must be made to the Commissioners by the person who signed the "order" for admission, and upon this application the Commissioners will communicate with the proprietor or superintendent as to the fitness of the patient for transfer.

A patient can be transferred from one asylum to another.

If this be satisfactory, the person making the application will receive from the Commissioners two copies of the "consent" and "order," the "consent" signed by two of the Commissioners, and the "order" by the person making application ; one of these documents is left with the proprietor or superintendent at the asylum from which the patient is removed, and the other copy, together with an exact copy of the original order, statement, and medical certificates, and endorsed by the proprietor or superintendent as being a true copy, is given to the proprietor or superintendent of the asylum to which the patient is transferred.

Consent and order for transfer.

COPY OF CONSENT AND ORDER FOR TRANSFER.

CONSENT.

We, the undersigned Commissioners in Lunacy, hereby consent to the removal, on or before the day of , 187 , of , a private patient in House, , to House, .

Given under our hands this day of , in the year of Our Lord One thousand eight hundred and seventy- .

     } Commissioners in Lunacy.

ORDER.

I, the undersigned, having authority to discharge , a private patient in House, , hereby order and direct that the said be removed therefrom to House, .

Given under my hand this day of , in the year of Our Lord One thousand eight hundred and seventy-

   (Signed)

   Place of abode,

Boarders in Asylums.

A person who has been under certificate can be received as a boarder.

A person having been a certified patient in an asylum, can be received as a boarder, provided he has been a patient in *any* asylum, hospital, or licensed house, or under care as a single patient, within five years from the time he wishes to become a boarder.

This is a very necessary and beneficial arrangement, for many persons who have been previously in asylums, conscious of a want of control, and recognising a recurrence of the malady, have an opportunity of voluntarily placing themselves under treatment.

Boarders must enter the asylum of their own free will, and while there are free agents, and are at liberty to leave whenever they please.

It was formerly required that the Commissioners in Lunacy should have a personal interview with the proposed boarder, before giving their sanction to his residence in an asylum.

The preparatory arrangements are simply these :— The person desirous of becoming a boarder makes a written application to the Commissioners, expressing his wish to reside in the asylum for a definite period. Two of the Commissioners, if they think proper, give their consent in writing. At the expiration of the time for which permission is given, a fresh application must be made to the Commissioners, and their consent obtained.

The medical superintendent cannot receive a boarder if he exhibits symptoms of mental unsoundness. Boarders do not count among the number of patients for which the house is licensed. If an asylum is licensed for twenty patients, and the house has sufficient accommodation, boarders can be received in excess of that number. *No person can be received as a boarder if he exhibits symptoms of mental unsoundness.*

Their names are not entered in the Case Book or Book of Admission.

" In very few cases as yet has advantage been taken of the provisions of the eighteenth section of the Lunacy Acts Amendment Act, 1862, legalising the reception into and the retention in licensed houses, as boarders, of persons who may have been within five years immediately preceding patients in any asylum, hospital, or licensed house, or under care as ' single patients.' As respects provincial licensed houses, the fact of the residence therein, with the assent of the visitors, of such voluntary boarders comes only to the knowledge of the Commissioners incidentally upon the occasion of their visits. *Remarks of the Commissioners on boarders.*

It is very desirable that in all cases of this kind

E

notice should be transmitted by the proprietors or superintendents to this office, and it is important that all boarders should be seen, whenever licensed houses are visited, with a view to ascertain beyond a doubt that they are of sound mind, and entirely free agents, and that they fully understand their position.

The necessity for such interviews with boarders has recently been strongly exemplified in the cases of two gentlemen in a metropolitan licensed house, to whose reception and residence as boarders our assent was duly given upon their written application. Both had been previously patients in the same house, and discharged therefrom as recovered.

Upon the occasion of a visit by two members of this Board, who conversed privately with the gentlemen referred to, it transpired that neither of them was aware of his being a free agent in all respects and at liberty to leave the house.

They both stated that they had been given by the proprietor and superintendent to understand that they were bound to remain and submit to the regulations of the establishment for the full period limited by the assent of the Commissioners. On enquiry it was found that the proprietor or superintendent had, in fact, so informed the gentlemen, and the explanation of so singular a misconstruction of the Act was, that the permission thereby given was to ' entertain and keep as a boarder.'

In the case of one of the gentlemen he was found to be in such a mental state as to be incapable of forming a rational wish upon the subject, and he was removed by his friends.

In the other case the permission to continue to reside as a boarder was, in compliance with the desire of the gentleman in question, for the remainder of the limited period left undisturbed; he, however, shortly afterwards relapsed into a state of mania, and was again placed under certificates." *

Correspondence of Patients.

All letters written by patients in asylums, hospitals, or licensed houses, or by a single patient, and addressed to the Commissioners in Lunacy, or to the Committee, and, in the case of houses within the immediate jurisdiction of visitors, to the visitors, must be forwarded unopened. All letters written by patients so confined, and addressed to other persons, must be forwarded to the persons to whom they are addressed, unless endorsed by the person who has charge of the patient, thus—*Not to be sent.* The letters are initialed, and must be placed before the visiting Commissioners, Committee, or visitors, as the case may be, at the next visitation.

Letters written by patients in asylums.

Any superintendent, proprietor, or person in charge of a single patient, failing to observe this provision is liable to a fine of 20*l.*

Ill-treatment or Neglect of Patients.

" If any superintendent, officer, nurse, attendant, servant, or other person employed in any registered hospital or licensed house, or any person having the care or charge of any single patient, or any attendant of any single patient, in any way abuse, ill-treat, or wilfully neglect any patient in such hospital or house, or such single patient, or if any person detaining, or taking or having the care or charge, or concerned or taking part in the custody, care, or treatment, of any lunatic or person alleged to be a lunatic, in any way abuse, ill-treat, or wilfully neglect such lunatic or alleged lunatic, he shall be guilty of a misdemeanour, and shall be subject to indictment for every such offence, or to forfeit for every

Any person who wilfully ill-treats a patient is liable to a fine.

* Commissioners' Eighteenth Report, 1864.

E 2

such offence, on a summary conviction thereof before two justices, any sum not exceeding twenty pounds."*

Unjust Confinement of Patients.

Any patient who has been discharged from an asylum, and who considers himself to have been unjustly confined, can apply to the Secretary of the Commissioners for a copy of the order and medical certificates upon which he has been detained, and he is furnished with such, without any fee.

If the Commissioners and visitors of an asylum report concerning the unjust confinement or ill-treatment of a patient, the Home Secretary is empowered to direct the Attorney-General to prosecute on the part of the Crown.

Search for Persons confined in Lunatic Asylums.

Any person desirous of ascertaining whether any particular patient is confined in a licensed house, the Commissioners have the power upon receiving an application to order their Secretary to examine and give information concerning the patient. This only applies to a person who has been confined as a lunatic within twelve months from the time of the application. Of course it is left entirely to the discretion of the Commissioners whether such information be given or refused.

In the case of patients who are not within the immediate jurisdiction of the Commissioners, application must be made to one of the visitors.

Visits of Friends to Patients.

In most private asylums the patients are allowed to be visited by their friends and relations at any hour during the day.

If access to the patients is refused, a Commissioner or visitor, as the case may be, is enabled, should it be

* *Lunacy Act*, 1853.

deemed desirable, to give an order for the admission of a friend to visit the patient at all reasonable times, and any person refusing to obey such order, or who endeavours to prevent these visits, renders himself liable to a fine not exceeding 20l.*

Temporary Leave of Absence of Patients.

It is lawful for the person who has signed the order for a patient's admission into an asylum, or for the person who made the last payment, to apply to the Commissioners for his temporary leave of absence under proper care. Before the Commissioners grant this request, the medical superintendent must state in writing that this change is for the benefit of the patient. It is customary for a written application to be made to the medical superintendent by the friends of the patient, and this application is forwarded to the Commissioners by the medical superintendent, with a letter from himself stating that the change will be beneficial, and also whether the person making the application, which is enclosed, signed the order, or made the last payment.

Patients on leave of absence.

Power of Commissioners to obtain Evidence.

The Commissioners have the power of summoning any persons before them, and examining them upon oath, concerning any matter relating to the Lunacy Acts.

Attendants.

One of the most important things connected with the management of asylums is to ensure a well-regulated staff of skilled attendants.

Attendants.

The Commissioners in Lunacy, with a view of assisting the proprietors of asylums and medical superinten-

* With regard to the advisability of seeing the patient the friend should be guided by the advice of the medical officer, as serious consequences often follow the injudicious visits of friends.

dents to obtain respectable and trustworthy attendants, forwarded a notice to the superintendents of all metropolitan asylums, requesting to be furnished with a list of attendants engaged since the commencement of the year.

This list must contain the age of each attendant, the time at which the attendant was engaged, and in what capacity he is to act, the wages he is to receive, the name of the place of his previous employment, and occupation.

The Commissioners require notice of the engagement or discharge of an attendant. I give below the form of notice which has to be sent to the Commissioners within three days of the admission or of the discharge of an attendant. It is filled up with the name of a fictitious person.

NOTICE OF THE ENGAGEMENT OF AN ATTENDANT.

Newton Asylum, Feb. 17, 1873.

Copy of notice to be sent to Commissioners on the engagement of an attendant.

I hereby give you notice that *William Thompson, aged 35,* was engaged by me as *attendant* on the 17*th day of February,* 1873, at the rate of 25*l. per annum, increasing 5l. per annum up to 50l.,* and that his previous occupation was *that of an attendant in Eltham House, Barnstaple, in December,* 1872.

(Signed) *William Wallace,*
Proprietor of Newton Asylum, Newton.

The Secretary,
Commissioners in Lunacy.

NOTICE OF THE DISCHARGE OF AN ATTENDANT.

Newton Asylum, March 4, 1873.

Copy of notice to be sent to Commissioners on the discharge of an attendant.

I hereby give you notice that *William Thompson,* an *attendant* in this house, who was engaged on the 17*th day of February,* 1873, was discharged on the 4*th day of March,* 1873, in consequence of *being intoxicated,* * and neglect of duty.*

(Signed) *William Wallace,*
Proprietor of Newton Asylum, Newton.

The Secretary,
Commissioners in Lunacy.

---

* The real cause for dismissal must be here definitely stated.

The Commissioners keep a record of the names of the attendants in the various licensed houses, and the facts relating to them, and this is at all times accessible to the proprietors of licensed houses. The wages in first-class private asylums, of a male attendant, generally commence at 30*l.* per annum, increasing 5*l.* per annum up to 50*l.*, with a certain extra allowance per month when the attendant is engaged on a call, i.e., upon attendance on a patient not residing in the asylum. In some asylums the wages are much less ; but if the wages are upon a low scale, the services of a high-class attendant cannot be obtained.

Record of attendants kept by Commissioners.

Wages of attendants.

The duties of an attendant, if properly and conscientiously performed, are arduous and responsible; and consequently they should be liberally remunerated.

Attendant's duties.

The Commissioners in Lunacy in their last report have drawn special attention to the small proportion of attendants in relation to the number of patients in public asylums.

CHAPTER V.

PRIVATE PATIENTS.

Proceedings necessary for Admission of Private Patients into Asylums.

Legal documents necessary for the reception of a patient into an asylum.

As previously stated, no person alleged to be insane or of unsound mind can be received into an asylum without an order, statement, and two medical certificates, as required by the Lunacy Act.

Order for Admission.

The order must be signed by a relative, friend, or some person authorised to place the patient under legal restraint; and as a rule it is desirable that this should be done by the nearest relative of the alleged lunatic.

The order can be signed either before or after the medical certificates, but it is necessary for the person who signs to have seen the patient within one month from the date of the order.

Persons who are prohibited from signing the order.

The following persons are prohibited from signing the order for admission :—

1. Any person receiving any percentage on or otherwise interested in the payments to be made by or on account of any patient received into a licensed or other house.

2. The term medical attendant is thus defined:— "Every physician, surgeon, and apothecary who shall keep any licensed house, or shall in his medical capacity

attend any licensed house, asylum, hospital, or other place where any lunatic shall be confined." *

3. The father, son, brother, partner, or assistant of either of the medical men who sign the certificates, or who himself has signed one of the certificates.

Legally the person signing the order is responsible for the maintenance of the patient during his residence in the asylum, and no patient can be discharged except by the direction of the Commissioners, without the authority of the person who signed the order. *The person who signs order can authorise patient's discharge.*

For example, if the order for admission be signed by a brother of the patient, neither the father nor any other relative can authorise his discharge without first obtaining the consent of the brother who signed the order.

There is a special provision by which, under certain specified circumstances, authority is given to other persons, who did not sign the order for admission, to discharge the patient.† If the person who signed the order be dead, mentally incapable, or absent from England, the person who made the last payment on account of such patient, or the husband or wife, or (if there be no husband, or the husband or wife be incapable as aforesaid), the father or (if there be no father, or he be incapable as aforesaid) the mother of such patient, or (if there be no mother, or she be incapable as aforesaid) then any one of the nearest of kin, for the time being, of such patient, may by writing, under his or her hand, give such directions as aforesaid, for the discharge or removal of such patient, and thereupon such patient shall be forthwith discharged or removed. *Provision where the person who signed the order for reception is dead or incapable of acting.*

The order for admission is in the form of a *request* made to the proprietor of the asylum to receive the patient, and not, as in the case of pauper lunatics, a *positive injunction.* *Order for admission is simply a request.*

* 8 and 9 Vict. c. 100, s. 114.
† 16 and 17 Vict. c. 97, s. 84.

The wording of the order for admission of a private patient is, "I request you to receive," whilst that of the order necessary for the reception of a pauper lunatic being "I hereby direct you to receive."

Order available for one month.

The order is available for one month from its date, and the patient can be admitted any time within this period.

Mistakes frequently made in filling up the order.

A mistake most generally made in filling up the order is the omission of the name of the patient, after the words "respecting the said" ——. The name has to be repeated *twice*; first, after the word "receive," and then again after the words "respecting the said."

All corrections in Order, Statement, or Medical Certificates must be initialed by the person who makes the alterations.

An omission of this kind destroys the legality of the document unless rectified.

The person who signed the order is required to make the necessary alterations, and these, as well as all erasures, or corrections, must be initialed.

Fourteen days from date of signing of medical certificates allowed for alterations.

Fourteen days from the signing of the medical certificates are allowed for alterations, and if not made in that time the documents cease to be valid, and the patient must be discharged from the asylum.

The order on the following page will illustrate what I mean by the alteration or correction being initialed.

It will be seen that the word "Solicitor" has been erased and consequently initialed. The words "mentally disordered" having been substituted for the terms used in the Act, "lunatic, idiot, *or* person of unsound mind," are erased and initialed, it being absolutely necessary for *one* of these terms to be used.

ORDER FOR THE RECEPTION OF A PRIVATE PATIENT.

Sched. (A) No. I., Sects. 4, 8.

I, the undersigned, hereby request you to receive *Thomas Wilson*, whom I last saw at 4, *Faversham Road, Kensington*, on the *third of unsound mind* day of *April*, 1873, (*a*) a (*b*) person ~~mentally disordered~~ (*H. W.*), as a patient into your house.

Subjoined is a statement respecting the said *Thomas Wilson*.

(Signed)　Name　*Henry Wilson*.　　　~~Solicitor~~ (*H. W.*)

Occupation (if any)　　　　*Solicitor*.

Place of Abode　.　　　4, *Faversham Road, Kensington*.

Degree of relationship (if any), ⎱
　or other　circumstances　of ⎰　　*Father*.
　connection with the Patient

Dated this *3rd* day of *April*, One thousand eight hundred and *seventy-three*.

To　　　　　*Dr. Wilkins*,

　(*c*) *Proprietor of* (*d*) *Eltham House, Barnstaple*.

(a) Within one month previous to the date of the order.

(b) Lunatic, *or* an idiot, *or* a person of unsound mind.

(c) Proprietor *or* superintendent of ——.

(d) Describing the house *or* hospital by situation and name (if any).

Statement.

Following the order is the "Statement," embodying a number of questions, all of which must be answered with the greatest care and truthfulness.

Statement.

It may be signed by the person who signed the order or by any other person.

Generally both order and statement are filled up and signed by the same person.

STATEMENT.

If any Particulars in this Statement be not known, the Fact to be so stated.

Name of patient, with Christian name at length . . . } *Thomas Wilson.*

Sex and age . . . . *Male. 26.*

Married, single, or widowed . *Single.*

Condition of life, and previous occupation (if any) . . } *Barrister-at-law.*

Religious persuasion, as far as known . . . . . } *Church of England.*

Previous place of abode . . *4, Faversham Road, Kensington.*

Whether first attack . . . *Yes.*

Age (if known) on first attack . *26.*

When and where previously under care and treatment . . } *Nowhere.*

Duration of existing attack . *One week.*

Supposed cause . . . . *Mental anxiety.*

Whether subject to epilepsy . *No.*

Whether suicidal . . . *Yes.*

Whether dangerous to others . *No.*

Whether found lunatic by inquisition, and date of commission or order for inquisition . . } *No.*

Special circumstances (if any) preventing the patient being examined, before admission, separately by two medical practitioners . . . } *None.*

Name and address of relative to whom notice of death to be sent . . . . . } *To myself, as below.*

(*e*) Where the person signing the statement is not the person who signs the order, the following particulars concerning the person signing the statement are to be added.

(Signed) Name (*e*) *Henry Wilson.*

Occupation (if any) *Solicitor.*

Place of Abode . *4, Faversham Road, Kensington.*

Degree of relationship (if any), or other circumstances of connection with the Patient } *Father.*

In order to assist us in forming a correct prognosis

of the case, it is desirable to know whether it is the first attack, or if not, how many previous attacks the patient has had ; the exact age on his first attack ; the duration of the existing illness, and whether there is any constitutional predisposition to insanity.

The statement, as is the case with the order, is often carelessly worded. In numerous instances the supposed cause is said to be *unknown*. This answer is not satisfactory, as it prevents the medical officers of the asylum from forming a correct diagnosis of the case.

If the statement is carefully and truthfully filled up, the medical officers connected with the asylum are materially aided in arriving at a right conclusion as to the origin of the mental disorder.

Take for illustration the case of Thomas Wilson, filled up in the "statement." The following answers to the questions would lead us to entertain a favourable prognosis :—

1. The patient having had no previous attack.

2. The short duration of the illness

3. The "supposed cause," mental anxiety. (A very common cause.) In such a case, *cæteris paribus*, the prognosis would be favourable.

4. The patient not being epileptic. In insanity associated with epilepsy or with epileptiform seizures, the prognosis as a rule is most unfavourable.

5. The age of the patient.

If these interrogatories are carefully answered, the medical officer is greatly assisted in forming an accurate opinion of the case.

One of the most important questions in the statement has reference to the "supposed cause" of the insanity. Great difficulty often exists in obtaining any information on this point from the patient's friends ; the answer given to the question is, that no cause can be assigned, or that the cause is unknown.

It rarely happens that a distinct cause cannot be discovered, although the friends object to mention it in the statement.

"Effect of an injury to the head," "sunstroke," "long exposure to a tropical climate," "intemperate habits," "loss of property," "domestic grief," "mental worry," "repeated attacks of delirium tremens," "effect of an acute attack of inflammation of the brain," or "softening or other organic disease of the brain," "long-continued epilepsy," "hereditary predisposition," "sudden accession of fortune," "mental shock," "deficient nutriment,"—any one of these causes would be a *proper* answer to the question.

Special circumstances in' which only one medical certificate is necessary. Another part of the statement requiring to be noticed alludes to the question relating to the special circumstances which have prevented the patient from being examined and certified by "*two*" medical men prior to admission. It is in some instances of the greatest importance to place a patient, in consequence of a sudden attack of mania, under immediate medical treatment. It occasionally happens that in such a case the two medical certificates required by the Act cannot be obtained. For example, in an acute case of insanity occurring in a small village, in which only one medical man resides, it may be found absolutely necessary for the patient to be placed without delay under care and treatment, and this can legally be done on the certificate of *one* qualified practitioner, but the special circumstances which have prevented the *second* certificate from being obtained must be clearly stated in the latter portion of the statement.

Proceedings subsequent to a patient's admission on one certificate. If a case is admitted into an asylum on one certificate, the patient must be examined by *two* medical men *within three clear days* from his admission into the asylum, and the two additional certificates must be forwarded to the Commissioners within that period. The medical men who sign the certificates, after the admission of the patient, must not be in partnership with each other, or connected with the medical man who signed the first certificate upon which the patient was received, or related to the proprietor or superintendent of the asylum, or interested in any way in such asylum. The examination, as in the case with ordinary medical certificates, is required to be made separately, and not in the presence of any other medical man.

The order, statement, and medical certificates need not necessarily be made on the printed form contained in the schedule of the Act, but may be written on ordinary paper, provided the exact and literal wording of the official documents is strictly adhered to ; it is, however, always desirable to use the printed form if one can be obtained. *Order and statement need not be printed.*

The statement should specify whether the patient is hereditarily predisposed to insanity. In the statement of pauper lunatics there is a special paragraph relating to this matter.

Medical Certificates.

No patient, except under special circumstances, previously referred to, can be admitted into an asylum without *two* medical certificates.* *Medical certificates.*

The medical certificates can be signed before or after the order and statement, but this must be done within seven clear days from the date of the examination of the alleged lunatic, and the patient can only be admitted within seven days from this examination. It may be dated and signed any time between the examination and reception of the patient. The medical men who sign the certificates must be in actual practice and duly registered, in order to render the certificates valid. *Signed before or after the order, and available for seven days from date of examination.*

* This does not apply to Chancery patients or pauper lunatics.

Persons prohibited from Signing Certificates in Lunacy.

Certain persons prohibited from signing the medical certificates.

There are certain persons who, although qualified to practise, are nevertheless prohibited from signing the medical certificates.*

1st. Any person receiving any percentage on, or otherwise interested in, the payments to be made by or on account of any patient received into a licensed or other house.

2ndly. Any medical attendant, as defined by the Lunacy Act.

3rdly. The medical men who sign must not be in partnership or professionally connected.†

4thly. The medical certificates cannot be signed by the father, brother, son, partner, or assistant of the person having the care or charge of the patient, and no physician, surgeon, or apothecary who, or whose father, brother, son, partner, or assistant shall have signed the order for admission can sign the certificate.

If a medical man desires to place his wife in an asylum, he can sign the order, but cannot, although a legally qualified practitioner, sign either of the medical certificates.

Remarks of Commissioners concerning medical certificates.

The Commissioners in their fifteenth Report (dated March 31, 1861, page 65) refer to the great care necessary in order to make these certificates legally valid. " Few of our duties require more vigilance than that of satisfying ourselves in all doubtful cases as to the validity of the orders and certificates on which patients are admitted into asylums, or become subject

---

* 25 and 26 Vict. c. 111, s. 114.

† It is not absolutely necessary that the medical man certifying should specify his medical or surgical degrees or qualifications, but he may describe himself as " a duly qualified registered practitioner."

to detention in any place. From time to time we have issued printed instructions with the view of ensuring, as far as possible, on the part of superintendents, proprietors, medical practitioners, and others an accurate compliance with the requirements of the law. Immediate steps are taken for correction upon discovery of defects or omissions; and where this is not found to be practicable, the substitution of new and valid certificates, or, as the unavoidable alternative, immediate discharge of the patient from illegal detention under certificates having no validity has been insisted on.

Among such cases of the past year one may be specially referred to because of the importance of the questions involved in it. By the statute the certifying medical man is required to set forth in the certificate not merely his opinion of the insanity of the person examined, but the specific fact or facts indicating insanity on which that opinion is formed ; in the body of the certificate the date and place of examination are to be exactly stated; each medical man, where two certificates are necessary, is to examine the patient separately and apart from the other practitioner; and, if such examination has taken place at any period beyond seven days before admission of the patient into the house or asylum where he is detained, the certificates are invalid, and detention under them becomes illegal. The object of all these precautions is to provide that no one shall be deprived of his liberty as a person of unsound mind except upon specific grounds, existing at the exact time when it is proposed to place such person under restraint. It would of course be impossible that any examining medical man should exclude from his consideration facts known to him of the antecedents of the patient, immediate or remote. These are entitled to their full influence; but the Legislature has been careful to guard against such facts exercising undue influence in the certificate he is

Discharge of a patient by Commissioners in Lunacy in consequence of insufficiency of facts, and inability to amend the certificates to their satisfaction.

called on to give, by requiring that this certificate shall be directly deducible from examination on a particular day and at a specified place, and that the opinion expressed therein as having been formed on such particular day shall be set forth as the result of his having observed at that time in the person under examination some specific fact indicating insanity.

In the case to which allusion has been made no such specific fact was stated in either certificate, and upon the necessary forms of amendment being suggested, it was found that the certificates of both the medical men were not given on what they observed on any particular day, but that, having attended the patient professionally for a considerable period, they had not any doubt from her ordinary course of conduct that the patient was of unsound mind, and that it was on this opinion they based their certificates. We had no alternative in these circumstances but to direct the discharge of the patient, in order to obtain a fresh examination and certificates in compliance with the law."

Mistakes render the certificates invalid if not amended within fourteen days from the reception of the patient.

It frequently happens that, in consequence of an apparently trifling mistake, the certificate becomes invalid, and, if not amended, the patient, though a dangerous lunatic, must be discharged.

As before mentioned, the certificate is only valid for seven days from the date of the examination of the patient. If a mistake is found in the certificate it will be returned by the Commissioners for alteration.

This alteration must be made within *fourteen* days from the reception of the patient, and if not done to their satisfaction the Commissioners, or any two of them, can authorise the discharge of the patient. Every alteration and correction, as is the case with the order and statement, must be initialed.

The medical certificates must *accurately* specify : 1st. The date and place of examination ; 2nd. The exact residence, with the number of the house, where the patient resides. These facts are of *great* importance, and without their specification the certificate is invalid. Serious inconvenience often results from these particulars being misstated and not properly corrected within the period allowed for amendments.

The medical men who sign the certificates are required to investigate the case thoroughly, so as not to state "facts" as delusions, without first assuring themselves that they are not based upon reality, but simply pure emanations from the insane imagination of the patient. For example, a person affirms that he is ruined, but before this can be stated as a delusion in the certificate certain enquiries must be made in order to ascertain whether there is any foundation for this impression.

Medical men are liable—and justly so—to an action at law on the ground of negligence if they sign a certificate without enquiring into the truth of the facts (should these facts admit of investigation) stated in their certificates as evidences of insanity necessitating restraint.

Of course there are ideas which are so obviously of an insane character, that it would be absurd to entertain any doubt as to their nature. They are *primâ facie* symptoms of mental aberration, and no questions need be asked about them. The certificate on the following page is given as an illustration.

Truth of the "facts" stated must be thoroughly enquired into.

MEDICAL CERTIFICATE.

Sched. (A) No. II., Sects. 4, 5, 8, 10, 11, 12, 13.

(a) Here set forth the qualification entitling the person certifying to practise as a physician, surgeon, or apothecary, ex. gra. :—Fellow of the Royal College of Physicians in London, Licentiate of the Apothecaries' Company (or as the case may be).

(b) Physician, surgeon, *or* apothecary (as the case may be).

(c) Here insert the street and number of the house (if any), or other like particulars.

(d) Insert residence and profession, or occupation (if any), of the patient.

(e) Lunatic, *or* an idiot, *or* a person of unsound mind.

I, the undersigned, being a (a) *Member of the Royal College of Surgeons, England,* and being in actual practice as a (b) *Surgeon,* hereby certify that I, on the *3rd day of April,* 1873, at (c) 4, *Faversham Road, Kensington,* in the county of *Middlesex,* separately from any other medical practitioner, personally examined *Thomas Wilson,* of (d) 4, *Faversham Road, Kensington, barrister,* and that the said *Thomas Wilson* is a (e) *person of unsound mind,* and a proper person to be taken charge of and detained under care and treatment, and that I have formed this opinion upon the following grounds, viz. :—

(f) Here state the facts.

1. Facts indicating insanity observed by myself: (f)

> *He is under the delusion that he is ruined, and that the sheriff's officers are waiting in the house to remove him. He is very desponding and low-spirited, and says his soul is completely lost, having committed the unpardonable sin.*

(g) Here state the information, and from whom.

2. Other facts (if any) indicating insanity communicated to me by others : (g)

> *His brother, John Wilson, tells me that the patient, Thomas Wilson, for the last few days has been in a desponding state of mind, and has made several attempts at self-destruction.*

(Signed) Name *Alfred Cowan.*

Place of Abode 44, *Faversham Road, Kensington.*

Dated this *third day of April,* One thousand eight hundred and *seventy-three.*

In signing a certificate there are two conclusions to be arrived at :— Conclusions to be arrived at before signing a certificate of lunacy.

1st. That the patient is a person of unsound mind.

2nd. That he is a proper person to be placed under restraint.

The medical men signing must consider carefully these two points before certifying.

Medical certificates are frequently carelessly written, and are, in consequence of inaccuracies, returned by the Commissioners for correction.

Mistakes in the certificates are often caused by the medical men omitting to read the marginal notes printed on the official document for their instruction. The following omissions are frequently made :—

1st. The name of the street and number of the house at which the examination of the patient is made. Omissions frequently made in certificates.

An omission of this kind renders the certificate invalid, and if it is not rectified within fourteen days the patient must be discharged.

Should there be no number to the house where the patient is examined the fact must be mentioned.*

2nd. A very common mistake is omitting to state the occupation (if any) and address of the patient.

3rd. The name of the informant in the second part of the certificate must be given.

It will not be sufficient to say, "His brother, wife, or his sister tells me so and so." If the name of the informant is not given, the certificate will be returned by the Commissioners.

Discharge of a Patient in consequence of Insufficient Facts.

I will cite one case from the 17th Report of the Commissioners in Lunacy, dated June 9, 1863.

---

* If there should be a particular name by which the house is known, it should be stated, as, for instance, "Ivy Cottage," "Holly Lodge," "Laburnum Villa," "The Firs," &c., &c.

Discharge of patient by Commissioners in Lunacy in consequence of defective certificate.

" We have had occasion in one case to exercise the powers vested in us by the 27th section of the ' Lunacy Acts Amendment Act 1862,' by ordering the discharge of a patient from a county asylum, on the ground of a defective medical certificate.

E. A., a female pauper lunatic, chargeable to the Bosmere and Claydon Union, was received into the Suffolk County Asylum, upon the usual order of a justice, and a medical certificate signed by Mr. J. Pennington, a surgeon, wherein under the head ' Facts indicating insanity, observed by myself,' he stated as follows :— ' None, but a stupid, sulky, obstinate temper.' The other facts indicating insanity, set forth as having been communicated to him by others, were the following :— ' Extremely indecent ; exposure of her person on all occasions, public as well as private ; attempting to cut her throat, as well as to strangle another girl ; these facts communicated to me by the nurse and deputy-matron.' In this certificate it will be noticed that the facts observed by Mr. Pennington himself, taken alone, were not indicative of insanity, and that what he had certified, therefore, did not satisfy the provisions of the ' Lunatic Asylums Act 1853,' s. 75, which declares that, ' No person shall be received into any asylum under any certificate which purports to be founded only on facts communicated by others.' The facts stated must plainly be of a kind indicating insanity, and no such facts were, according to his averment, observed by Mr. Pennington.

In these circumstances, the Board felt that they had no option in the case, and were bound to insist upon an amendment of the certificate.

It is not necessary to set forth in detail the correspondence which passed upon the subject, and which extended over a period of three months. Every effort was made on the part of this Board to procure a substantial compliance with the Act. The visitors of the asylum declined to interfere, and Mr. Pennington ultimately stated that he had nothing to add to his certificate. This was after the Commissioners had communicated to the visitors their opinion, that it was impossible legally to detain E. A. under the certificate of Mr. Pennington, and had said that, unless a valid certificate were procured in its place, they would be obliged to exercise the power conferred on them by the recent Act and order her discharge.

Accordingly an order for that purpose was made by two members of the Board on January 3, and, in obedience thereto, E. A. was discharged, and removed on the 16th, a fortnight having been allowed for that purpose. Dr. Kirkman, the superintendent of the asylum, to whom the order was transmitted, was informed that, considering the nature of the case (which was reported to be one of epileptic mania), the Commissioners had made the order with great reluctance ; but that the manifest defect in Mr. Pennington's certificate, and the neglect either to amend the same or to procure a fresh one in its place, left them no choice in the matter. He was at the same time requested at once to communicate on the subject with the relieving officer, in order that, with the least possible disturbance to the patient, she might be readmitted into the asylum on a fresh order and certificate. No notice has been received of her readmission."

" Facts of Insanity observed by myself."

The most important part of the certificates relates to the evidence of insanity observed by the medical men who sign them. The facts therein stated must clearly establish the existence of mental unsoundness, and such unsoundness of mind as to justify the confinement of the

Facts of insanity must be clearly stated in the medical certificates.

patient in an asylum or elsewhere. It will not be sufficient
for the person signing to say, he *thinks* So-and-so to be
insane, or *believes* him to be so, or that he has the
appearance of being of unsound mind, or that his
actions indicate the presence of insanity, or that he
hears that the person alleged to be insane has been guilty
of conduct not consistent with the supposition of his mind
being in a sound state; that his general conversation is
symptomatic of insanity, or that he is wasting his property, and is unable to take care of himself or to
manage his affairs.   Facts referable to all these points
no doubt are important, particularly when considered in
relation to actual mental delusions or other evidences of
alienation of mind, but *per se* they do not justify a certificate or legal confinement.   All vague, hypothetical,
and loose generalisations should be studiously avoided
when signing the certificates.

   Facts, specific facts only—*which the medical man himself has observed* at the time of signing—should be clearly
stated.   If this injunction is not strictly acted upon, the
certificate will be valueless.   It should be the medical
man's object to discover, if practicable, the presence of
defined delusions, hallucinations, or illusions.   In some
cases it may be extremely difficult to detect the insane
idea inciting the patient to overt acts of madness jus-
tifying restraint.   It may be cunningly concealed for a
purpose, or the lunatic may obstinately refuse to give
utterance to his insane thoughts, and be doggedly silent
when closely questioned on the subject.   Again, there
are states of mental unsoundness which apparently are
unconnected with any perceptible delusions or insane
impressions—such as in some cases of acute melancholia,
imbecility, or homicidal mania.   But as a rule, morbid
delusions may be detected in nearly all cases of insanity
requiring restraint.   One distinctly defined fact indicative of insanity will be more valuable than whole

pages of ambiguous speculations or loose surmises. For example, a belief in the commission of the " sin against the Holy Ghost," or the " unpardonable sin" (common delusions among the insane), or the existence of a delusion that the patient has come into the possession of, or is entitled to, a fabulous amount of wealth, or that his relatives or friends are conspiring against him, that the police are in search of him and are about to arrest him for committing some imaginary crime, or that he (although in the possession of ample means) believes himself to be ruined, and that consequently he is to be placed in the workhouse. In numerous cases of acute melancholia delusions will be found relating to religious subjects, such as the patient believing that his soul is lost, that God has forsaken him, that he is satanically possessed, that he is in hell and doomed to everlasting torment, or that he has received a direct command from God to do certain things—such as to commit suicide, or to kill his wife or one of his children.

Insanity is often shown by a perversion of scriptural texts. Many a lunatic has mutilated himself by literally acting under what he conceives to be a Divine command, such as " If thine eye offend thee, pluck it out." *Insanity shown by perversion scriptural texts.*

In many cases the patient shows his insanity by his unnatural and morbid hatred to his wife or some of his children, either under the delusion of his wife's infidelity or that his children are conspiring against or robbing him.

These hallucinations occasionally lead to serious acts of murderous violence; and, if clearly proved to be creations of a diseased imagination, justify restraint. In numerous cases it is sufficient to certify that the patient is labouring under general paralysis of the insane, accompanied with great mental excitement and exaltation, and insane ideas of exalted rank and position. Clearly manifested symptoms of softening of the brain,.

associated with imbecility and incoherent conversation, are sufficient to justify a certificate; but no physical disease or disordered conditions of the brain and nervous system, even if associated with paralysis or convulsive disorders, such as epilepsy, will warrant a certificate of insanity, unless the patient shows symptoms of positive *mental* derangement, with or without delusions. Acts of reckless extravagance, violent deportment, cruelty, brutality of conduct, or gross immorality, are not by themselves sufficient to authorise a certificate, unless it can be clearly established that these states of mind are the *effect* of some disorder of the brain deranging or impairing the intellect, and are likely to incite to mischievous acts.

Chronic intemperance will not of itself be sufficient to warrant a certificate, unless connected with some symptoms of disease of the brain, or disorder of the mind. The existence of what is termed "moral insanity" will not alone justify a certificate or the imposition of legal restraint.

The moral sense is often morbidly perverted and deranged. In many of these cases no actual mental delusions are detected. This condition of mind is often fraught with serious mischief to the patient and his family, and such patients require control and treatment. Persons so afflicted present great difficulties to the medical man, when called upon to certify, for the purpose of placing them under restraint. No certificate would be justifiable unless there can be detected with the so-called "moral insanity" a clearly manifested disorder of those powers of the mind which are involved in the exercise of the judgment and reasoning faculties, and which disorder is likely to impel the patient to the commission of some insane and mischievous act to himself or family. The line of demarcation between vice and insanity is most difficult to perceive or define.

[margin note: Chronic intemperance will not per se justify a certificate.]

[margin note: Difficulty of dealing with patients with moral insanity.]

In conclusion, the medical men who sign the certificates must remember that only "facts" observed on the *day of their examination* of the patient are admissible.

Facts only observed on day of examination of the patient are admissible.

" *Other Facts (if any) indicating Insanity communicated to me by Others.*"

In order for a certificate to be legal, the facts of insanity observed by the medical men who sign must be stated.

Other facts of insanity.

The second part of the certificate has reference to other facts communicated to the medical men by the attendant of the patient, the relatives, or friends. It is always most desirable for the certificate to contain some facts obtained from those who have been in immediate attendance on the patient during his illness. Besides strengthening the certificate, those who are to have the charge of the patient will have these important facts for their guidance in the management of the case.

Facts communicated by others, though not compulsory, in order for the certificate to be legal, are notwithstanding very desirable.

At the time of the examination the patient may, though labouring under delusion, be calm and quiet. The friends of the patient may be enabled to tell the medical men that at certain times the patient is very noisy and excited, and will then, if not prevented, destroy whatever comes in his way. This is an important fact "communicated by others."

" His sister (Jane Wilson) informs me that he has threatened several times to commit suicide."

Examples of "other facts."

" His brother (John Wilson) informs me that he refuses his food, and that during the last few days he has not eaten sufficient to support life."

" His attendant (William Jennings) tells me that the patient is very cunning, and will endeavour to conceal anything with which he can do injury to himself, and that last evening a knife was found concealed underneath his pillow."

The name of the informant *must* always be given.

The following instructions relating to the signing of medical certificates were drawn up by Mr. Commissioner Phillips during the time he acted as Secretary.

MEDICAL CERTIFICATES.

Instructions.

Instructions for filling up medical certificates.

Every medical certificate must, in order to its validity, be according to the subjoined form, prescribed by the "Lunatics' Care and Treatment" and "Lunatic Asylums" Acts, 1853.

In filling up the certificate the medical practitioner signing is requested especially to observe the following *essential* particulars, viz.:—

1. After the words "being a" he is required to insert, not the word "physician," "surgeon," or "apothecary," but the legal qualification, diploma, or licence entitling him to practise as such within the United Kingdom.

The words of the interpretation clause are as follows:—"'Physician,' 'surgeon,' or 'apothecary' shall respectively mean a physician, surgeon, or apothecary, duly authorised or licensed to practise as such by or as a member of some college, university, company, or institution legally established and qualified to grant such authority or licence in some part of the United Kingdom, or having been in practice as an apothecary in England or Wales on or before the 15th day of August, 1815, and being in actual practice as a physician, surgeon, or apothecary, and registered under the Medical Act."

2. He is required to insert:—1. The date of examination. 2. The place, with "*the street and number of the house (if any), or other like particulars,*" where the patient was examined. 3. The patient's ordinary place of residence. 4. The patient's profession or occupation, if any.

3. In any case where more than one medical certificate is required by the Act he should insert before the words "personally examined" the words "separately from any other medical practitioner."

4. He is required, in order that his certificate may have any validity in law, to set forth some fact or facts, or symptoms, indicating insanity, *observed by himself* at date of examination.

5. The certificate need not be drawn up or dated on the day of examination, but the patient *must be examined within seven clear days prior to admission.*

6. Every certificate should be an independent and complete document, and no reference should be made therein to another.

7. In case of a private patient, the medical practitioners certifying may not be in partnership, or in the position of principal and assistant.

Note.—Medical officers of unions or parishes are no longer prohibited from signing certificates in the cases of pauper lunatics belonging thereto.

CHARLES P. PHILLIPS,
Secretary.

Office of Commissioners in Lunacy.

The following table contains a complete list of all metropolitan and provincial asylums in England and Wales. By this will be seen the various towns in which asylums are situated, the name of the asylum, to whom licensed, the number of patients, whether male or female, residing in the asylum, and the average number resident during the previous year.

Metropolitan Licensed Houses.

Town	Name of House	To whom Licensed	Number for which Licensed			Average number resident during the year 1871			
			M.	F.	Total	M.	F.	Total	
Acton	Derwentwater House	Miss Benfield	—	12	12	—	5	5	
Bethnal Green	Bethnal House	Dr. John Millar	164	246	410	129	203	332	Pauper and private patients.
Bow	Grove Hall	Mr. E. H. Byas, surgeon, and Dr. Mickle	302	150	452	299	115	414	Pauper and private patients.
Brixton	Effra Hall	Mr. C. A. Elliott, Dr. W. H. Diamond	—	26	26	—	20	20	
Brompton	Clarence Villa	Mr. G. F. Bloxsome, surgeon	2	—	2	2	—	2	
"	Earls Court House	Miss Burney and Dr. R. G. and Mrs. Hill	—	30	30	—	28	28	
Brook Green	Montague House	Mrs. Roy	13	—	13	12	—	12	
Camberwell	Camberwell House	Dr. J. H. Paul and Dr. F. Schofield	184	269	453	145	236	381	Pauper and private patients.
Chelsea	Blacklands House	Mr. A. C. Sutherland and Mr. E. Hall, surgeon	35	—	35	16	—	16	
"	Elm House, 149 Church Street	Mr. F. A. B. Bonney, surgeon	—	10	10	—	8	8	
Chiswick	Manor House	Dr. Tuke	20	20	40	13	13	26	
Clapham	The Retreat Union Road*	Mr. John Bush, surgeon (deceased)	—	—	—	6	6	12	

* This establishment is now closed.

METROPOLITAN LICENSED HOUSES—*continued.*

Town	Name of House	To whom Licensed.	Number for which Licensed			Average number resident during the year 1871		
			M.	F.	Total	M.	F.	Total
Clapton Upper	Brooke House	Dr. H. Monro and J. O. Adams, surgeon	44	46	90	40	37	77
Fulham	Munster House *	Dr. Blandford, Mr.J.F.Hemming, Mr. C. Williams	35	—	35	27	—	27
,,	Normand House	Miss Talfourd	—	15	15	—	8	8
,,	OttoHouse North End	Mr. A. C. Sutherland and Miss E. Dixon	—	35	35	—	32	32
Hackney	London House	Mrs. Ayre	—	15	15	—	12	12
Hammersmith	Upper Mall House	Mrs. Cotes	—	10	10	—	5	5
,,	Sussex and Brandenburg Houses	Drs. F., H. F., and L. S. Winslow	42	22	64	36	21	57
HamptonWick	Normansfield	Mrs. Down	25	25	50	19	15	34
Hanwell	Lawn House	Dr. H. Maudsley	—	10	10	—	6	6
,,	Kent Lodge	Mr. F. Waite	3	2	5	3	1	4
,,	Vine Cottage, Norwood Green	Mr. and Mrs. Chalk	—	12	12	—	11	11
Hayes	Hayes Park	Mr. and Mrs. Benbow	—	19	19	—	15	15
,,	Wood End Grove	Dr. H. Stilwell, Mr. J. Elliott and Mrs. Spence	—	19	19	—	18	18
Hendon	Hendon House	Miss Dence	—	10	10	—	8	8
Hillingdon	Moorcroft House	Dr. H. Stilwell and H.Elliott,surgeon	46	—	46	45	—	45
Hoxton	Hoxton House	Dr. W. J. Hunt	94	231	325	84	173	257
Isleworth	Wyke House	Dr. E. S. Willett	25	20	45	23	15	38
Kensington	Kensington House †	Dr. Wood and T. Bigland, surgeon	30	·33	63	17	23	40
Kilburn	51 Priory Road	Mr. G. Moseley, surgeon	—	2	2	—	2	2
Leyton	Great House	Mrs. Davey	—	15	15	—	13	13
Norwood Lower	Colville House,Norwood Lane	Mrs. Foreman	4	1	5	4	1	5
Peckham	Peckham House	Mr. E. H. Byas and Dr. A. H. Stocker	105	225	330	78	154	232
Peckham Rye	Silverton House, Linden Grove	Mrs. Fruin	—	8	8	—	6	6
Southall	Southall Park	Dr.Steward andMrs. Vickers	15	12	27	13	11	24
,,	The Shrubbery	Dr. and Mrs. Steward	—	4	4	—	3	3
,,	South Lodge	Mr. E. Harvey	—	2	2	—	2	2
Stoke Newington	Northumberland House	Dr. and Mrs. Sabben	40	45	85	36	36	72
Sunbury	Halliford House	Dr. Seaton	12	16	28	9	13	22
Twickenham	Twickenham House	Dr. H. W. and Mrs. Diamond	1	14	15	2	14	16
Totals			1241	1631	2872	1058	1289	2347

Left margin: Pauper and private patients.　　Private and pauper patients.

* New licensees since Commissioners' Report, 1872.
† Dr. Wood has transferred his patients to the Priory, Roehampton.

Provincial Licensed Houses.

County	Houses	To whom Licensed.	Number for which Licensed M.	F.	Total	Average number resident during the year 1871 M.	F.	Total	
Beds.	Springfield House, near Bedford	Dr. H. Harris, (Surg.)	20	20	40	10	11	21	
Chester	Hollingworth Hall, Motham, Manchester	Mr. E. Rowlands .	8	2	10	4	2	6	
Derby	Wye House, Buxton .	Drs. T. and F. K. Dickson .	24	20	44	15	17	32	
Devon	Kenton House, Kenton	Miss E. A. Teage .	–	6	6	–	2	2	
,,	Plympton House, Plympton .	Mr. S. Langworthy(Surg.)	17	17	34	14	9	23	
Durham	Dinsdale Park, near Darlington .	Dr. J. W. Eastwood	28	22	50	21	13	34	Pauper and private patients.
,,	Dunston Lodge, near Gateshead .	Mr. W. Garbutt .	30	25	55	27	14	41	
Essex	Essex Hall, near Colchester .	Mr. W. Millard .	66	33	99	66	30	96	
,,	Witham . .	Mr. T. M. Tomkin (Surg.) .	15	10	25	9	5	14	
Glamorgan	Vernon House, Briton Ferry .	Mr. Chas. Pegge (Surg.) .	80	80	160	27	53	80	Pauper and private patients.
Gloucester.	Northwoods, near Bristol	Dr. J. G. Davey .	15	15	30	7	10	17	
,,	Fairford House, Fairford .	Messrs. D. D. and H. Iles .	35	35	70	21	23	44	
,,	The Croft House, Fairford .	Mrs. Iles .	–	4	4	–	3	3	
,,	Sandywell Park, Dowdeswell, near Cheltenham	Dr. W. H. O. Sankey	17	17	34	12	15	27	
,,	Tusculum House, Mitcheldean .	Mrs. Powell .	–	3	3	–	2	2	
Hants	Westbrook House, Alton .	Mrs. E. J. Burnett	25	25	50	14	15	29	
Herts	Harpenden Hall, near St. Albans	Mr. A. G. Rumball	7	3	10	3	1	4	
,,	Hadham Palace, Much Hadham .	Dr. F. M. Smith .	12	8	20	6	4	10	
Kent	North Grove House, Hawkhurst .	Mr. W. Harmer and Dr. W. M. Harmer .	16	8	24	12	6	18	
,,	Tattlebury House, Goudhurst .	Mr. R. S. Newington (Surg.).	4	4	8	2	–	2	
,,	West Malling Place, near Maidstone .	Dr. T. H. Lowry .	18	14	32	9	11	20	
Lancaster.	Marsden Hall, Burnley	Mr. E. A. Bennett (Surg.) .	15	13	28	12	9	21	
,,	Clifton Hall, near Manchester .	Mrs. Lomas and Mr.D.H.Lomas	15	15	30	10	10	20	
,,	Haydock Lodge, Ashton, Newton-le-Willows .	Dr. E. Lister .	105	145	250	101	140	241	Pauper and private patients.
,,	Tue Brook Villa, near Liverpool .	Mr. H. Owen (Surg.) .	26	26	52	15	19	34	

PROVINCIAL LICENSED HOUSES—*continued.*

Pauper and private patients.

—			Number for which Licensed			Average number resident during the year 1871		
County	Houses	To whom Licensed	M.	F.	Total	M.	F.	Total
Norfolk .	Heigham Hall, near Norwich .	Mr. W. P. Nichols, and Mr. J. F. Watson (Surgeons) . .	35	35	70	31	31	62
"	The Grove, Catton, near Norwich .	Mr. T. J. C. Rackham . .	11	13	24	9	9	18
Northampton	Abington Abbey Retreat, near Northampton .	Dr. Thos. Prichard	24	17	41	18	16	34
Shropshire	Stretton House, Church Stretton	Mr. W. Hyslop .	40	–	40	33	–	33
"	Grove House, All Stretton . .	Mrs. Bakewell .	–	45	45	–	31	31
Somerset .	Brislington House, near Bristol. .	Drs. F. K. and C. H. Fox .	56	50	106	52	38	90
"	Longwood House, near Bristol .	Dr. G. Rogers .	30	20	50	26	16	42
"	Bailbrook House, Bath Easton .	Mr. J. Terry (Surg.)	20	20	40	15	10	25
"	Upper House, Combe Down, Bath . . .	Miss B. Long .	5	5	10	4	3	7
"	Amberd House, near Taunton .	Dr. F. H. Woodforde . .	–	20	20	–	16	16
"	Downside Lodge, Midsomer Norton	Miss M. Short .	–	7	7	–	5	5
Stafford .	Moat House, Tamworth . . .	Mr. J. F. Woody (Surg.) . .	–	10	10	–	3	3
"	Barr House, Great Barr, near Birmingham . .	Mrs. Moore . .	–	10	10	–	6	6
Suffolk .	Aspall Hall, near Debenham . .	Miss I. J. Chevallier . .	5	5	10	4	2	6
"	The Grove, Ipswich .	Dr. B. Chevallier .	8	2	10	6	–	6
"	Belle Vue House, Ipswich . .	Miss S. A. F. Walter	3	5	8	2	3	5
Surrey .	Lea Pale House, near Guildford . .	Mr. T. J. Sells (Surg.) . .	8	–	8	5	–	5
"	Church Street, Epsom	Mr. G. Stilwell (Surg.) .	–	10	10	–	8	8
Sussex .	Ticehurst Asylum .	Dr. Samuel Newington .	44	30	74	41	24	65
"	Church Hill House, Brighton * . .	Mrs. Foreman .	–	–	–	–	–	–
"	St. George's Retreat, Ditchling, Burgess Hill . . .	Miss Eccles, &c. .	10	24	34	2	11	13
Warwick .	Driffold House, Sutton Coldfield .	Dr. G. F. Bodington	12	18	30	7	12	19
"	Burman House, Henley in Arden	Dr. Wade and Dr. S. H. Agar .	17	13	30	14	7	21
"	Arden House, Henley in Arden .	Mr. G. R. Dartnell (Surg.) . .	4	2	6	1	–	1

* Patients removed to Colville House, Lower Norwood.

Provincial Licensed Houses—*continued*.

County	Houses	To whom Licensed	Number for which Licensed			Average number resident during the year 1871		
			M.	F.	Total	M.	F.	Total
Warwick	Hurst House, Henley in Arden	Mrs. Phillips	–	8	8	–	3	3
"	Midland Counties Idiot Asylum, Dorridge Grove, Knowle Common	Dr. T. B. E. Fletcher and Mrs. Stock	8	12	20	6	10	16
Wilts	Laverstock House, near Salisbury	Mr. J. Haynes & Mr. H. Manning (Surg.)	35	35	70	24	27	51
"	Fisherton House, near Salisbury	Mr. W. C. Finch (Sur.) and Dr. J.A.Lush,M.P.	338	278	616	183	191	374
"	Fiddington House, Market Lavington, Devizes	Dr. C. Hitchcock	20	20	40	15	13	28
"	Kingsdown House, Box	Dr. Jos. Nash	17	23	40	16	22	38
Worcester	Droitwich Asylum	{ Mr. F. J. Bennett (Surg.). }	–	–	–	8	6	14
York, E.R.	Marfleet Lane Retreat, Sculcoates, Hull	Mr. J. Brown	–	11	11	–	10	10
"	Dunnington House, near York	Mr. R. H. Hornby	24	16	40	21	13	34
York, N.R.	Terrace House, Osbaldwick	Dr. J. Ure	–	10	10	–	7	7
York,W.R.	Mount Stead, near Leeds	Dr. G. P. Smith and Mrs. Smith	15	15	30	9	11	20
"	Greta Bank, Barnoldswick, near Bentham	Mrs. J. Parker	5	5	10	3	2	5
"	Grove House, Acomb,near York	Mr. Robt. Pearson.	14	17	31	13	13	26
"	Lime-tree House, Acomb,near York	Mr. Samuel Nelson	12	6	18	4	–	4
"	The Grange, Kimberworth, Rotherham, (late St. John's House, Wakefield)	Dr. J. G. Atkinson	–	12	12	–	7	7
York City	Lawrence House,York	Mr. W. Pumphrey	4	8	12	4	5	9
	Totals		1422	1407	2829	993	1015	2008

Right margin notes:
Pauper and private patients.
Pauper and private patients.
Pauper and private patients.

CHAPTER VI.

SINGLE PATIENTS CONFINED IN UNLICENSED PRIVATE HOUSES.

It is illegal to take charge of, for profit, a person of unsound mind without first obtaining the necessary documents.

No person, except a Committee appointed by the Lord Chancellor, who derives profit from the charge of a lunatic, can receive him into his house without an order, statement, and medical certificates, similar to those required previous to the admission of a patient into an asylum.

Single Patients.

The number of private patients under single care, in pursuance of the 90th section of the Act 8 and 9 Vict. c. 100, on Jan 1, 1872, was 420, and the changes which have taken place in the past year are shown in the following table, taken from the Commissioners' last report:—

				Males.	Females.	Total.
Number on January 1, 1871 . .				160	232	392
Registered during the year . .				79	109	188
				239	341	580
Discharged and died				71	89	160

	Recovered.	Not Recovered.	Died.	Total.
Males . .	6	49	16	71
Females .	13	66	10	89
	19	115	26	160

	Males.	Females.	Total.
Remaining, January 1, 1872 . .	168	252	420
Of whom found lunatic by inquisition and not visited by the Commissioners	57	64	121

If a person is desirous to place any relative alleged to be insane under care and treatment, and has arranged for some one to admit him into his house, it is advisable for the person who is about to receive the patient to call at the office of the Commissioners in Lunacy,* and obtain from the Secretary copies of the necessary legal documents, which have to be properly filled up before the patient can be received. *(margin note: Proceedings prior to the reception of an insane person into a private house.)*

The order and statement can be signed by the father or any other relative or friend of the patient who is authorised to act. *(margin note: Order.)*

The order is addressed either to the person receiving the patient as "*proprietor*," or to the attendant under whose charge the patient is, as "*superintendent*."

The patient will have to be examined by two medical men, who will sign the certificates. *(margin note: Medical Certificates.)*

Legal authority is now given to the proprietor or superintendent to receive the patient into his house within seven days from the date of the certificates.

He is required to transmit to the Commissioners in Lunacy an accurate copy of the order, statement, and certificates within twenty-four hours from the reception of the patient into his house. *(margin note: Copies of legal documents sent to Commissioners.)*

The person selected to act in the capacity of medical attendant (who is appointed either by the person signing the order for the patient's admission or by the proprietor of the house or lodgings) must send to the office of the Commissioners a statement respecting the bodily health and mental state of the patient, and regularly visit him, and make the proper entries in the "Medical Visitation Book" † (as required by Act of Parliament) at least once a fortnight. *(margin note: Medical Attendant. ... Statement.)*

The examination for the statement must be made

* 19 Whitehall Place, S.W.

† This book, as well as all official documents, can be obtained at Shaw & Sons', Fetter Lane; and Knight & Co's., 90 Fleet Street.

after the expiration of two, and before the expiration of seven clear days from the patient's reception, and can be sent to the Commissioners any time within that period.

Single patients visited by Commissioners.

All single patients are visited at least once a year by one or more of the Commissioners.

Single Chancery patients are visited four times a year by the Chancery visitors.

No licence is required for one patient.

No licence is required for one patient, but if more than one is confined in the house the proprietor must have a licence, and the house becomes for the time being an asylum, and subject to the same rules and regulations.

I have thought it advisable to give the regulations referring to single patients as laid down by the Commissioners in Lunacy in the appendix of their seventeenth Report. By this it will be clearly seen what is required from all who undertake the responsibility of admitting single patients in their houses for profit.

TO ALL PERSONS HAVING CHARGE OF SINGLE INSANE PATIENTS.

The Law relating to Single Insane Patients, and defining the duties and responsibilities of those who undertake to receive such Patients to reside with them, being in general very imperfectly understood, and frequently violated, your attention is urgently requested to the subjoined statement of the various provisions of the Statutes, which the Commissioners intend, in future, most strictly to enforce.

PROVISIONS OF THE LAW AS TO SINGLE PATIENTS.

Order and Certificates. 8 & 9 Vic. c. 100, s. 90, and 16 & 17 Vic. c. 96, ss. 4, 8.
Copies, &c., to be sent to Commissioners. 25 & 26 Vic. c. 111, s. 28.

No person deriving profit from the charge can receive into any house, or take care or charge of, a patient, as a lunatic, or alleged lunatic, without an order, and two medical certificates.

Within one clear day after receiving a patient, true copies of the order and certificates, together with a statement of the date of reception, and of the situation and designation of the house into which the patient has been received, as well as of the Christian and surname of the owner or occupier thereof, must be forwarded to the Office of the Commissioners in Lunacy, No. 19, Whitehall Place, London, S.W.

In addition to these documents, there must now be forwarded to the office of the Commissioners a statement of the condition of the patient, signed by his medical attendant, after two clear days and before the expiration of seven clear days from the day of reception, according to the form in Schedule F to chapter 100. *Statement. 25 & 26 Vic. c. 111, s. 41.*

The order and certificates must not be signed by any person receiving a percentage on or otherwise interested in the payments for the patient, nor by the medical attendant, as defined by the Lunacy Act, chapter 100 ; nor must the certificates be signed by the father, brother, son, partner, or assistant of the person having the care or charge of the patient. *Persons disqualified from signing. 25 & 26 Vic. c. 111, s. 24. 16 & 17 Vic. c. 9, s. 12.*

The patient must be visited, at least once in two weeks, by a physician, surgeon, or apothecary who did not sign either of the certificates of insanity, and who derives no profit, and who is not a partner, father, son, or brother of any person deriving profit, from the care or charge of the patient. *Fortnightly visits. 8 & 9 Vic. c. 100, s. 90.*

Such medical man must at each visit enter in a book to be kept at the house, according to the subjoined form, and to be called the "Medical Visitation Book," a statement of the condition of the patient's health, both mental and bodily, and also of the condition of the house. *Entries.*

These visits may, by special permission of the Commissioners, be made less frequently than once in every two weeks ; but in such case, where the patient is under the care or charge of a medical man, such medical man must himself make an entry once at the least in every two weeks in a book to be called the "Medical Journal." *Less frequent visits. 16 & 17 Vic. c. 96, s. 14.*

Every physician, surgeon, or apothecary who visits a single patient, or under whose care a single patient may be, must, on the 10th of January, or within seven days thereof, in every year, report in writing to the Commissioners the state of health, mental and bodily, of the patient, and such other circumstances as he may deem necessary to be communicated. Each annual report should give all these particulars fully, even although no change may have occurred since the previous report. *Annual Reports. 16 & 17 Vic. c. 96, s. 16.*

"The Medical Visitation Book" and "Medical Journal," and the order and certificates, must be so kept that they may be accessible to the Commissioners whenever they may visit the patient. *"Medical Visitation Book," &c. 8 & 9 Vic. c. 100, s. 90, and 16 & 17 Vic. c. 96, s. 14.*

Notice must be forwarded to the Office of the Commissioners in case of the death, discharge, removal, escape and re-capture of a patient. *Notices. 8 & 9 Vic. c. 100, ss. 53, 54, 55 and 90. Continued and extended. 16 & 17 Vic. c. 96, s. 21-22.*

Notice of the death of the patient must also be forwarded to the Coroner of the district. *25 & 26 Vic. c. 111, s. 44.*

Transfers.
16 & 17 Vic.
c. 96, s. 20.
If it is proposed to remove the patient to the care or charge of another person, the consent to an order of transfer must previously be obtained from the Commissioners, otherwise a fresh order and certificates will be necessary.

Changes of Residence.
16 & 17 Vic.
c. 96, s. 22.
When any person having the care of a single patient proposes to change his residence, and remove the patient to such new residence, seven clear days' notice of the proposed change, with the exact address and designation of the new residence, must be sent to the Commissioners, and to the person who signed the order for reception of the patient.

Removals for Health.
If it should be desired to give the patient liberty of absence anywhere, for a definite time, for improvement of his health, or for a trial of his powers of self-control, the consent of the Commissioners must first be obtained; the written consent of the person who signed the order must accompany the application, as well as a statement by the medical attendant showing the fitness of the patient for such trial.

Penalties for neglect or violation of the law.
8 & 9 Vic.
c. 100, s. 90.
The attention of every person having charge of a single patient is specially drawn to the concluding paragraphs of the 90th section of the 8 and 9 Vict. cap. 100, by which he will see that if he shall receive a patient without a proper order and certificates; or if, having such certificates, he neglect to transmit copies to the Commissioners in Lunacy; or if he fail to cause such patient to be visited fortnightly by a medical man (not disqualified as above); or if he make any untrue entry in the "Medical Visitation Book," he shall be guilty of a misdemeanour.

N.B.—A licence for the house becomes necessary only where more than one patient is received.

FORM OF MEDICAL VISITATION BOOK, OR MEDICAL JOURNAL.

Date.	Mental State and Progress.	Bodily Health and Condition.	Restraint or Seclusion since last entry. When and how long? By what means, and for what reasons?	Visits of Friends.	State of House, Bed, and Bedding, &c.

FORM OF NOTICE OF DEATH.

I hereby give you Notice, That_____
a Private Patient, received into this house on the_____
day of_____18___, died therein on the_____
day of_____187___; and I further certify, that_____
_____ was present at the death of the said
_____ and that the apparent cause of
death of the said_____(*)
_____was_____
   Signed, _____
    (†) _____

Dated this_____day of_____One
Thousand Eight Hundred and Seventy _____
 To the Commissioners in Lunacy.

(*) Ascertained by *post-mortem* examination, *if so.*
(†) Medical proprietor of ———— house, or medical attendant.

FORM OF NOTICE OF DISCHARGE.

I hereby give you Notice, That_____
a Private Patient, received into this house on the_____
day of_____18___, was discharged therefrom (*)
_____ by the authority of_____
on the_____day of_____187_____
   Signed, _____
    (†) _____

Dated this_____ day of _____One
Thousand Eight Hundred and Seventy_____
 To the Commissioners in Lunacy.

(*) Recovered, *or* relieved, *or* not improved.
(†) Proprietor of ———— house.

The Commissioners in Lunacy are constantly en-
forcing compliance with the law relating to single insane

Remarks by
Commis-
sioners on
single
patients.

patients, and the following remarks, taken from their twenty-fifth Report, clearly show the necessity of strictly complying with the law: " We have during the past year continued to use all available means to promulgate and enforce compliance with the law applicable to the insane under single private care, and have availed ourselves of all sources of information with a view to discover cases of violation of its provisions. The result has been to extend to a considerable number under illegal charge (some of whom were greatly neglected) the benefits of proper medical supervision and treatment.

In some cases the information upon which we acted was communicated to us voluntarily by the persons having charge of the patients, who, influenced by fears of prosecution, pleading ignorance, and desiring instructions, thus disclosed the facts.

In such cases we have had to consider whether, regard being had to all the circumstances, including the position in life of the parties implicated, the plea of ignorance could properly be entertained.

Whenever after due enquiry we saw good reason to be satisfied upon the points, we have simply required an immediate compliance with the Lunacy Acts by placing the patients under certificates, and providing for their future medical visitation and care.

In several other cases we have imposed, as a condition for foregoing prosecution, a public apology in the London and provincial papers and medical periodicals.

The publication of such apologies being much dreaded, we have been strongly appealed to not to insist upon them, but to such appeals we have never yielded.

We never adopt this intermediate and lenient course without very careful consideration, nor have we applied it in any case which essentially, in our judgment, called for criminal proceedings and punishment.

We have always borne in mind the encouragement it might give to wilful offenders."

The Commissioners in Lunacy having had frequent occasion to consider the legal construction of the 90th section of the 8th and 9th Vict. c. 100, which refers to single patients, thought it desirable in 1870 to submit a case for the law officers of the Crown, through the Home Secretary.

Case and Opinion on Construction of 90th Section of 8th and 9th Vict. c. 100. *

Counsel are requested to consider the letter and spirit of the stringent statutory provisions for the reception or charge of the insane, and especially the language of the 90th Section of the Act 8th and 9th Vict. c. 100, and to advise the Commissioners in Lunacy upon the following points :—

QUESTION.	ANSWER.	Opinion of Counsel taken on certain statutory provisions relative to single patients.
1. Is the word "profit" in that section to be read as synonymous with "payment?" If not, how is that word to be construed?	1. We are of opinion that "payment" is not absolutely synonymous with "profit." Profit is the larger term, and may include other advantages besides pecuniary.	
2. Is receiving "to board or lodge" in that section to be read as a proceeding distinct from taking the "care or charge" of a lunatic? If so, where a lunatic is received to board or lodge in the house of one person, and another takes the "care or charge" of him, by which person should the statutory documents be obtained; and are both punishable for neglect in obtain-	2. We are of opinion that receiving to board or lodge must be read as distinct from taking care or charge. The duty in question is imposed by the statute on both, and both are punishable if they neglect it.	

* Appendix N, Commissioners' Report, 1870.

ing the same, and supplying copies to the Commissioners?

3. What is the full force and meaning of the words in the 90th section, "as a lunatic or alleged lunatic," and by whom must the lunatic be alleged to be so?

3. We think the words "lunatic or alleged lunatic" are used for the purpose of ensuring the protection of the law not only to lunatics in fact, but to all persons who, without being lunatics, are treated as lunatics. No one in particular need "allege" the person to be a lunatic for the purposes of s. 90. It is enough if the person is received, or taken charge of, as being, or as being represented to be a lunatic.

4. If a wife become lunatic, and be removed by her husband from home to a house elsewhere taken for her exclusive accommodation, and she be there placed in the charge of a resident medical man or paid attendant, are an order and certificates under the 90th section requisite for her reception or charge; and if so, to whom should the order of reception be addressed?

4. In the case of a husband, he will very seldom be within s. 90 at all, because he very seldom derives any profit from the charge. In the case supposed, the resident medical man is, however, we think, bound to have the order and certificates, and to transmit them under s. 90.

5. Is the last question affected, and in what way, by the fact that the house to which the lunatic is so removed is not a house specially hired for the lunatic, but the property or former residence of the husband?

5. No.

6. Does the residence in that house of the husband, or of any and what number of the patient's family, affect, and in what way, that question? Are occasional visits to the wife there, by

6. We think the residence of the husband in the house would render any order or certificates unnecessary, if he, in fact, took the care and charge of his own wife, without placing her under

the husband or relative, tantamount to residence by him?

the care or charge of any one
else; otherwise it would not affect the question. Occasional
visits by the husband or other
relation would not, in our
opinion, amount to residence, or
to taking care and charge.

7. Is an insane person remaining at home and alone, in
consequence of having no relations, but placed in the charge
of a resident medical man or
attendant paid for his services,
subject to the provisions of the
Act 8 and 9 Vict. c. 100?

7. We are of opinion that
this question must be answered
in the affirmative.

8. Is the case of a lunatic
husband, or any other and what
lunatic member of a family, dealt
with, as stated in query 4, by
his wife, or any and what near
relative, equally within the provisions of the Act 8 and 9 Vict.
c. 100, as that of a wife?

8. We give the same answer
to this question.

9. Can a person sign an order
of reception under the Act expressly as an agent, and can he
thereby avoid individual responsibility in the proceeding save to
his principal?

9. We think not. The order
is to be "under the hand" of
some person; and the signing
person seems to us, therefore, to
be a principal, and cannot sign
as agent for another.

10. If a husband deny the
lunacy of his wife, may another,
being the husband's solicitor, or
styling himself to be so, sign an
order for her reception under the
Act as a lunatic?

10. We think he may, and
that such order would *primâ
facie* be good, if it purported to
be made by the solicitor acting
for himself, and not as attorney
or agent for another person. The
matter of fact would, in regular
course, if disputed, come to be
tried.

11. If the copy of an order
signed by the solicitor, and so
described at the foot of the
order, be sent to the Commis-

11. If the order purported to
be signed by the solicitor, *qua*
solicitor or agent, it would be
invalid; if on. his own behalf,

sioners, what is their proper course ? and the statutory forms were complied with, it should be dealt with by the Commissioners as a valid order. The peculiar circumstances would, of course, suggest the strictest possible enquiry.

(Signed)   R. P. COLLIER.
J. D. COLERIDGE.

Temple, April 25, 1870.

Persons guilty of any infringement of the law relating to single patients are liable to criminal indictment. Opinion expressed by Lord Shaftesbury on the subject of "single patients."

All persons violating the provisions of the law enacted respecting single patients, are liable to an action for misdemeanour.

With regard to the advisability of recommending the confinement of single patients at their own residence or in unlicensed houses, in preference to sending them to an asylum, there is a diversity of opinion, but into the consideration of this subject I do not propose to enter. I would, however, *en passant* refer to the views of the Earl of Shaftesbury on this vexed point, as expressed by his lordship when examined in 1859 before the Committee of the House of Commons.

In reply to the question, asked by the Chairman of the Committee, "You do not know how many houses there are with single patients ?" Lord Shaftesbury said: "We * have no sufficient knowledge of that, and we have spent years and years in endeavouring to learn it. I am certain that there are hundreds of persons called single patients of whom we have no knowledge whatever; and during the early periods of legislation single patients were hardly ever mentioned. By Act of Parliament no one was compelled to send a record to the Secretary unless a patient was under his charge eleven months; and we found this to be the consequence, that they kept a

* I.e., the Commissioners in Lunacy.

patient under their charge for ten months or so, and then shifted him to another house."

"Do you think the single system an advantageous one for patients ?"—"No, it is in many instances the very worst, and from the bottom of my heart I would advise anybody, if it should please Providence to afflict any member of his family, to send him or her to a private asylum; for if my own wife or daughter were so afflicted, and if I could not keep her in my own house under my own eye, I would send her to a private asylum—to a good private asylum, because there are most remarkable examples of excellence and comfort among them. So long as a patient is kept within the walls of his own house, under the care of his wife; or, if it be a wife, under the charge of her husband, I do not think that public opinion is ripe for allowing anyone to go into it. If relatives choose to take charge of patients themselves, they are right, if it is necessary for their own happiness and comfort; but if they put them under the charge of another, then I think the law has a right to see that there is no undue power exercised over the personal liberty and comfort of the sufferer."

CHAPTER VII.

PAUPER LUNATICS.

1. IN County and Borough Asylums.
2. In Licensed Houses.
3. In Workhouses.

Having considered in detail the course to be pursued in dealing with private, I next proceed to a consideration of pauper lunatics.

Definition of "Pauper."

A pauper lunatic is thus defined by the Act:—" Every person maintained wholly, or in part, at the expense of any parish, union, county or borough."

Preliminary steps previous to the admission of a pauper lunatic.

Previously to placing a patient in a county asylum information must be given to the medical officer of the parish or union in which the lunatic resides ; the subsequent proceedings are as follows :—

Notice in writing is to be given by medical officer of the parish to the relieving officer if a lunatic is resident in the parish. This is required to be done within three days from receiving the information.

* " Every medical officer of a parish or union who shall have knowledge that any pauper resident in such parish, or in any parish within the district of such medical officer, is, or is deemed to be a lunatic, and a proper person to be sent to an asylum, shall, within three days after obtaining such knowledge, give notice† thereof in writing to a relieving officer of such parish, or if there is no relieving officer, then to one of the overseers of such parish, and every relieving officer of any parish within a union or under a board of guardians, and every overseer of a parish of which there is no relieving officer, who shall have knowledge, either by such notice

* 16 and 17 Vict. c. 97, s. 67.

† All forms and orders referred to in this chapter will be found at the end of the book.

or otherwise, that any pauper resident in such parish is or is deemed to be a lunatic (*and a proper person to be sent to an asylum*), shall within three days after obtaining such knowledge give notice thereof to some justice of the county or borough within which such parish is situate; and thereupon the said justice shall, by an order under his hand and seal, require such relieving officer or overseer to bring such pauper before him or some other justice of the said county or borough, at such time and place, within three days from the time of such notice being given to such justice, as shall be appointed by the said order ; and the said justice before whom such pauper shall be brought, shall call to his assistance a physician, surgeon, or apothecary, and examine such person ; and if such physician, surgeon, or apothecary shall sign a certificate with respect to such pauper, according to the form in schedule (F) No. 3, to this Act annexed, and such justice be satisfied, upon view or personal examination of such pauper, or other proof, that such pauper is a lunatic, and a proper person to be taken charge of and detained under care and treatment, he shall, by an order under his hand, according to the form in the said schedule (F) No. 1, to this Act annexed, direct such pauper to be received into such asylum, as hereinafter mentioned, or, where hereinafter authorised in this behalf, into some hospital registered or some house duly licensed for the reception of lunatics, and such relieving officer or overseer shall immediately convey or cause the said lunatic to be conveyed to such asylum, hospital, or house, and such lunatic shall be received and detained therein : provided always, that it shall be lawful for any justice, upon notice being given to him as aforesaid, or upon his own knowledge, without any such notice as aforesaid, to examine any pauper deemed to be lunatic, at his own abode or elsewhere, and to proceed in all respects as if such pauper were brought before him in

Justice orders the lunatic to be brought before him.

pursuance of an order for that purpose ; provided also, that in case any pauper deemed to be lunatic cannot, on account of his health or other cause, be conveniently taken before any justice, such pauper may be examined at his own abode or elsewhere by an officiating clergyman of the parish in which he is resident, together with a relieving officer, or, if there be no relieving officer, an overseer of such parish ; and such officiating clergyman, together with such relieving officer or overseer, shall call to their assistance a physician, surgeon, or apothecary ; and if such physician, surgeon, or apothecary shall sign a certificate with respect to such pauper, according to the said form in the said schedule (F) No. 3, and if, upon view or examination of such pauper, such officiating clergyman and such relieving officer or overseer be satisfied that such pauper is a lunatic, and a proper person to be taken charge of and detained under proper care and treatment, such officiating clergyman, together with such overseer or relieving officer, shall, by an order under their hands, according to the said form in the said schedule (F) No. 1, direct such pauper to be received into such asylum as hereinafter mentioned, or, where hereinafter authorised in this behalf, into some such registered hospital or licensed house as aforesaid, and such relieving officer or overseer shall immediately convey or cause such pauper to be conveyed to such asylum, hospital, or house, and such pauper shall be received and detained therein ; provided also, that if the physician, surgeon, or apothecary, by whom any such pauper shall be examined, shall certify in writing that he is not in a fit state to be removed, his removal shall be suspended until the same or some other physician, surgeon, or apothecary shall certify in writing that he is fit to be removed; and every such physician, surgeon, and apothecary is required to give such last-mentioned certificate as soon as in his judgment it ought to be given ; provided also, that where a certificate in the form in the said schedule (F) No. 3, is signed by the medical officer of the parish or union in which the pauper named therein is resident, as well as by some other person, being a physician, surgeon, or apothecary, called to the assistance of the justice or clergyman and overseer or relieving officer, as hereinafter mentioned, such joint certificate or such two certificates [as the case may be] shall be received by the justice or clergyman and overseer or relieving officer by whom such person is examined, as hereinbefore mentioned, as conclusive evidence that the person named therein is a lunatic, and a proper person to be taken charge of and detained under care and treatment, and he or they shall make an order in the form in the said schedule (F) No. 1, accordingly.''

I give below a short summary of the chief sections of the Act referring to pauper patients :—

1st. The medical officer of a district must under a penalty of 10*l.* give within three days from his receiving information written notice to the relieving officer, or, if there be no relieving officer, to the overseers, if there is any pauper lunatic resident in his parish, and deemed to be a proper person to be sent to an asylum.

Notice given by medical officer to relieving officer that a lunatic is resident in his parish.

2nd. The relieving officer or the overseers, as the case may be, must within three clear days from his receiving information give notice thereof to some justice of the county or borough, who will thereupon deal with the case.

Notice given by relieving officer to the justice.

3rd. In the event of the pauper patient not being able to be conveniently taken before a justice, an officiating clergyman of the parish (in priest's orders), in conjunction with the relieving officer or overseers, as the case may be, may examine him, and, if satisfied as to his state of mind, sign the order for his admission into the asylum.

The lunatic can be examined by the clergyman of his parish, who, if satisfied, may sign the order for his admission into an asylum.

4th. The justice upon receiving notice from the

Justice
orders
lunatic to
be brought
before him.
relieving officer (or overseer) orders the pauper patient to be brought before him, or before some other justice within three days

In the
examination
of the
lunatic the
justice may
have the
assistance
of a medical
man.
If the patient is unable to be brought before him, or if the justice or officiating clergyman prefers it, he can visit the patient at his own home or wherever he may be, and examine him there. The justice during the examination of the patient can have the assistance of a medical man.

One certifi-
cate only is
required,
provided the
justice is
satisfied
himself as
to the
insanity.
5th. One medical certificate filled up in the ordinary way is sufficient for the reception of the patient into the asylum, accompanied by an order. This is, provided the justice himself is satisfied that the person is of unsound mind.

On the other hand, supposing the justice is not convinced of the person's insanity, and refuses to give an order for the admission, he can be compelled to do so if two medical certificates are given, the one signed by the medical man called in by the justice, and who examined the patient with the justice, and the other signed by the medical officer of the parish.

Relieving
officer,
except under
special cir-
cumstances,
must cause
the lunatic
to be taken
to an asylum
immedi-
ately.
The relieving officer is required under a penalty to convey the patient, or cause him to be taken immediately to an asylum (or other establishment), unless the medical man who examined him certifies that he is in an unfit state for removal; in which case the removal is postponed until he is well enough to be removed.

Patient
may be first
taken to
workhouse.
6th. If the patient cannot be brought forthwith to the asylum, he can be taken to the workhouse.*

The lunatic
must be
taken to the
County or
Borough
asylum of
the parish
or place
from which
he has
been sent,
except under
7th. The lunatic must be taken to the county or borough asylum connected with the parish or place from which he is sent, unless, in consequence of deficiency of room or other special circumstances, he cannot be received therein.

If he is unable to be admitted into the county or

* 25 and 26 Vict. c. 111, s. 20.

borough asylum, or if there be no county or borough special circumstances. asylum, then the law does not prohibit him from being admitted into any other asylum in which pauper lunatics are received; but the special circumstances, &c., which have prevented him from being received into his own county asylum must be clearly stated in the order; for instance, "*Deficiency of room,*" "*No asylum in his own county,*" &c. It must also be stated that the justices are satisfied with this arrangement; but no pauper can be received into an asylum without the proper order, statement, and certificate, and these will authorise his detention in the asylum until he is duly removed or discharged.

Pauper patients are permitted to go on leave of Leave of absence for a stated time, permission being granted by absence. any two of the visitors of the asylum, the medical officer first advising the proceeding in writing.

In the event of the patient not returning within the stated time he can be recaptured and brought back within fourteen days.

The discharge of a pauper patient rests with the visi- Visitors of asylums can tors of the asylum. The medical officer of the asylum authorise the patient's having first given his advice in the matter in writing, any discharge. two of the visitors can authorise the discharge, and any three of them can do so without obtaining the advice of the medical officer.

The relatives or friends of a pauper patient can re- The relatives can receive ceive the patient home, provided they give a satisfactory the pauper guarantee to the visitors that the patient will be no home. longer chargeable to any parish, union, or county, and shall be properly looked after and taken care of, and prevented from doing injury to himself or others.

A pauper patient dying in the asylum is buried at Death and expenses of the expense of the union, parish, or county to which burial. the deceased pauper is chargeable.

Any person wishing to obtain information concern-

ing a pauper relative confined in an asylum can obtain
it upon reference to the Commissioners in Lunacy, 19
Whitehall Place, S.W.

In Licensed Houses.

Pauper lunatics can be received into licensed houses on one medical certificate.

If in consequence of deficiency of room, or from any
other special circumstances the patient is unable to be
sent to a county or borough asylum, an order and
medical certificate must be obtained, and upon these he
can be received into a licensed house, such "special
circumstances" being stated in the order.

The order, statement, and certificate are similar to
those made use of in the case of private patients admitted
into asylums.

The order can be signed by the same person who is
authorised to sign the order for admission into a county
asylum.

"It shall not be compulsory on the superintendent
of any registered hospital or the proprietor of any licensed
house to receive any lunatic under any such 'order'
except in pursuance of any subsisting contract." *

Guardians of the parish can discharge any pauper lunatic confined in a licensed house.

The guardians of the parish or union are empowered
to discharge or remove a pauper patient confined in a
licensed house, and may order such. If the medical
superintendent or proprietor receive a written direction
from the guardians, he shall discharge the patient, unless
the patient is dangerous or unfit to be at large. The
Commissioners or visitors can give their consent in
writing in these cases to removal.

The officiating minister and one of the overseers or
any two of the justices will authorise the discharge in
the case of parishes which possess no board of guardians
and visitors. The Commissioners in Lunacy of course
have power to discharge any patient.

The superintendent or proprietor of a licensed asylum

---

* 16 and 17 Vict. c. 97, s. 78.

containing pauper patients must, in the event of the recovery of a patient, send such notice to the guardians, overseers, or clerk of the peace, as the case may be, and the patient must be discharged or removed within fourteen days. Notice of recovery is given to guardians, overseers, or clerk of the peace.

If the patient is not discharged within that time notice must be sent to the Commissioners in Lunacy and to the visitors. Of course all notices of removal or discharge must be sent to the Commissioners and visitors.

In Workhouses.

On January 1, 1872, there were thirteen thousand six hundred and eight pauper lunatics in workhouses, showing an increase of one thousand four hundred and forty-seven over the preceding year. Lunatics confined in workhouses.

The number of workhouses visited during the year 1871 by the Commissioners in Lunacy was two hundred and nineteen.

No dangerous lunatic, insane person, or idiot can be detained in a workhouse beyond fourteen days. "And be it further enacted that nothing in this Act contained shall authorise the detention in any workhouse of any dangerous lunatic, insane person, or idiot for any longer period than fourteen days, and every person wilfully detaining in any workhouse any such lunatic, insane person, or idiot for more than fourteen days shall be deemed guilty of a misdemeanour: provided always that nothing herein contained shall extend to any place duly licensed for the reception of lunatics and other insane persons, or to any workhouse, being also a county lunatic asylum."* Dangerous lunatics cannot be detained in a workhouse beyond fourteen days.

This applies not only to dangerous lunatics, but also to other insane persons, except under special circumstances.

* 4 and 5 William IV., c. 76, s. 45.

Lunatic pauper to be sent to asylums. (25 & 26 Vict. c. 111, s. 20.)

"No person shall be detained in any workhouse, being a lunatic or alleged lunatic, beyond the period of fourteen days, unless in the opinion, given in writing, of the medical officer of the union or parish to which the workhouse belongs, such person is a proper person to be kept in a workhouse, nor unless the accommodation in the workhouse is sufficient for his reception; and any person detained in a workhouse in contravention of this section shall be deemed to be a proper person to be sent to an asylum, within the meaning of section 67 of the Lunacy Act, chapter 97; and in the event of any person being detained in a workhouse in contravention of this section, the medical officer shall, for all the purposes of the Lunacy Act, chapter 97, be deemed to have knowledge that a pauper resident within his district is a lunatic and a proper person to be sent to an asylum, and it shall be his duty to act accordingly, and further to sign such certificate as is contained in Schedule F to the said Act, No. 3, with a view to more certainly securing the reception into an asylum of such pauper lunatic as aforesaid."

The Commissioners can themselves order any patient confined in a workhouse to be removed to a licensed house or asylum, as they may think proper.

Lunatics wandering at large.

Lunatics wandering at large.

I refer to private as well as pauper patients. It often happens that insane people are found wandering at large in the streets or public thoroughfares. A lunatic found thus wandering is taken before a justice of the peace.

This is done by a constable, relieving officer, or overseer of the district, and if any of these officials are informed of the fact that a lunatic is at large they are legally bound to take the patient before a magistrate. Any person may give information relating to lunatics wandering at large either to the relieving officer, overseer constable, or to the justice himself.

The lunatic having been brought before a justice, a medical man is called in, and upon his signing one medical certificate, according to the Act, an order will be given by the justice for the reception of the lunatic into an asylum or licensed house. The justice can also act upon his own knowledge and examine the lunatic at his own abode, or wherever he thinks proper to conduct his examination.

" Every constable of any parish or place, and every relieving officer and overseer of any parish, who shall have knowledge that any person wandering at large within such parish or place (whether or not such person be a pauper) is deemed to be a lunatic, shall immediately apprehend and take, or cause such person to be apprehended and taken before a justice ; and it shall also be lawful for any justice, upon its being made to appear to him by the information upon oath of any person whomsoever that any person wandering at large within the limits of his jurisdiction is deemed to be a lunatic, by an order under the hand and seal of such justice, to require any constable of the parish or place, or relieving officer or overseer of the parish where such person may be found, to apprehend him and bring him before such justice, or some other justice having jurisdiction where such person may be found ; and every constable of any parish or place, and every relieving officer and overseer of any parish who shall have knowledge that any person in such parish or place, not a pauper and not wandering at large as aforesaid, is deemed to be a lunatic, and is not under proper care and control, or is cruelly treated or neglected by any relative or other person having the care or charge of him, shall, within three days after obtaining such knowledge, give information thereof upon oath to a justice, and in case it be made to appear to any justice, upon such information or upon the information upon oath of any person whomsoever,

Provision as to lunatics wandering at large, not being properly taken care of, or being cruelly treated, &c. (16 & 17 Vict. c. 97, s. 68.)

that any person within the limits of his jurisdiction
not a pauper, and not wandering at large, is deemed
to be a lunatic, and is not under proper care and
control, or is cruelly treated or neglected by any
relative or other person having the care or charge
of him, such justice shall, either himself visit and examine such person and make inquiry into the matters so
appearing upon such information, or by an order under
his hand and seal direct and authorise some physician,
surgeon, or apothecary to visit and examine such person,
and make such inquiry, and to report in writing to such
justice his opinion thereupon; and in case upon such
personal visit, examination, and inquiry by such justice,
or upon the report of such physician, surgeon, or apothecary it appear to such justice that such person is a
lunatic, and is not under proper care and control, or is
cruelly treated or neglected by any relative or other
person having the care or charge of him, it shall be
lawful for such justice, by an order under his hand and
seal, to require any constable of the parish or place, or
any relieving officer or overseer of the parish, where such
person is alleged to be, to bring him before any two
justices of the same county or borough; and the justice
or justices (as the case may be) before whom any such
person as aforesaid in the respective cases aforesaid is
brought, under this enactment, shall call to his or their
assistance a physician, surgeon, or apothecary, and shall
examine such person, and make such inquiry relative to
such person as he or they shall deem necessary; and if
upon examination of such person or other proof such
justice be satisfied that such person so brought before
him is a lunatic, and was wandering at large, and is a
proper person to be taken charge of and detained under
care and treatment, or such two justices be satisfied
that such person so brought before them is a lunatic,
and is not under proper care and control, or is cruelly

treated or neglected by any person having the care or charge of him, and that he is a proper person to be taken charge of and detained under care and treatment, and if such physician, surgeon, or apothecary sign a certificate with respect to every such person so brought either before one justice or two justices, according to the form in schedule (F) No. 3 to this Act, it shall be lawful for the said justice or justices, by an order under his or their hand and seal or hands and seals, according to the form in schedule (F) No. 1 to this Act, to direct such person to be received into such asylum as hereinafter mentioned, or, whereinafter authorised in this behalf, into some hospital registered or house licensed for the reception of lunatics, and the said constable, relieving officer, or overseer who may have brought such person before the said justice or justices, or any constable whom such justice or justices may require so to do, shall forthwith convey such person to such asylum, hospital, or house accordingly: provided always that it shall be lawful for any justice, upon such information on oath as aforesaid, or upon his own knowledge, and alone, in the case of any such person as aforesaid wandering at large and deemed to be a lunatic, or with some other justice, in any other of the cases aforesaid, to examine the person deemed to be a lunatic, at his own abode or elsewhere, and to proceed in all respects as if such person were brought before him or them as hereinbefore mentioned ; provided also, that it shall be lawful for the said justice or justices to suspend the execution of any such order for removing any such person as aforesaid to any asylum, hospital, or house for such period not exceeding fourteen days as he or they may deem meet, and in the meantime to give such directions or make such arrangements for the proper care and control of such person as he or they shall consider necessary : provided also, that if the physician, surgeon, or apothecary by whom such person

County and Borough Asylums.

United Counties and Boroughs	Where Situate	Superintendents and Medical Officers	PRIVATE Patients remaining on January 1, 1872			PAUPER Patients remaining on January 1, 1872			Total Lunatics on Jan. 1, 1872
			M.	F.	Total	M.	F.	Total	
Beds, Herts, and Hunts	Arlesey, Baldock	W. Denne (Surgeon)	—	—	—	290	328	618	618
Berks	Cholsey, near Wallingford	Dr. R. B. Gilland	—	—	—	116	132	248	248
Bucks	Stone, near Aylesbury	John Humphry (Surgeon)	6	4	10	135	207	342	352
Cambridge and Isle of Ely	Fulbourn	Dr. G. M. Bacon	—	—	—	125	136	261	261
Carmarthen, Cardigan, Pembroke, and Haverfordwest	Carmarthen	Dr. G. J. Hearder	—	—	—	125	126	251	251
Chester	Chester	Dr. J. H. Davidson	—	—	—	210	194	404	404
„	Parkside, nr. Macclesfield	Dr. P. M. Deas	—	2	2	132	161	293	295
Cornwall	Bodmin	Dr. Richard Adams	21	27	48	182	233	415	463
Cumberland and Westmoreland	Near Carlisle	Dr. T. S. Clouston	10	7	17	213	174	387	404
Denbigh, Anglesea, Carnarvon, Flint, and Merioneth	Denbigh	G. T. Jones (Surgeon)	13	11	24	178	189	367	391
Derby	Mickleover, near Derby	Dr. J. Hitchman	1	—	1	181	206	387	388
Devon	Exminster	Dr. G. J. S. Saunders	—	—	—	268	436	704	704
Dorset	Near Dorchester	J. G. Symes (Surgeon)	14	9	23	218	260	478	501
Durham	Sedgefield, near Ferry Hill	Dr. R. Smith	2	5	7	329	271	600	607
Essex	Brentwood	Dr. Donald Campbell	—	—	—	303	390	693	693
Glamorgan	Bridgend	Dr. D. Yellowlees	—	—	—	224	203	427	427
Gloucester	Gloucester	E. Toller (Surgeon)	1	2	3	274	311	585	588
Hants	Knowle, near Fareham	Dr. J. Manley	1	6	7	286	335	621	628
Hereford	Hereford	Dr. T. A. Chapman	—	—	—	104	—	104	104
Kent	Barming Heath, near Maidstone	Dr. W. P. Kirkman	—	—	—	527	710	1,237	1,237
Lancaster	Lancaster Moor	J. Broadhurst (Surgeon)	—	—	—	533	494	1,027	1,027
„	Rainhill, near Prescot	Dr. T. L. Rogers	—	—	—	321	355	676	676
„	Prestwich, nr. Manchester	H. R. Ley (Surgeon)	—	—	—	476	527	1,003	1,003
Leicester and Rutland	Leicester	J. Buck (Surgeon)	16	25	41	190	195	385	426
Lincoln	Bracebridge, near Lincoln	Dr. E. Palmer	—	—	—	284	305	589	589
Middlesex	Colney Hatch	Dr. E. Sheppard / W. G. Marshall (Surg.)	—	—	—	827	1,243	2,070	2,070

COUNTY AND BOROUGH ASYLUMS—*continued.*

United Counties and Boroughs	Where Situate	Superintendents and Medical Officers	Private — Patients remaining on January 1, 1872 M.	F.	Total	Pauper — Patients remaining on January 1, 1872 M.	F.	Total	Total Lunatics on Jan. 1, 1872
Middlesex	Hanwell	{ Dr. W. C. Begley / Dr. J. M. Lindsay }	—	—	—	701	1,096	1,797	1,797
Monmouth, Hereford, Brecon, and Radnor	Abergavenny	Dr. D. M. McCullough	—	—	—	209	283	492	492
Norfolk	Thorpe, near Norwich	Dr. W. C. Hills	—	—	—	179	261	440	440
Northumberland	Cottingwood, nr. Morpeth	R. Wilson (Surgeon)	1	—	1	185	168	353	354
Notts	Nottingham	Dr. W. P. Stiff	—	—	—	173	200	373	373
Oxford	Littlemore, near Oxford	R. H. H. Sankey (Surg.)	—	—	—	199	261	460	460
Salop and Montgomery	Bicton, near Shrewsbury	Dr. A. Strange	—	—	—	234	280	514	514
Somerset	Wells	Dr. C. W. C. M. Medlicott	4	9	13	235	275	510	523
Stafford	Stafford	Dr. M. N. Bower	—	—	—	265	236	501	501
"	Burntwood, nr. Lichfield	Dr. R. A. Davis	2	1	3	245	210	455	458
Suffolk	Melton, near Woodbridge	Dr. J. Kirkman	—	—	—	181	243	424	424
Surrey	Near Tooting	Dr. J. S. Biggs	—	—	—	406	544	950	950
"	Brookwood, near Woking	Dr. T. N. Brushfield	—	—	—	295	333	628	628
Sussex	Hayward's Heath	Dr. S. W. D. Williams	2	—	2	259	341	600	602
Warwick	Hatton, near Warwick	Dr. W. H. Parsey	4	4	8	230	250	480	488
Wilts	Near Devizes	Dr. J. Thurnam	—	—	—	204	252	456	456
Worcester	Powick, near Worcester	Dr. J. Sherlock	5	11	16	285	324	609	625
York, N. Riding	Clifton, near York	Dr. J. T. Hingston	4	7	11	205	212	417	428
York, W. Riding	Wakefield	Dr. J. C. Browne	—	—	—	701	786	1,487	1,487
York, E. Riding	Beverley	Dr. N. G. Mercer	—	1	1	114	81	195	196
Birmingham	Birmingham	T. Green (Surgeon)	27	23	50	243	309	552	602
Bristol	Stapleton, near Bristol	G. Thompson	3	8	11	126	132	258	269
Hull	Hull	P. W. Casson (Surgeon)	—	—	—	82	62	144	144
Ipswich	Ipswich	C. F. Long (Surgeon)	—	8	8	71	83	154	162
London (City of)	Stone, near Dartford	Dr. O. Jepson	—	—	—	116	159	275	275
Leicester	Humberstone	J. B. M. Finch (Surgeon)	—	—	—	133	140	283	283
Newcastle-on-Tyne	Coxlodge	R. H. B. Wickham (Surg.)	1	8	9	118	138	256	265
Norwich	Norwich	F. Sutton (Surgeon)	—	—	—	50	51	101	101
Total . . .			138	167	305	12,495	16,841	29,336	29,641

Counties, United Counties, and Boroughs.	Where Situate	Total Average Weekly Cost per Head	Weekly Charge for Paupers from Counties or Boroughs to which Asylum belongs.	Weekly Charge for Paupers from other Counties or Boroughs	Weekly Charge for Private Patients.
		s. d.	s. d.	s. d.	s. d.
Beds, Herts, and Hunts	Arlesey, Baldock	8 11	(a)8 10½	14 0	—
Berks	Cholsey, near Wallingford	10 7¼	13 0	—	—
Bucks	Stone, near Aylesbury	10 1¼	9 4 and 9 11	14 0	12 0 to 21 0
Cambridge and Isle of Ely	Fulbourn	10 2½	9 11	14 0	—
Carmarthen, Cardigan, Pembroke, and Haverfordwest	Carmarthen	9 6¾	9 4 and 9 11	13 11 and 13 4	—
Chester	Chester	9 0¾	7 7	14 0	—
"	Parkside, near Macclesfield	11 3	9 11	14 0 and 12 0	15 0 to 20 0
Cornwall	Bodmin	10 4	9 6¾	10 6	10 0 to 84 0
Cumberland and Westmoreland	Near Carlisle	9 0½	8 9 and 9 4	14 0	14 0
Denbigh, Anglesea, Carnarvon, Flint, and Merioneth	Denbigh	8 10½	8 2	12 10 to 14 0	12 6 to 126 0
Derby	Mickleover, near Derby	9 10¾	9 9	12 9 to 14 0	14 0
Devon	Exminster	8 3⅝	9 0	12 6	—
Dorset	Near Dorchester	6 11½	7 0	11 6 to 12 0	10 0 to 14 0
Durham	Sedgefield, near Ferry Hill	9 5½	9 9	14 0	16 0
Essex	Brentwood	9 10½	10 0	14 0	—
Glamorgan	Bridgend	8 11¾	9 0	14 0	—
Gloucester	Gloucester	8 10½	8 6	12 0 and 14 0	12 0 and 16 0
Hants	Knowle, near Fareham	8 11¾	9 0½	11 0 to 14 0	14 0
Hereford	Hereford	13 3	10 6	—	—
Kent	Barming Heath near Maidstone	10 0	9 11	14 0	—
Lancaster	Lancaster Moor	7 9¼	7 7	14 0	—
"	Rainhill, near Prescot	9 4½	9 4	14 0	—
"	Prestwich, nr. Manchester	9 0½	8 9 and 9 4	14 0	—
Leicester and Rutland	Leicester	9 6¼	9 0	14 0	9 11

a Average.

Counties, United Counties, and Boroughs	Where Situate	Total Average Weekly Cost per Head	Weekly Charge for Paupers from Counties or Boroughs to which Asylum belongs	Weekly Charge for Paupers from other Counties or Boroughs	Weekly Charge for Private Patients
		s. d.	s. d.	s. d.	s. d.
Lincoln . . .	Bracebridge, near Lincoln	8 8¼	8 8¼	—	—
Middlesex . .	Colney Hatch .	9 8	9 4	14 0	—
" . .	Hanwell . .	10 0¼	10 2½ and 9 7½	14 0	—
Monmouth, Hereford, Brecon, and Radnor .	Abergavenny. .	9 0¾	9 0	12 0 and 14 0	—
Norfolk . .	Thorpe, near Norwich .	8 7	9 0	14 0	—
Northumberland .	Cottingwood, near Morpeth	11 0¾	9 4	14 0	15 (min.)
Notts . . .	Nottingham . .	9 1	8 6	14 0	—
Oxford . . .	Littlemore, near Oxford .	9 9½	9 3¼	11 7	—
Salop and Montgomery . .	Bicton, near Shrewsbury	9 2½	8 9	14 0	—
Somerset . .	Wells	9 1¼	8 9	11 11½ to 14 0	11 11½ to 21 0
Stafford . .	Stafford . . .	8 10¾	8 9	14 0	—
" . . .	Burntwood, near Lichfield	8 8	8 8	14 0	14 0
Suffolk . . .	Melton, near Woodbridge	9 0¾	9 6	11 11¼	—
Surrey . . .	Near Tooting. .	10 8	10 0	14 0	—
" . . .	Brookwood, near Woking	10 3¾	10 6	14 0	—
Sussex . . .	Hayward's Heath .	9 8	9 3	14 0	16 0
Warwick . .	Hatton, near Warwick .	9 2	9 11 and 9 7½	14 0	11 8½ to 14 0
Wilts . . .	Near Devizes .	8 3	7 7	10 7 and 11 7	—
Worcester . .	Powick, near Worcester .	8 5¼	8 2	14 0	8 2 to 15 0
York, N. Riding .	Clifton, near York	10 2¾	8 9	13 5 to 15 9	14 0 to 31 6
" W. Riding .	Wakefield . .	9 6¼	(a)9 7½	14 0	—
Birmingham		7 8½	8 0	14 0	8 9 to 21 0
Bristol (Stapleton, near Bristol) . .		12 0¼	12 0	14 0	20 0
Hull		14 4¾	10 6	15 0	—
Ipswich		11 6	13 0	15 2 and 16 0	20 0
London (City of), Stone, near Dartford		12 0	14 0	14 0	—
Leicester (Humberstone) . . .		10 7	10 6	10 6 to 14 0	—
Newcastle-on-Tyne (Coxlodge) . .		10 6¾	12 0 and 11 0	16 0 and 14 0	14 0 to 29 0
Norwich (the return from Norwich Infirmary has not been received) . .		—	—	—	—

a Average.

CHAPTER VIII.

COMMISSIONS IN LUNACY, AND CHANCERY LUNATICS.

THE ancient mode in dealing with the property of persons of unsound mind, was for the King, upon a petition being presented to the Lord Chancellor, accompanied by affidavits of facts relating to the insanity, to issue a writ to the Sheriff or Escheator of the county, so that the case might be tried by jury, and so ascertain by personal examination whether the person was of unsound mind.

The Escheator was an ancient officer, so called because the nature of his office was to look to escheats, wardships, and other casualties belonging to the Crown. The writs, which were returnable into the Court of Chancery, were of various forms, one writ being whether the lunatic has had no understanding from his nativity, and consequently an idiot, and so presumed by law never to attain any mental capacity.

The Sheriff or Escheator before whom the alleged lunatic was examined, having come to a decision that the person was of unsound mind, the lunatic was entitled personally, or through his friends, to come into the Court of Chancery or before the Chancellor, or the "*coram rege in concilio*" (King's council), and, having placed the matter before them, he might petition to be examined by them as to whether he was *compos* or *non compos mentis*; or might issue a writ out of Chancery to certain individuals, to bring him who had been so found lunatic before the King in his council at Westminster, and there be examined.   If upon examination he was found to be *compos mentis*, notwithstanding the Sheriff or Escheator had given his verdict of *non compos mentis*, the verdict would, of course, be upset or traversed in consequence of that given by the Councillors at Westminster.

Persons of unsound mind were divided into two classes, idiots and lunatics, and a distinct commission was required for each of these individual classes.   In the first the commission was *de idiotâ inquirendo*, and in the other *de lunatico inquirendo*.   Three of the regular Commissioners appointed by the Lord Chancellor were authorised to execute a commission in the nature of a writ *de lunatico inquirendo*; this was returned to the Lord Chancellor duly signed and sealed, after the jury had held their inquisition.

By virtue of the royal prerogative, all persons pronounced of unsound mind and incompetent to take care of themselves or manage their property, are placed under the protection of the Crown.

Four classes of persons *non compos mentis*, according to Coke.

Lord Coke mentions four classes of persons *non compos mentis*, to whom the royal prerogative extends.

1st. Idiot, or fool natural.

2nd. He who was of good and sound memory, but, by the visitation of God, has been deprived of it.

3rd. *Lunaticus qui gaudet lucidis intervallis* and sometimes is of good and sound memory, and sometimes *non compos mentis*.

4th. He that is so by his own act, as a drunkard.

The distinction between an idiot and a lunatic was formerly of great importance.

In former times the distinction between an idiot and a lunatic was important.

The care of the person and estate of the born idiot was entrusted to the lord of the fee, whereas that of the lunatic was under the prerogative of the King; but in the present day, whether the person is an idiot or a lunatic, his person and estate are under the protection of the Crown, but though it has the protection of the person and estate in both instances, the interest possessed by the Crown is different. In that of a lunatic the Crown has simply the duty of acting as a trustee, and taking care of the person and property for the sole benefit of the particular individual. In the case of an idiot the Crown has both a trust and an interest; and after making provision sufficient for the requisite wants of the idiot and his family, it can take the profit of the estate for its own use.

The Crown, in the event of the recovery of its charge, restores the estate to him, or, in the event of his death, to such members of the family as are legally entitled to it, in as nearly the same condition as when it first took the management of it. *Upon the death or recovery of the lunatic, the estate is no longer under the jurisdiction of the Chancellor.*

There are two ways of dealing with the property of a lunatic : *Two modes of dealing with property of lunatics.*

1st. When the property exceeds 1,000l. or the income is more than 50l. per annum.

2nd. When the property does not exceed 1,000l. or the income 50l. per annum.

Let us consider the first of these.

Mode of Procedure, and Object of Enquiry.

The object of a Commission in Lunacy is to enable the Crown, or the Lord Chancellor, as its representative, to protect, and deal with as he may think proper, the property of persons of unsound mind. *Why a commission in lunacy is held.*

The Lord Chancellor will appoint committees of the lunatic's person and estate, who are the representatives of the lunatic in all matters.

Mode of Procedure prior to Commission.

It is customary for one or more members of the family of the alleged lunatic to present a petition to the Lord Chancellor. *Preliminaries prior to commission.*

I

This is signed by the petitioners, and attested by a solicitor duly admitted into the Court of Chancery.

I give below a form of petition.

PETITION OF ENQUIRY.

In the matter of L. B., a supposed Lunatic.

To THE RIGHT HONOURABLE THE LORD CHANCELLOR OF GREAT BRITAIN.

Petition for enquiry.

The humble petition of W. H. of   and H. I. of
showeth that L. B., now residing at
is now, and for the space of   last past, hath been of unsound mind, and altogether unfit and unable to govern herself or to manage her affairs, as by the (accompanying affidavits or the) affidavits hereto annexed appears.

That your petitioner, W. H., is the paternal nephew of M. B., the late husband of the said L. B.

Your petitioners therefore humbly pray your Lordship, that the Masters in Lunacy, or one of them, may be directed to enquire and certify concerning the lunacy of the said L. B.

And your petitioners shall ever pray, &c.

W. H.
H. I.

Witness to the signing by the said W. H. and H. I.
     R. H., Solicitor of   (Address.)

Medical and other affidavits must accompany petition.

These petitions must be accompanied by affidavits of medical men, and of members of the lunatic's family, and others to whom he is known.

They must contain facts relating to the alleged unsoundness of mind, and the reasons for coming to this conclusion, and state the symptoms of mental aberration.

All affidavits made in lunacy must be made and expressed in the first person of the deponent, divided and numbered in paragraphs consecutively, and respectively confined as nearly as possible to distinct portions of the subject-matter.

AFFIDAVIT OF MEDICAL MAN IN SUPPORT OF COMMISSION.

I, William Pemberton, of 42, Glasgow Square, London, Doctor of Medicine of the University of Edinburgh, and Fellow of the Royal College of Physicians of Edinburgh, have this day personally examined John Smith, a person residing at 12, Egan Road, London.

I consider him to be a person of unsound mind, and quite incapable of managing himself or his affairs.

I have arrived at this conclusion from the consideration of the following facts :—

1. He is under the delusion that his food is poisoned by his relatives, and consequently he refuses to eat.

2. He is quite ignorant of the amount or the value of his property.

3. He cannot tell me where he is, and the day of the week, month, or year.

4. His conversation is incoherent and irrational.

(Signed)
W. PEMBERTON, M.D., F.R.C.P.E.

42, Glasgow Square, London.
June 4, 1872.

This affidavit is sworn before a Commissioner authorised to administer oaths in Chancery ; and, having been returned to the solicitor who is conducting the case, is forwarded, with the petition, to the Lord Chancellor.

The nature and amount of the alleged lunatic's property must be stated in the affidavits made by the members of the family, and the names of his nearest relatives are required to be given.

These affidavits must not be sworn before the solicitor of the petitioner, but before some other solicitor authorised to administer oaths in Chancery.

The petition, with the affidavits, is now filed with the Registrar in Lunacy, who prepares office copies of them for the persons concerned in the enquiry.

The Registrar marks upon the original petition the

date of its presentation, and then returns it to the solicitor, who will serve it upon the alleged lunatic.

It is requisite, in the case of a lunatic who is married, and whose husband or wife does not petition the Court, that evidence should be given in writing, and proved by affidavits, that the husband or wife, as the case may be, consents or is acquainted with the proposed enquiry. The affidavit of assent must be lodged with the Registrar.

Particulars relating to the notice of enquiry being sent to the lunatic.

The alleged lunatic must have notice sent him of the intended enquiry.*

"Where the alleged lunatic is within the jurisdiction he shall have notice of the presentation of the petition for enquiry, and may, by a notice, signed by him, and attested by his solicitor, and filed with the Registrar, either before the presentation of the petition, or within seven days after such notice had by him as aforesaid, or at or within such other time as the Lord Chancellor, entrusted as aforesaid, shall order in the particular case, demand an enquiry before a jury." †

We do not often find a patient demanding to be tried before a jury, as the majority of cases are incurable lunatics, who, upon the presentation of the citation to them, will either not look at it or tear it up immediately.

Enquiry conducted by jury.

Let us suppose the alleged lunatic, upon receiving the citation, demands a jury.

"Where the alleged lunatic demands an enquiry before a jury, the Lord Chancellor, entrusted as aforesaid, shall, in his order for enquiry, direct the return of a jury, unless he be satisfied, by personal examination of the alleged lunatic, that he is not mentally competent to form and express a wish for an enquiry before a jury; and the Lord Chancellor entrusted as aforesaid may, where he shall deem it necessary, after presentation of the petition

---

* The solicitor, or one of his clerks, will call upon the lunatic and show him the original petition, and present him with a copy of it.

† 16 and 17 Vict. c. 70, s. 40.

for enquiry, and for the purpose of personal examination, require the alleged lunatic to attend him at such convenient time and place as he may appoint." *

If the lunatic does not demand a jury, or the Lord Chancellor, as before mentioned, is satisfied that the patient is not mentally competent to form and express a desire in that behalf; and if there is no opposition to the enquiry being held, and the Chancellor is satisfied with the evidence and propriety of the enquiry, and also satisfied that due notice has been given to the alleged lunatic, and that the time in which a jury could have been demanded has expired, the affidavit of service having been duly filed with the Registrar, an order for the enquiry is given. *(margin: No jury demanded.)*

Order for the enquiry having been given, the special order is prepared by the Registrar in Lunacy, who delivers it to the solicitor who has the charge of it. It is signed by the Lord Chancellor or Lords Justices, and is on a paper impressed with a 2l. Chancery stamp. *(margin: Order for enquiry.)*

I here give a form of the order without a jury :—

That F. B. and S. W., Esquires, the Masters in Lunacy, or one of them, do, in pursuance of the General Commission under the Great Seal of Great Britain to them for that purpose directed, enquire by the oath of good and lawful men concerning the alleged lunacy of the said H. K., now residing at, &c.; that the said enquiry be held at the place of abode of the said H. K., or as near thereto as conveniently may be.

Where a jury is directed, the order is as follows :—

That F. B. and S. W., Esquires, the Masters in Lunacy, or one of them, do, in pursuance of the General Commission under the Great Seal of Great Britain to them for that purpose directed, enquire by the oath of good and lawful men concerning the alleged lunacy of the said J. N., now an inmate of, &c., at, &c., and that the said enquiry be held at the place of abode of the said J. N., or as near thereto as conveniently may be, and that a good jury of the said county and of the neighbourhood where the said J. N. resides be returned to enquire of his lunacy.

---

* 16 and 17 Vict. c. 70, s. 41.

Power of the Court to grant or refuse order.

The Court has power to refuse or grant the order for enquiry at its discretion. It sometimes happens that *more* than *one* petition is presented to the Chancellor; but it is usual to give preference to the petitioner whose petition was first presented.

The petitioner may be called upon to defray all expenses connected with the enquiry; and if he die before the execution of the order, a new order or petition must be obtained, stating by whom the enquiry is to be presented.

The lunatic in the meantime remains within the jurisdiction of the Court pending the commission.

The commission will now have to be held, and any person preventing such enquiry is liable to a contempt of court.

Opposition of Commission.—Caveat.

Caveat.

If the petition is opposed, or a caveat lodged, or the application is made by a stranger or relative, without the assent of the husband or wife, the petition will be set down for hearing before the Lord Chancellor or Lords Justices.

IN LUNACY.

In the matter of L. B. of

Form of caveat.

Caveat against the petition of enquiry in lunacy herein, without notice to C. of, &c., Solicitor on behalf of

Dated this   day of   1873.

(Signed)

If the petition is presented by a stranger, it must be served, when answered, upon the nearest relative of the alleged lunatic; or if it is presented without the consent of husband or wife, it must be served on the husband or wife, as the case may be. After the serving of the petition, and after the service or consent has been proved by affidavit, the matter is heard in court, and an order pronounced thereon.

Power of Commissioners in Lunacy to enquire into Lunatics' Property.

When the Commissioners have reason to believe that the property of the alleged lunatic is not duly protected, they are empowered to report to the Lord Chancellor.*

Property of lunatics not properly protected.

" Where the Commissioners in Lunacy for the time being shall, after the commencement of this Act, by virtue of any authority for the time being enabling them in that behalf, report to the Lord Chancellor, entrusted as aforesaid, that they are of opinion that the property of any person alleged to be a lunatic, or detained or taken charge of as a lunatic, but not so found by inquisition, is not duly protected, or that the income thereof is not duly applied for his benefit, or to the same effect, the report shall be filed with the Registrar, and shall be deemed and taken to be tantamount to an ordinary petition for enquiry, supported by evidence ; and the alleged lunatic shall have notice of the report from such person as the Lord Chancellor, entrusted as aforesaid, shall from time to time direct ; and the case shall proceed and be conducted, as nearly as may be, in all respects as is hereinbefore directed, upon the presentation of a petition for enquiry."

A lunatic residing in England, and who possesses property in Jamaica, where he was found lunatic, in order to obtain protection from the Lord Chancellor, must nevertheless be the subject of an enquiry in England.

Previous to the commission being held, funds are directed by the Court to be placed at the lunatic's disposal to defray the expenses of the enquiry ; and during

Expenses connected with enquiry.

* 16 and 17 Vict. c. 70, s. 54.

the time it is pending, necessary arrangements are made by the Court for protection of the alleged lunatic's estate.

Procedure of enquiry. The enquiry into the state of mind of the alleged lunatic is conducted by one of the Masters in Lunacy, unless the Lord Chancellor shall order it to be held before a jury, or the alleged lunatic demand one, or the Master considers a jury necessary, or the alleged lunatic is not placed within their jurisdiction, or resides abroad.

The order for the enquiry, when issued, must be taken, with the office copies of the affidavits, to the office of the Masters in Lunacy, 45, Lincoln's-Inn-Fields.

Place for enquiry. The solicitor conducting the enquiry must, at his interview with the Master, inform him of a fit and convenient place to hold it.

It is customary for the enquiry to be held at the residence of the alleged lunatic, or at some adjoining court or inn, or where a room can be found sufficiently large to accommodate the witnesses, or a jury, if one is required. The Master will then appoint a day and place for holding the enquiry.

Evidence proving the insanity must be in readiness. Previous to the enquiry being held, the solicitor is required to have prepared evidence of the alleged lunatic's insanity, and to be able to state who are the heirs and next of kin, the amount of the property, and who are the proper persons to be appointed committees of the person and estate, and the sum proposed for the alleged lunatic's maintenance.

If a verdict of unsoundness of mind is given, the Master will, by *vivâ voce* evidence, enquire into these particulars.

Witnesses are summoned. The attendance of witnesses on the enquiry is obtained by a summons, given under the hand and seal of the Master.

Subpœnas issued. The solicitor conducting the case can obtain from the Master's office copies of the subpœnas; and having inserted the names of the several witnesses he proposes to call, the Master will attach his signature to each subpœna. If any doubt arise as to the production of the alleged lunatic at the time of the enquiry, the Master issues a summons for his appearance, and this is served upon the person in whose charge the lunatic is.

SUMMONS TO PRODUCE ALLEGED LUNATIC.

L. S. By virtue of Her Majesty's General Commission, under the Great Seal of Great Britain, bearing date, &c., directed to, &c., the Commissioners therein named, and an order of, &c., made, &c., to enquire whether   , of   , in the county of be a lunatic or not :

These are to will and require you to produce before the said Commissioners, or one of them, the said   at the execution of the said enquiry, at the house commonly called, &c., situate at, &c., on, &c., there to be examined touching the matters aforesaid. And you are to give (*him*) notice accordingly, as also to any other person or persons who are guardians of (*him*), or trustees of (*his*) estate, that they may appear in (*his*) defence if they shall think fit. Given under the hand and seal of me,   , one of the said Commissioners, this   day of, &c.

L. S.

To   or such other person or persons as now have the said   in their custody or power.

Form of summons to produce lunatic.

Any person refusing to produce the alleged lunatic, when summoned to do so by the Master, can be committed for contempt of court.

When the enquiry is held, the evidence must be confined to the question whether or not the alleged lunatic is *at the time* of such enquiry of unsound mind and incapable of managing himself or his affairs; and no evidence of anything done or said by him any time more than two years previous to the enquiry can be received as proof of insanity, unless the Judge or Master shall otherwise direct.

Detention of lunatic after summons has been issued is a contempt of court.

Evidence must be of recent date.

Lunatic may be present at enquiry.

The alleged lunatic has the power and right to be present at the enquiry ; he is personally examined by the Master, who will call and examine such witnesses as he may think proper, and ask for such information as he may think desirable to further the ends of justice.

Master empowered to order the enquiry before a jury.

If the case is a very difficult or complex one, the Master has power, having duly considered the evidence adduced, to certify to the Lord Chancellor that an enquiry before a jury would be desirable ; and he can, without further notice, issue his precept to the Sheriff, and the enquiry will be proceeded with in the same manner as if the Lord Chancellor had ordered a jury in the first instance.

The room in which the enquiry is held is an open court for the time being.

Evidence of witnesses residing abroad.

When the commission is held upon a person who is abroad, and consequently out of the jurisdiction of the Court, it may be necessary to obtain the evidence of witnesses abroad.

Permission to procure such evidence may be obtained, the Court being first petitioned for the purpose, and duly supported by proof of its necessity.

The Master will attend on the day fixed for the enquiry, and it will be conducted in precisely the same way as if a jury were present.

If the enquiry is held by jury, the Sheriff empannels persons whose names appear on the special jury list, and are resident in the immediate neighbourhood of the alleged lunatic's house.

The case is conducted before the jury by the Master explaining to them the object and nature of the enquiry, together with the principles of the law respecting it and the several points to which the jury must direct their attention.

If a counsel in support of the enquiry is engaged, he opens his case by informing the jury what he intends

to prove; and having done this, he calls his witnesses.

When no counsel appears in support of the enquiry the Master states to the jury, as far as he is able, from the affidavits on which the enquiry has been granted, the nature of the case at issue. Case stated by Master.

The witnesses are examined by the Master, or by the solicitor for the enquiry; and having personally examined the alleged lunatic, he sums up the case, and directs the jury to consider their verdict.

If the enquiry is opposed, the counsel cross-examines the witnesses; and after their examination the Master examines the alleged lunatic, and the case is summed up by the counsel for the enquiry.

The counsel for the opposition then states his observations upon the case, and produces evidence endeavouring to show the sanity of the person.

The counsel for the enquiry now replies, and the Master sums up the case, and directs the jury to consider their verdict.

The jury never come to a decision without personally examining the alleged lunatic, except when the lunatic resides abroad; but in these cases the evidence must be most conclusive. When no jury is assembled, the Master, having pronounced his verdict of the lunatic's inability to manage himself and his affairs, fills up and signs the necessary document, and attaches the seal to the parchment. Examination of
alleged
lunatic by
jury.

Appointment of Committee or Guardian of the Patient's Estate and Person.

The person having been pronounced by the Master to be of unsound mind and incapable of managing him-
self and his affairs, he will become a Chancery lunatic; and the next thing to be considered is the appointment of committees. This is occasionally settled in court Committee.

immediately succeeding the enquiry, or by the Master in chambers, in consultation with the solicitor.

Proceedings after enquiry.

Immediately after the inquisition the Master will enquire and report on the following matters :—

1. The lunatic's situation.

2. The nature of his lunacy.

3. Who are the persons most fit to be appointed committees of the person and estate.

4. Of what the lunatic's property consists.

5. The amount of income.

6. In what manner and at what expense, and by whom and where, he has been maintained; what sum is to be allowed for his past maintenance; whether anything, and what, is due, and to whom, in respect thereof; and to whom and out of what fund the same ought to be paid.

7. What is a proper allowance for his future maintenance, and from what time this is to commence, and from what fund the same ought to be paid.

Facts and proposals to be considered.

A statement of facts and proposals is usually placed before the Master, relating to—

1. The nature of the enquiry lately held.

2. Who is the heir-at-law and next of kin to the lunatic.

3. The situation of the lunatic, including age, position in life, profession, and residence.

4. The nature of the lunacy.

5. The amount and nature of his income, verified usually by affidavits; and how the money is invested.

6. The maintenance of the lunatic.

Here must be stated the annual amount paid up to the present time for the maintenance of the lunatic, who has defrayed the expense; and the sum due for the maintenance. A scheme must also be drawn up, with suggestions for the lunatic's future maintenance.

7. Debts.

All moneys due to others besides those who have supported the patient previous to the commission must be stated, and the names of the creditors given, with the respective amounts.

8. Committee of person and estate.

State residence and condition in life of the person or persons who are proposed as committee or committees of the lunatic's person and estate, and of their willingness to act ; and that the committee of the estate is prepared to give the necessary security, and that the committee of the person is prepared to visit the patient periodically.

The consent of the committees should be produced in writing.

Affidavits should be produced by some independent person, stating the respectability and fitness for committeeship of the proposed committees.

9. Proposal.

Here is given the names of the proposed committee or committees, together with the proposed sum for maintenance, and from what time it is to commence.

The Master, having been furnished with evidence in support of these facts, will at a convenient time proceed into the questions of the property, maintenance, and appointment of committees.

Committees.

The heir-at-law, if willing to act, will have the preference of being appointed committee of the estate ; and the next of kin committee of the person, provided the Master approve of such appointments.   In the selection of committees it is customary to give the preference to relations before strangers.

Persons to act as committees.

The committees are required to reside within the jurisdiction of the Lord Chancellor ; and in the appointment of such committees special attention is given to persons who are expected to make the best provision for the lunatic's welfare and comfort, and to take care of and protect his property.

The petitioners for the commission have the privilege of nominating persons as committees, though it does not necessarily follow that the Master will appoint them.

The solicitors engaged in the case are objected to as committees, as also any officer connected with the Court of Chancery.

The Duties of Committees.

Duty of a committe

A person who is found lunatic by inquisition usually will have two committees appointed—

1. Committee of the person.
2. Committee of the estate.

I. Committee of the Person.

We will first consider briefly what are the duties of the committee of the person.

The committee of the person superintends the personal care of the lunatic, such charge being committed to him by grant when the appointment is determined.

It is his duty to determine the residence of the lunatic, and to make all other necessary arrangements for his care and comfort; and to endeavour to carry out to the letter the scheme originally drawn up for the lunatic's maintenance. He must visit the lunatic periodically, these visits being usually fixed by the Court or Master; and at these visits he must see that the lunatic is properly taken care of, and that his bodily as well as mental state is attended to.

If the allowance for the maintenance of the lunatic is "so much as shall be expended not exceeding a certain sum," the committee of the person is required to place before the Master a yearly account of the expenditure.

If the fixed sum allowed for the maintenance of the lunatic is not expended, the balance must be placed to the credit of the lunatic's estate.

The committee of the person must send to the Visitors in Lunacy a half-yearly report, in which is stated the mental and bodily condition of the patient, and any important change that has occurred in his health since the last visit. The custody of the lunatic being placed in his hands, he is at liberty to place him where he likes, and vary the residence of the lunatic as often as he may think proper. If the residence of the lunatic has been fixed by the Lord Chancellor, permission from the Master must first be obtained before making any change.

If the committee is desirous to place the lunatic in an *unlicensed* house as a *single* patient, no medical certificates are required ; an order signed by the committee, having an office copy of such appointment annexed, is sufficient authority for the reception of such patient. The fortnightly medical visitations as required in the case of ordinary single patients confined in unlicensed houses are dispensed with. *Chancery lunatics in private houses.*

The committee of the person is required to send to the Visitors in Lunacy immediate notice of any change in the lunatic's residence, whether the removal is temporary or permanent. And he must also give to the Board of Visitors his own direction and the name of the medical attendant of the lunatic.

It is left to the discretion of the committee of the person to decide what friends may be allowed to visit the lunatic.

II. *Committee of the Estate.*

The duty of the committee of the estate is to receive the income of the lunatic's estate and pay everything becoming due from it. He must arrange the proper in-

vestment of the money and manage everything connected
with the lunatic's property; but before taking any *extraordinary* step in the management he must obtain the
consent of the Lord Chancellor or Master. He must
see that the lunatic's estate is properly taken care of, and
that the houses, buildings, and structures belonging to
the lunatic are sufficiently repaired, and so kept and
maintained, during the continuance of the grant. All
legal documents, title-deeds, &c., are taken care of by
him, but he is at liberty to deposit these at the Master's
office.

The committee of the estate will have the absolute
power to arrange for the letting, by yearly tenancy, but
not on lease, of any houses or land that belong to the
lunatic, and he, if authorised by an order of the Lord
Chancellor, can execute deeds in the name of the lunatic.
He must collect the rent and money due from the estate,
and pay to the committee of the person the sum for the
lunatic's maintenance, as well as other money allowed by
the Lord Chancellor for the maintenance of his family.

If any alteration is necessary in the scheme of maintenance, the committee of the estate and person must
consult together, and the matter is referred, through
their solicitor, to the Master, to be dealt with by him as
he may think proper.

Accounts must be kept by the committee of the
estate, and he is required to pass his annual accounts at
a certain time appointed by the Master; and any balance
due after the passing of the accounts must be paid into
Court and invested for the interest of the lunatic's estate.

He must be very particular and precise in dealing
with receipts and payments and other moneys, as he is
liable to be discharged for any irregularity; and in the
event of the death of the lunatic he may be called upon
by a suit of Chancery to produce an account of his
dealings.

If an action at law is commenced, the lunatic, and not the committee of the estate, is the plaintiff, as also in an action brought against the lunatic, he and not the committee is made the defendant.

In equity the lunatic and committee of the estate are both made parties.

Under the sanction of the Lord Chancellor, the committee of the estate, as representative of the lunatic, is enabled to institute proceedings in the Divorce Court for a judicial separation on the ground of adultery of the lunatic's wife.

If the lunatic is patron of a vacant benefice, the committee of the estate is *not* empowered to deal with the presentation; it is his duty, through his solicitor, to communicate with the Secretary of Presentations of the Lord Chancellor, who is enabled to make the presentation; but, of course, in doing so due regard is paid to the interests of the lunatic's family.

If the lunatic be an incumbent of a parish, the committee of the estate should communicate with the bishop of the diocese, whose duty it will be to nominate a curate to do the lunatic's duty, the stipend of the curate being paid by the committee of the estate out of the lunatic's estate.

All reasonable expenses incurred by the committee of the estate are allowed; but irrespective of this there is no remuneration attached to the office.

On Death or Retirement of Committees.

Before a committee is allowed to retire, permission must first be obtained from the Lord Chancellor, by petition or application to the Master, and his report confirmed by fiat.

Upon the death or retirement of a committee a statement of facts is brought into the Master's office proposing a new committee.

Appointment of new committees in the case of death.

K

If the proposal be made for a new committee of the estate, a statement must be given as to the extent of the lunatic's property.

If a committee of the person is required, the amount lately allowed and the scheme for maintenance must be stated; and if it is then found that a larger sum can be allowed than has been previously done, it is taken into consideration whether the lunatic is able to enjoy greater comforts.

Evidence must be given of the retirement or death of the committee, and of the fitness of the proposed successor. The Master will sometimes require the committee to personally appear before him, and require evidence of his willingness to act and visit the patient at stated times; and evidence must be given that he is a fit person to superintend the person or estate of the lunatic.

Death of the Lunatic.

Death of lunatic; power of the Master to deal with the documents deposited at his office.

If the will has been deposited at the Master's office, he is empowered to open it; and having ascertained whether any particulars are therein directed relative to the interment, and who the executors are, it will be deposited in the Court of Probate.

The Masters, on being satisfied of a lunatic's death, may, without order, open and read any paper deposited at their office purporting or alleged to be the will, in order to ascertain who is therein nominated executor, and whether there are any and what directions concerning the funeral or place of interment, and afterwards deliver the same to the Registrar or other officer of the Court of Probate.

Before the Master will return any papers or documents which have been deposited at his office, he must have a statement of facts placed before him showing the nature of the said documents, the interest which the lunatic had in them, and who is entitled to them. The Master will draw up his report, and it is filed with the Registrar for confirmation. If a special order is obtained for this purpose, a copy of it is left with the Master, and a summons taken out for comparing the deeds with the schedule of them.

This examination having been made, the papers and deeds will be delivered over as directed.

If the person to whom an order has been given for the delivering of the documents is unable to attend in person to receive them, he must give a written authority to some person to act for him; and his signature must be sworn to by two witnesses, one of whom is required by affidavit to identify the person giving the authority with the person named in the order to receive the docu-- ments, and prove the signatures of such person, and the witnesses' also. *Order for delivering up the lunatic's documents.*

The person to whom this authority is given must attend in person and give a proper receipt for them.

As mentioned before, the Crown, on the death of the lunatic, renders back the estate to those members of his family who are entitled to it, and has no further juris- diction in the affairs of the late lunatic.

Proceedings necessary when the property does not exceed 1,000l., or the income is not more than 50l. per annum.

I have considered, in the first part of this chapter, the necessary steps to be taken in dealing with the property of lunatics that exceeds 1,000l., or is more than 50l. per annum.

I will now pass on briefly to consider the legal steps to be pursued in dealing with the property of a lunatic amounting to 1,000l., or not exceeding 50l. per annum.

In section 12 of the Lunacy Regulation Act 1862, we see—

"Where, by report, one of the Masters in Lunacy or *Proceedings for dealing*

with the
property of
lunatics not
exceeding
1,000*l.* or
50*l.* per
annum.

of the Commissioners in Lunacy, or by affidavit or otherwise, it is established to the satisfaction of the Lord Chancellor entrusted as aforesaid that any person is of unsound mind and incapable of managing his affairs, and that his property does not exceed 1,000*l.* in value, or that the income thereof does not exceed fifty pounds per annum, the Lord Chancellor entrusted as aforesaid may, without directing any enquiry under a commission of lunacy, make such order as he may consider expedient for the purpose of rendering the property of such person, or the income thereof, available for his maintenance or benefit, or for carrying on his trade or business : Provided nevertheless that the alleged insane person shall have such personal notice of the application for such order as aforesaid as the Lord Chancellor shall, by general order to be made as after mentioned, direct."

In cases where the property is of the amount abovementioned no enquiry takes place before the Master, but conclusive evidence of the invested property must be given.

The mode of proceeding is as follows :—

If it be established to the satisfaction of the Lord Chancellor, by medical affidavits or otherwise, that the person is of unsound mind and incapable of managing his own affairs, and that his property does not exceed one thousand pounds, or his income fifty pounds per annum, the Lord Chancellor can then make an order as he may think proper for the purpose of rendering the property of such person or the income thereof available for the maintenance of the person.

The patient must have had a notice of the application for such order.*

---

* 25 and 26 Vict. c, 86, s. 12.

Single Chancery Patients.

It is enacted that the person who undertakes the care of a Chancery patient in his house for profit is liable to the same responsibilities and duties as are enforced in the case of a single private patient. Single Chancery patients.

If the committee takes care of the patient, he is not affected by this clause.

The fortnightly visitation, as required in the case of private patients, is dispensed with.* The patient is subject to visitation, both by the Commissioners in Lunacy and also by the Lord Chancellor's visitors.

Visitors of Chancery Lunatics.

All Chancery lunatics are visited once in every year, and sometimes more frequently, by one or more of the Lord Chancellor's visitors, who report upon each case separately to the Chancellor. Visitation of Chancery patients.

The Lord Chancellor's visitors consist of one legal and two medical visitors. The legal visitor is William Norris Nicholson, Esq.; the two medical visitors are John Bucknill, Esq., M.D., and Lockhart Robertson, Esq., M.D.

Their salary is 1,500l. per annum, exclusive of travelling expenses.

The two Masters in Lunacy are, by virtue of their appointments, visitors of lunatics.

The visitors are not allowed to engage in private practice.

They at the time of their visit are furnished with a statement of the income of the lunatic, the scheme of allowance for maintenance, and they have to consider whether the means provided for the comfort are sufficient for the sum allowed for the maintenance, and that he has such comforts as his mental condition and

* 25 and 26 Vict. c. 111, s. 22.

income will allow of, or whether anything can be done to further the enjoyment of the same, or any alteration made in the scheme drawn up for his maintenance.

If the visitors are of opinion that a change in any of these respects is desirable, the Board, having considered the matter, will take such steps as appear necessary, or the visitors may refer to the Masters, who, having investigated it, will summon the committee before them to give any explanation that may be required.*

Visitors may order a change in the lunatic's residence.

No person shall be appointed to be a visitor if he is, or has been within two years preceding his appointment, interested directly or indirectly in an asylum, and if any of the visitors becomes after his appointment so interested, his appointment as visitor shall *ipso facto* cease. The visitors hold their appointment during their good behaviour, and may be removed therefrom by the Lord Chancellor in case of misconduct or neglect of duty.

Lunatics not within the Jurisdiction of the Court.

Lunatics possessing property in Ireland.

A lunatic residing in England, in which country an inquisition has been held, but whose property is in Ireland, a committee of the person and estate is nevertheless appointed by the Lord Chancellor of England in the same way as if the lunatic's property was in England.

A copy of the inquisition is ordered to be sent to Ireland, and proceedings are taken out in the Irish Chancery Court with reference to his estates and the sum allowed for maintenance as if he were residing in Ireland.

Inquisition and *supersedeas* may be trans-

" Where it is desired that an inquisition taken on a commission issued under, or a writ of *supersedeas* thereof issued under, the great seal of the United Kingdom, or under the great seal of Ireland respectively, should be

---

* The visitors have no legal power to authorise the discharge of a Chancery patient; they can only recommend his removal to the Committee and to the Lord Chancellor.

acted upon in Ireland or in England respectively, the proper officer may, under order of the Lord Chancellor of Great Britain or the Lord Chancellor of Ireland, as the case may be, transmit a transcript of the record of the inquisition, or of the writ to the Chancery of Ireland or of England, as the case may be, which transcript shall thereupon be entered, and be of record there respectively, and shall when so entered of record, and if, and so long only, as the Lord Chancellor of Ireland entrusted as aforesaid, and the Lord Chancellor of Great Britain entrusted as aforesaid, as the case may be, shall see fit, may be acted upon by them respectively, and be of the same validity and effect to all intents and purposes as if the inquisition had been taken on a commission issued under, or the writ of *supersedeas* had been issued under, the great seal of Ireland, or of the United Kingdom respectively." *

Similar proceedings are adopted when the lunatic resides in Ireland, and the inquisition is held there, but has property in England.

The Lord Chancellor is generally unwilling to admit a lunatic, found so by inquisition, to reside out of the jurisdiction of the Court.

Nevertheless, sometimes in exceptional cases, when it has been clearly established that a change of residence is for the lunatic's benefit, permission is given for removal to Scotland or Ireland, but in a case like this the committee is required to bring the lunatic within the jurisdiction of the Court at such a time and place as may be directed, and also to send periodical reports respecting the lunatic's bodily and mental state, and to comply with any other directions made by the Court.

Mr. Dyce Sombre was allowed, after being found lunatic by inquisition, to reside in Paris.

* 16 and 17 Vict. c. 70, s. 52.

' *Supersedeas* ' of the Inquisition.

When a person has been found lunatic by inquisition and the question of mental unsoundness is disputed, a *supersedeas* may be applied for.

A petition accompanied with medical and other evidence of the recovery must be left with the Registrar, and a copy of the petition endorsed with the order for hearing be delivered to the committees and next of kin.

The Lord Chancellor having appointed a day for hearing the application personally examines the lunatic either at the hearing of the petition or at some other appointed time. Except under very special circumstances the personal examination of the lunatic is indispensable.

If the Lord Chancellor is satisfied that the lunatic has recovered, an order for the *supersedeas* and the writ of *supersedeas* resulting thereupon are drawn up by the Registrar in the usual way.

WRIT OF SUPERSEDEAS OF COMMISSION (or Fiat) AND INQUISITION.

Victoria, by the Grace of God, of the United Kingdom of Great Britain and Ireland, Queen, Defender of the Faith.

To all to whom these our present Letters shall come Greeting. *Whereas*, by a certain Inquisition taken at, &c., on, &c., by virtue, &c., in that behalf duly made and issued to enquire amongst other things of the lunacy of A. B., of, &c., *it was found* (amongst other things) that the said A. B., at the time of taking the said Inquisition, was a *person of unsound mind*, so that he was not sufficient for the government of himself and his estate, as by the same Inquisition (amongst other things) remaining on record may more fully appear. *But* upon full examination in our Court of Chancery before us, had in this behalf, it sufficiently appears to us, that the said A. B. is recovered of his unsoundness of mind aforesaid, and is of sound mind, memory, and understanding, so that he is sufficient for the government of himself and his estate.

And we in this behalf being willing that what is just and right be done to the said A. B.: *Know ye, therefore*, that we, for and in consideration that the said A. B. now is not lunatic, but of sound mind, sane memory, and understanding, and for divers other good causes and considerations, us in this behalf especially moving, *Have superseded* and determined, and by these presents *Do supersede* and determine the aforesaid Commission (or, &c.), &c., the aforesaid Inquisition, and all other proceedings thereupon had and made, and all and singular the same, to all intents and purposes whatsoever, we annul, make void, and fully discharge by these presents. *In testimony* whereof we have caused these our Letters to be made Patent.

Witness ourself at Westminster the   day of
in the   year of our reign.

The Lord Chancellor is empowered to supersede an inquisition upon certain terms and conditions; this is done when the Lord Chancellor is of opinion that it is not for the benefit of the lunatic for the commission to be superseded unconditionally. He must first obtain the consent of the lunatic and also of other persons whom the Lord Chancellor may think necessary.

If the Lord Chancellor think proper, instead of immediately superseding the commission he may for a time suspend the proceedings under it in order to test the effect of removing the previous surveillance.

Traverse of Inquisition.

Any person who is desirous to traverse the inquisition is required to present a petition within three months from the time of its being held. [Proceedings necessary for traverse.]

The case is heard within six months from the date of the petition; the petition is presented to the Registrar, and having been answered in the usual way is set down for hearing before the Lord Chancellor, who will appoint a time for examining the lunatic, adopting such a course as he may think proper.

No person is allowed to traverse more than once. Notice of the trial is given by the solicitor, and the case is heard at the next assizes, either in the county where the inquisition was held, or in which the petitioner is then residing, as the Chancellor may direct. [Only one traverse is allowed.]

If the verdict is against the lunatic, the result of the inquisition remains the same, and committees are appointed in the usual manner; but if, on the other hand, the verdict is for the lunatic, proceedings are immediately taken for restoring the patient to the enjoyment of his liberty and rights.

I give a form of petition for traverse presented by the lunatic. This must be accompanied by medical affidavits of his mental condition and capacity to manage his affairs.

Form of petition for traverse.

FORM OF PROCEEDINGS AS TO A TRAVERSE.

PETITION FOR LEAVE TO TRAVERSE INQUISITION.

In the matter of O. E. W., a person found to be of unsound mind.

To the Right Honourable the Lord High Chancellor of Great Britain.

The humble petition of the said O. E. W. *showeth,*

That by an Order for Inquiry made in this matter on, &c., it was ordered that, &c., should enquire of the lunacy of your petitioner.

That by the Inquisition taken on the execution of the said Order on, &c., it was found that your petitioner was a person of unsound mind, &c.

That your petitioner has been informed, and believes that (*state grounds of Traverse*).

That your petitioner is advised that the said finding was contrary to the evidence adduced on the part of your petitioner.

That your petitioner is greatly aggrieved and prejudiced by the issuing of the said Fiat (or Commission), and the return of the said Inquisition.

And that your petitioner is of sound mind, and perfectly competent to the government of himself and his property.

That the proceedings to appoint committees of the person and estate of your petitioner, and to enquire who are the heir-at-law and next of kin of your petitioner, and other matters under the General Orders in Lunacy are now pending before the Master in Lunacy.

Your petitioner, therefore, humbly prays your Lordship that he may be at liberty to traverse the aforesaid Inquisition, and that your Lordship will stay in the meantime all further proceedings going before the Master.

Or that your Lordship will be pleased to make such further or other order in the premises as to your Lordship shall seem just.

And your petitioner will ever pray, &c.

Signature of petitioner

Witness to the signing hereof

By the said O. E. W.

J. B., of   Solicitor.

Answer.

(Date.) Let all persons concerned attend me on the matter of this petition on   next, the   instant, hereof give notice forthwith.

Admission of Chancery Patients into Licensed Houses.

A person who has been found of unsound mind by inquisition can be received into an asylum * *without* medical certificates. " An ' Order ' signed by the Committee appointed by the Lord Chancellor, and having an office copy of such appointment annexed, is a *sufficient* authority for his reception into any hospital or licensed house without any further order or medical certificate."

[margin note: No certificates required previous to the admission of Chancery patients into asylums.]

I cannot conclude this chapter without acknowledging the great assistance I have derived from Elmer's *Practice in Lunacy* in enabling me to arrange concisely the facts I have mentioned in connection with Commissions in Lunacy and Chancery lunatics, and I strongly recommend all who are interested in this subject, or who desire more information than I have given, to carefully peruse the pages of this valuable work.

* *Removal, Change of Address, Visits to the Seaside, &c., &c.*— The Committee of the person, or any person in whose private house, or asylum, a Chancery lunatic resides, is required to send notice to this office, three days previous to any intended change of residence, of the exact address where the patient is to be found. A similar notice three days before the return home is also to be sent. Such notices are to be posted unpaid, addressed " Lunatics Visitors' Office, 45 Lincoln's Inn Fields, London, W.C."

By order of the Board,

EASTON COX, *Secretary.*

CHAPTER IX.

REGULATIONS RESPECTING THE ADMISSION OF PATIENTS INTO
ST. LUKE'S HOSPITAL AND BETHLEHEM HOSPITAL.

St. Luke's Hospital for Lunatics.

THIS hospital is situated in Old Street, in the parish of St. Luke's, and is exclusively for private patients who are unable to avail themselves of the advantages of a private asylum. The average number of patients during the year 1871 was 144; of this number 93 were females, and 51 males. The total number of patients admitted during the year 1871 was 24 males, and 45 females. The number discharged was 35 males, and 62 females; and out of this number 16 males and 32 females were discharged as "recovered."

Prelimi-
naries
previous to
admission.

In order to obtain admission into this hospital it will be necessary for a friend or relative of a patient to go to St. Luke's, and he will then procure a form of admission, containing the order, statement, and medical certificates; these have to be properly filled up and signed before the patient can be received. The form of admission is nearly the same as that required for an ordinary patient; but there are a few additional facts to be stated, for the guidance of the authorities of the hospital.

Patients have to be presented to the Board for admission on Friday morning, at half-past ten, with the form of admission properly filled up, as mentioned in the preceding paragraph. If this is satisfactory, the patient will be admitted; but the medical officer of the hospital has the power to receive a patient on any day, if the case be an urgent one and the certificates are correct. The patient being then only received conditionally, the Board at their meeting must formally sanction the admission before the patient is considered as duly admitted.

At the last visit of the Commissioners in Lunacy to this hospital there were 156 patients on the books. Of this number 24 were maintained free of charge, 26 were received at the rate of seven shillings per week, 19 received at fourteen shillings per week, 56 at twenty-one shillings per week, and 2 at thirty shillings. We see, therefore, that the patients are charged according to their means. Any case which the Board considers a proper one is admitted free of all charge. *{Number on books at Commissioners' visit.}*

The medical superintendent is Dr. Eager, who is always ready and willing to give any information respecting the hospital.

The patients have the use of a billiard-room. They have weekly entertainments, consisting of concerts and dances, at which those patients who are capable and in a fit state are present. *{Amusements of the patients.}*

ST. LUKE'S HOSPITAL, LONDON, E.C.*

————————————————187

As it will materially assist the Committee in their consideration of the eligibility for admission or otherwise of the patient on whose behalf you apply, and also tend to save the friends trouble and expense, you or some of the friends or relations are requested to furnish answers to the following questions, and forward them to me.

I am,

Your obedient Servant,

GEORGE SEYMOUR,

Secretary.

To ————————————————

————————————————

* This must be sent to the Secretary *previous* to forwarding the Certificates.

Name and Age.	Married or Single	No. of Children	Occupation	Degree of Education

How long has Patient been Insane?	
Is this the first attack? if not, how many previous attacks?	
If previously under treatment state as follows: 1. Where treated? . . 2. In what year? . . . 3. If discharged cured?	
Mention the insane peculiarities of action or fancy .	
Is Patient 1. Noisy? . . . . . 2. Dirty in habits? . . 3. Destructive? . . . 4. Suicidal? and how? . 5. Violent to others? .	
Does Patient refuse food? and if so, how long abstinent?	
Does Patient sleep well? . .	
Does Patient suffer from any, and if so, what bodily illness?	
Is Patient subject to Fits of Epilepsy? or if Paralytic say so	
State previous habits of life .	
Here state means of support of Patient, or what amount the Friends are in a position to contribute towards the Patient's maintenance . .	

Name _____
Address _____
Business or Profession _____

SAINT LUKE'S HOSPITAL FOR LUNATICS.

ESTABLISHED A.D. 1751.

Instructions to Persons applying for the Admission of Patients.

1.—A Committee of Governors assembles at the Hospital every Friday Morning, at Eleven o'clock precisely, for the purpose of considering applications for the admission of Patients ; but urgent cases are, subject to the approval of the Committee, admissible during the week.

2.—All Insane Persons whose friends cannot afford to make any payment, are eligible for admission free, except Chronic cases, and the following, *who are inadmissible under any circumstances :—*

    A.—Persons in regular receipt of Parochial Relief, or who, in the opinion of the Committee, are proper objects for it.

    B.—Idiots, Persons suffering from Epilepsy, from certain forms of Paralysis, from Infectious Disease; being pregnant; in a condition which threatens a speedy dissolution of life ; in a dirty state, or unprovided with the requisite Clothing.

3.—Persons who have been Insane for Twelve Months, or whose cases are considered by the Committee to be Chronic, can only be admitted on payment.

4.—The amount of payments, in all cases, will be arranged by the Committee.

Notice.—Every Person who, through mistake, misinformation, or otherwise, shall have been received into the Hospital as a Patient, shall be discharged therefrom immediately on a discovery of any of the above disqualifications.

Special Directions.

The Order, Statement, and Medical Certificates properly filled up and signed, must, *on Thursday*, be forwarded to the Secretary at the Hospital, and the nearest Relation or Friend, accompanied by the Patient, must attend on *Friday Morning*, at Half-past Ten o'clock at latest, to be examined respecting the Case; and the Committee will then admit the Patient, if a fit object.

N.B.—The Medical Certificates will be invalid, if not filled up in strict accordance with the printed instructions.

Clothing.—Every Patient must, on admission, be provided with articles of apparel, according to the List subjoined, and the same must be kept supplied from time to time as required :—

FOR A MALE PATIENT.

1 Coat, ⎫
1 Waistcoat, ⎬ Sunday Suit.
1 Pair Trousers, ⎭
1 Coat, ⎫ Working, or
1 Waistcoat, ⎬ Every-day
1 Pair Trousers, ⎭ Suit.
1 Pair Braces.
6 Day Shirts.
3 Night Shirts.
6 Pocket Handkerchiefs (cotton).
2 Neck Ties.
4 Pairs of Socks.
2 Pairs of Shoes or Boots, without tips and nails.
2 Pairs Flannel Drawers, ⎫
2 Night Caps, ⎬ If worn usually by the Patient.
2 Flannel Waist-coats, ⎭
1 Hat.
1 Cap.
4 Chamber Towels.
1 Hair Brush and Comb.
1 Pair Leather Slippers, without heels or nails.
6 Collars.

FOR A FEMALE PATIENT.

4 Long Night-gowns.
4 Night Caps.
2 Day Caps or Head Dresses.
4 Chemises.
2 Flannel Petticoats.
2 Stuff Upper Petticoats.
1 Pair of Stays.
4 Pairs of White Stockings.
6 Handkerchiefs.
4 Collars.
2 Black Aprons.
3 Dresses.
1 Shawl.
1 Bonnet.
2 Flannel Waist-coats, ⎫
4 Pairs Drawers, ⎬ If worn usually by the Patient.
2 Pairs of Shoes or Boots. ⎭
4 Chamber Towels.
1 Hair Brush and Comb.
6 Diapers.
4 Bodices.

Two substantial Housekeepers must bind themselves by Bond, in the penalty of One Hundred Pounds, to make such Weekly Payment for the Patient as may be arranged; to provide sufficient Linen and Clothing; to pay for all damage done by the Patient whilst in the Hospital; and to remove the Patient from the Hospital on Seven Days' notice.

₊ It being very important in the treatment of insanity generally, and conducive to the recovery of those afflicted with that distressing malady, that the physical condition of the Brain, as well as the cause of the disorder, should be ascertained, in cases of death,—the Committee have directed that, should a Patient die while in the Hospital, the Medical Officers of the Establishment be

authorised to examine the body, unless an objection shall have been made in writing to the Secretary previous to the decease of such patient.

N.B.—The following Order and Statement *must be very carefully filled up* by a Relative or Friend of the Patient.

"ORDER" FOR THE RECEPTION OF A PRIVATE PATIENT.

*I, the undersigned, hereby request you to receive*_____
  *whom I last saw at*_____
  (*a*) *on the*_____*day of*_____ (*a*) Within
  a Lunatic, as a Patient into your Hospital. Subjoined is a one month
  *Statement respecting the said*_____ previous to
                                                                the date of
        (Signed) Name .   .   ._____ the order.
                Occupation (if any)_____
                Place of Abode ._____
        Degree of Relationship (if ⎫
        any) or other circumstances ⎬ _____
        of connection with the Pa- ⎪
        tient .   .   .   . ⎭

  Dated this_____day of_____One Thousand
Eight Hundred and Seventy_____

To the President, Vice-Presidents, Treasurer, and Governors
        of St. Luke's Hospital *for* Lunatics, London.

"STATEMENT."

If any particulars in this Statement be not known, the Fact to be so stated.

Name of Patient, with Christian name at ⎫
  length .   .   .   .   .   . ⎭ _____
Sex and age .   .   .   .   . ._____
Married, Single, or Widowed .   . ._____
Condition of life, and previous occupation ⎫
  (if any) .   .   .   .   . ⎭ _____
The religious persuasion, as far as known_____
Previous place of abode .   .   . ._____
Whether first attack .   .   .   . ._____
Age (if known) on first attack .   . ._____
When and where previously under care ⎫
  and treatment .   .   .   . ⎭ _____

L

Duration of existing attack . . . _____

Supposed cause . . . . . . _____

Whether subject to Epilepsy . . _____

Whether Suicidal . . . . _____

Whether Dangerous to others . . _____

Whether found Lunatic by Inquisition, ⎫
and date of Commission or order for ⎬ _____
Inquisition . . . . . ⎭

Special circumstances (if any) preventing ⎫
the Patient being examined before ⎪
admission, separately by two Medical ⎬ _____
Practitioners . . . . ⎭

Name and Address of Relative to whom ⎫ _____
Notice of Death to be sent . . ⎭

How many previous attacks? . . . _____

Have any Relatives of the Family been ⎫ _____
similarly affected? . . . . ⎭

State in what degree of relationship . _____

Has the Patient been of sober habits? . _____

Number of Children? (if any) . . _____

Age of youngest? . . . . _____

Degree of Education? . . . _____

(e) Where the person signing the statement is not the person who signs the order, the following particulars concerning the person signing the statement are to be added.

(Signed)   Name, (e) . _____

Occupation (if any) . _____

Place of Abode . . . _____

Degree of Relationship (if ⎫
any) or other circum- ⎪
stances of connection with ⎬ _____
the Patient . . ⎭

The Medical Gentlemen certifying, must not be Assistant one to the other, nor in Partnership with each other, nor in Partnership with, nor nearly related to, the Person signing the annexed Order. They are required to state the Facts on which their Opinion has been formed, *e.g.*: delusions (specifying the nature of the delusions), incoherence, imbecility, fatuity, alteration of conduct and affections, dirty habits, &c., and the Certificates must not have reference to each other.

N.B.—It is indispensably 'necessary that the Patient be brought to the Hospital for admission within Seven Days from the date of signature of the Medical Certificates, or the Patient cannot be received except upon new Certificates; and a Statement of the Patient's Case from one of the Medical Gentlemen who has attended the Patient, should be sent to the Hospital, directed to "Dr. Monro," or "Dr. Wood" (the Physicians), previous to the admission of the Patient.

Should either of the Medical Certificates be signed by members of the profession *not* on the last issued Medical Register, it will be necessary to afford evidence to the Secretary, that they have subsequently *duly registered*, otherwise the Certificate will be illegal.

(See Clause 37—21 & 22 Vict., Cap. 90.)

A Medical Certificate is invalid if there be not inserted therein " *the Street and Number of the House (if any) or other like particulars* " where the Patient was examined.

[See Mr. Justice Coleridge's decision *in re* Greenwood, 12th February, 1855.]

FIRST MEDICAL CERTIFICATE.

* State here your precise legal qualification to practise, &c.

I, the undersigned, being a *_____ and being in actual practice as a_____ † hereby Certify, that I, on the_____ day of_____18____, at ‡_____ in the County of_____, separately from any other Medical Practitioner, personally examined_____

* State occupation of patient.

of §_____ a *_____ and that the said_____ is a Lunatic, and a proper Person to be taken charge of, and detained under care and treatment : and that I have formed this opinion upon the following grounds, viz :—

1. *Facts indicating Insanity observed by myself,*—

* Here set forth the qualification entitling the person certifying to practise as a physician, surgeon, or apothecary, ex. gra. *being a Fellow of the Royal College of Physicians in London.*

† Physician, surgeon, or apothecary, *as the case may be.*

‡ Here insert the street and No. of the house (if any), or other like particulars.

§ Insert residence and profession or occupation, if any.

Here state the facts.

2. *Other facts (if any) indicating Insanity communicated to me by* ¶

Here state the information, and from whom.

¶ Christian and surname of informant must be given here.

(Signed)_____

Place of Abode_____

Dated this_____ day of_____18

L 2

SECOND MEDICAL CERTIFICATE.

* Here set forth the qualification entitling the person certifying to practise as a physician, surgeon, or apothecary, ex. gra. *being a Fellow of the Royal College of Physicians in London.*

† Physician, surgeon, *or* apothecary, *as the case may be.*

‡ Here insert the street and No. of the house (if any), or other like particulars.

§ Insert residence and profession or occupation, if any.

I, the undersigned, being a * _____ and being in actual practice as a _____† hereby Certify, that I, on the _____ day of _____18____, at ‡ _____ in the County of _____, separately from any other Medical Practitioner, personally examined _____ of § _____ a * _____ and that the said _____ is a Lunatic, and a proper Person to be taken charge of, and detained under care and treatment: and that I have formed this opinion upon the following grounds, viz:—

* State here your precise legal qualification to practise, &c.

* State occupation of patient.

1. *Facts indicating Insanity, observed by myself,—*

Here state the facts.

_____
_____
_____

Here state the information, and from whom.

¶ Christian and surname of informant must be given here.

2. *Other facts (if any) indicating Insanity, communicated to me by* ¶

_____
_____
_____

(Signed) _____

Place of Abode _____

Dated this _____ day of _____ 18

══════════

I do hereby certify that the above-named _____ is NOT in the receipt of Parochial Relief or Alms from his (or her) Parish.

To be Signed by the Overseer, or Relieving Officer _____

I, the undersigned, a Governor of SAINT LUKE'S HOSPITAL, desire the said Lunatic may be admitted if a fit Object.

_____

[This is sent] "To the Secretary, St. Luke's Hospital, Old Street, London, E.C."

BOND.

Know all Men by these Presents That We (¹)_____

_ _____ of (²) _____

_____ in the County of_____

(³)_____ and (¹) _____

of (⁵)_____

in the County of_____ (⁶) _____

are jointly and severally held and firmly bound, as Principals, to the President, Vice-Presidents, Treasurer, and Governors of Saint Luke's Hospital (hereinafter mentioned or referred to as "the said Corporation"), in the sum of one hundred pounds of lawful money of Great Britain, to be paid to the said Corporation, or their certain Attorney, Successors, or Assigns, for which payment, to be well and faithfully made, we bind ourselves, and each of us, as Principals, our and each of our heirs, executors, and administrators, firmly by these Presents, sealed with our Seals. Dated this day of   in the year of our Lord One thousand eight hundred and seventy

Whereas

of   in the County of hereinafter called or referred to as "the said Lunatic," was, on the day of   187   , received as a Patient into the Hospital of the said Corporation, known as St. Luke's Hospital, situate in Old Street, St. Luke's, in the County of Middlesex, upon the condition of our entering into the above Bond subject to the conditions hereinafter set forth. *Now therefore the Condition* of the above written Bond or Obligation is such that if we or either of us do and shall from time to time, during all the time in which the said Lunatic shall continue to be an inmate of the said Hospital, well and truly pay, or cause to be paid, unto the said Corporation, or unto the Treasurer for the time being of the said Corporation, money at the rate or scale of   shillings per week as and by way of contribution towards the board and maintenance of the said Lunatic during h   continuance in the said Hospital, the same to be always paid in advance at that rate by payments at intervals of four weeks each, the first payment thereof to commence and be made on the   day of   187   : *And also* if we or either of us shall, from time to time, find and provide, and keep supplied, for the said Lunatic, sufficient and decent linen and clothing, according to the list set out in the Schedule hereto, during all the time that   h   continues a Patient in the said Hospital, or shall, from time to time, on demand in writing signed by the Treasurer or the Secretary for the time being of the said Corporation, and left at the last or last known place of abode or of business of us, or of either of us, repay unto the said Corporation or unto the Treasurer for the time being of the said Corporation, all such moneys as may have been from time to time expended by the said Corporation in providing and supplying such sufficient and decent linen and clothing as aforesaid, for the said Lunatic whilst a patient in the said Hospital: *And also* if we or either of us do and shall from time to time, on demand in writing, signed by the Treasurer or the Secretary for the time being of the said Corporation, and left at the last or last known place of abode or of business of us, or of either of us, pay unto the said Corporation or unto the Treasurer for the time being of the said Corporation, all the costs, outlay, and expenses from time to time incurred by the said Corporation in reinstating, repairing, or otherwise making .good all furniture, bedding or other clothing, glass, china, or other property of the said Corporation, which may at any time or times be destroyed, torn, broken, or otherwise damaged by the said Lunatic during h   stay in the said Hospital: *And also* if we or either of us do and shall within seven days next after we or either of us shall be thereunto required by notice in writing, signed by the Treasurer or the Secretary for the time being of the said Corporation, and left at the last or last known place of abode or of business of us, or of either of us, remove and take away the said Lunatic from the said Hospital, at our, or one of our, costs and charges : *Then* the above obligation shall be void.

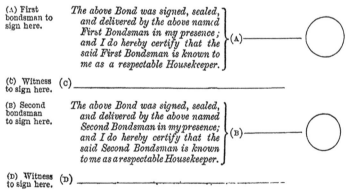

(A) First bondsman to sign here.

The above Bond was signed, sealed, and delivered by the above named First Bondsman in my presence; and I do hereby certify that the said First Bondsman is known to me as a respectable Housekeeper. (A)————— ◯

(C) Witness to sign here.   (C) ————————————————

(B) Second bondsman to sign here.

The above Bond was signed, sealed, and delivered by the above named Second Bondsman in my presence; and I do hereby certify that the said Second Bondsman is known to me as a respectable Housekeeper. (B)————— ◯

(D) Witness to sign here.   (D) ————————————————

The Schedule referred to in the above-written Bond :—

CLOTHES FOR A MALE PATIENT.	CLOTHES FOR A FEMALE PATIENT.

CLOTHES FOR A MALE PATIENT.

1 Coat, ⎫
1 Waistcoat, ⎬ Sunday Suit.
1 Pair Trousers, ⎭
1 Coat, ⎫ Working or
1 Waistcoat, ⎬ Every-day
1 Pair Trousers, ⎭ Suit.
1 Pair Braces.
6 Day Shirts.
3 Night Shirts.
6 Pocket Handkerchiefs.
2 Neckties.
4 Pairs Socks.
2 Pairs of Shoes, or Boots, without tips or nails.
2 Pairs Flannel ⎫
  Drawers, ⎪ If worn usu-
2 Night Caps, ⎬ ally by the
2 Flannel ⎪ Patient.
  Waistcoats, ⎭
1 Hat.
1 Cap.
4 Chamber Towels.
1 Hair Brush and Comb.
1 Pair Leather Slippers.
6 Collars.

CLOTHES FOR A FEMALE PATIENT.

4 Long Night-gowns.
4 Night Caps.
2 Day Caps or Head Dresses.
4 Chemises.
2 Flannel Petticoats.
2 Stuff Upper Petticoats.
1 Pair of Stays.
4 Pairs of White Stockings.
6 Handkerchiefs.
4 Collars.
2 Black Aprons.
3 Dresses.
1 Shawl.
1 Bonnet.
2 Flannel Waist- ⎫ If worn
  coats, ⎬ usually
4 Pairs Drawers, ⎪ by the
  ⎭ Patient.
2 Pairs of Shoes or Boots.
4 Chamber Towels.
1 Hair Brush and Comb.
6 Diapers.
4 Bodices.

BETHLEHEM HOSPITAL.

Bethlehem Hospital is situated in the St. George's Road, Lambeth, in the county of Surrey. It contains on an average about 270 patients, of both sexes.

At the time of the Commissioners' visit in 1871, the number on the books was 258, classified as follows:—

—	Males	Females	Total
Curables	88	114	202
Incurables	25	30	55
Criminals	—	1	1
Total	113	145	258

Admissions during the year.

The admissions during the year were 76 male and 128 female patients, the discharges 201, out of which number 37 males and 72 females were discharged recovered.

Dr. W. R. Williams, the resident medical officer, is always willing to give any information respecting the hospital, and does all in his power to promote the comfort and happiness of his patients.

INSTRUCTIONS FOR PERSONS APPLYING FOR THE ADMISSION OF PATIENTS INTO BETHLEHEM HOSPITAL.

1. All poor lunatics, presumed to be curable, are eligible for admission into this hospital, for maintenance and medical treatment, except—

1. Those who have sufficient means for their suitable maintenance in a Private Asylum.

2. Those who have been Insane more than twelve months, and are considered by the Resident Physician to be Incurable.

3. Those who are in a state of Idiocy, or are subject to Epileptic Fits, or whose condition threatens the speedy dissolution of life, or requires the permanent and exclusive attendance of a Nurse.

N.B.—" A preference will be given to Patients of the educated classes—to secure accommodation for whom, no Patient will be received who is a proper object for admission into a County Lunatic Asylum."

Certificate to be signed by the Minister and Parish Officers, and also by some Relation or Friend of the Lunatic.

We whose Names are hereunder subscribed, being the Minister and the Churchwarden, or the Overseer of the Parish of_____ in the County of_____and *_____ of the Parish of_____in the County of_____the †_____ of_____in whose behalf the present petition is presented, having carefully read over the foregoing Three Regulations, and the annexed Certificates signed by Medical Practitioners, do hereby Certify to the best of our knowledge and belief, that _____who has resided in this Parish for_____or upwards now last past, is a Lunatic, and has ‡_____ received Alms from such Parish—is not in any of the states or conditions above named—but is in every respect a proper object for Bethlehem Hospital. And _____humbly pray that the said Lunatic, who is _____Years of Age, who has been disordered in_____Senses_____Months and no longer, may be admitted into the said Hospital for Medical treatment.

† Here insert the degree of relationship (if any).

‡ Here insert whether the lunatic has or has not received parochial support.

* The petitioner must be as near a relation of the lunatic as possible, but in default of such relation, then some friend of the patient, or officer of the parish in which such patient resides, will suffice.

Witness our hands, this_____day of_____18

_____} Minister.

_____} Churchwarden
                                                  or
_____} Overseer.

_____} Relation or Friend.

I, the undersigned, a Governor of Bethlehem Hospital, desire that the above-named Lunatic may be admitted, if a proper object.

_____

If the parties do not happen to know any governor—this signature may be omitted.

BOND.

Whereas petition hath been made to the Governors of Bethlehem Hospital, for the admission of _____ as a Patient therein : *Now* we do hereby jointly and severally undertake, promise, and agree, that in case the Lunatic above-named shall be received as a Patient in the said Hospital, that we, or one of us, will, within seven days next after we shall be thereto required, by notice in Writing, to be signed by the Steward for the time being of the said Hospital, remove and take away the said Lunatic from the said Hospital, at our, or one of our Costs and Charges ; and at the like Costs and Charges bury such Lunatic, in the event of Death ; and also that we, or one of us, will pay to the said Steward the Costs and Charges of clothing the said Lunatic, during the term of such Lunatic's continuance in the said Hospital. And in case of any default in the Premises, we do hereby jointly and severally undertake, promise and agree to pay to the Treasurer of the said Hospital for the time being, the sum of One Hundred Pounds, on Demand, together with all Costs of Suit to be incurred in respect thereof. As witness our hands this   day of
18

Signatures of the two Securities	Residence	Occupation

I, the undersigned, the officiating Minister of the Parish of , do hereby certify that the above signatures were made in my presence ; and that the parties so signing are respectable Housekeepers residing in this Parish_____

The following is a List of the several Articles of Clothing required to be brought for the use of the Patient ; and the Friends of the Patient will take notice, that, during the abode of the Patient in the Hospital, they are not to furnish any further Articles of Clothing unless by the written request or permission of the Steward or Matron. The Friends of the Patient are also strictly prohibited from giving Money to the Servants, to purchase any Articles of Clothing for the Patient ; and they are not to offer or give any Fee, Gratuity, or present to any of the Servants under any pretence whatever. The infringement of these Regulations will involve not only the dismissal of the Servant, but *the discharge of the Patient* from the Hospital.

Articles Required	For Male Patient	Articles Required	For Female Patient
1	Coat ⎫	2	Night-gowns
1	Waistcoat ⎬ Sunday suit	2	Night-caps
1	Pair of trousers ⎭	2	Day caps
1	Coat ⎫ Working or	4	Shifts
1	Waistcoat ⎬ every-day	2	Flannel petticoats
2	Pairs of trousers ⎭ suit	2	Upper petticoats
4	Shirts	1	Pair of stays
3	Pocket handkerchiefs (cotton)	3	Pairs of stockings
2	Neckerchiefs or stocks	3	Handkerchiefs
3	Pairs of stockings	2	Neckerchiefs
2	Pairs of shoes or boots	2	Aprons
3	Nightcaps ⎫ If worn	2	Gowns
3	Flannel waistcoats ⎬ usually	1	Shawl
3	Pairs of flannel ⎬ by the	1	Bonnet
	drawers ⎭ patient	2	Flannel ⎫ If worn
3	Night shirts		waistcoats ⎬ usually
1	Hat	2	Pairs of ⎫ by the
1	Garden cap or hat		drawers ⎭ patient
1	Pair of thin shoes or slippers	2	Pairs of shoes or boots

N.B.—When the Petition, Bond, and Certificates shall have been filled up, and answers written to the following enquiries in the " *Statement*," this Paper must be forwarded to the Resident Physician of Bethlehem Hospital, and notice will be returned when the Patient may be brought up for examination, at which time the Patient must be accompanied by some relative or friend able to give information as to the circumstances and previous history of the case

*N.B.—Under all circumstances the " Order " and " Statement " below
to be filled up by the Patient's Relatives or Friends.*

Lunatics
(16 and 17
Vict. c. 96.)
PRIVATE
PATIENT.

" ORDER " FOR THE RECEPTION OF A PRIVATE PATIENT.

Schcd. (A) No. 1, Sects. 4, 8.

I, the undersigned, hereby request you to receive
_____whom I last saw at _____

(*a*) Within one month previous to the date of the order.

(*b*) Lunatic, or an idiot, or a person of unsound mind.

on the (*a*)_____day of_____18
a (*b*)_____ as a Patient into your Hospital.
Subjoined is a Statement respecting the said_____

(*Signed*) *Name*, _____

Occupation (*if any*) _____

*Place of Abode*_____

Degree of Relationship (*if any*),
or other circumstances of connection with the Patient \}_____

Dated this   day of
One Thousand Eight Hundred and

To the

*Superintendent of
Bethlehem Hospital, St. George's Road, Lambeth, S.*

" STATEMENT."

*If any Particulars in this Statement be not known, the Fact to be so
stated.*

Name of Patient, with Christian Name
at length   .   .   .   .   . \} _____
Sex and age .   .   .   .   . ._____
Married, single, or widowed .   .   . _____
Condition of Life, and previous occupation (if any)   .   .   .   . \} _____
Religious Persuasion, as far as known   ._____
Previous Place of Abode   .   . ._____
Whether First Attack .   .   . ._____
Age (if known) on First Attack   .   ._____
When and where previously under Care
and Treatment .   .   .   . \} _____
Duration of existing Attack .   .   ._____
Supposed cause .   .   .   . ._____
Whether subject to Epilepsy .   .   ._____

Whether suicidal . . . . ._____

Whether dangerous to others . ._____

Whether found lunatic by Inquisition, ⎤
and Date of Commission, or Order ⎬ _____
for Inquisition . . . . ⎦

Special Circumstances (if any) prevent- ⎤
ing the Patient being examined ⎟
before Admission, separately by Two ⎟ _____
Medical Practitioners . . ⎦

Name and Address of relative to whom ⎱ _____
Notice of Death to be sent . . ⎰

How many previous attacks ?

Have any relatives of the family been similarly affected ?

State in what degree of relationship.

Has the patient been of sober habits ?

Number of children ?

Age of youngest ?

Degree of education ?

(*Signed*) *Name* (e) _____

    Occupation (*if any*) _____

    Place of Abode _____

Degree of Relationship (*if any*), ⎤
or other circumstances of ⎬ _____
connection with the Patient ⎦

(e) The " Statement "
must be signed, but where
the person signing the statement is not the person who
signs the order, the following particulars concerning
the person signing the statement are to be added.

8 AND 9 VICT. CAP. 100, SEC. 45.

N.B.—Medical Certificates of Patient's Examination, and the
Signatures, are required, by the above Statute, to be dated *within
Seven clear Days* of the Patient's Reception.—In stating the Residence the *number* of the House must be specified, when there is
any.

The Medical Men signing the Certificates must not be in Partnership, nor one an Assistant to the other.

By Order of the Commissioners in Lunacy.

1.—It is absolutely necessary that the Medical Men should write
their Certificates legibly, so as to afford the opportunity of an exact
copy being made.

2.—" All alterations in the original Certificates, *unless by the
certifying Medical Men*, invalidate them ; and *the initials of the
latter* must be placed to every change or addition made."

3. " If a Registered Medical Man describes himself as ' A duly
qualified *Registered* Practitioner,' it is not necessary that he should
specify his Medical Qualifications in full, in addition."

MEDICAL CERTIFICATE.

Sched. (*A*) *No.* 2, *Sects.* 4, 5, 8, 10, 11, 12, 13.

(*a*) Here set forth the qualification entitling the person certifying to practise as a physician, surgeon, or apothecary, ex. gra. : —*Fellow of the Royal College of Physicians in London.*

(*b*) Physician, surgeon, *or* apothecary, *as the case may be.*

(*c*) Here insert the street, and number of the house (if any), or other like particulars.

(*d*) A. B. of —— insert residence and profession, or occupation (if any).

(*e*) Lunatic, *or* an idiot, *or* a person of unsound mind.

I, the undersigned,_____
being a (*a*)_____
and being in actual practice as a (*b*)_____
hereby certify, that I, on the_____ day of
_____ 18 at (*c*) *Here insert the street,
and number of house* (*if any*)_____
in the County of_____separately
from any other Medical Practitioner, personally
examined _____ of (*d*) (*State
address and occupation, if any*)_____
and that the said_____is a (*e*)_____
and a proper Person to be taken charge of and
detained under care and treatment, and that I
have formed this opinion upon the following
grounds ; viz. :—

(*f*) Here insert the facts. Some definite fact or facts must be specified.

1. Facts indicating Insanity observed by myself (*f*) (*Some definite fact or facts must be specified*)

Please to write the facts legibly, and on the lines.

_____
_____

(*g*) Here state the information and from whom received.

2. Other facts (if any) indicating Insanity communicated to me by others (*g*) (*State the name of the person giving the information*)

_____
_____

(*Signed*) Name_____
       Place of Abode_____

Dated this   day of   One
Thousand Eight Hundred and

MEDICAL CERTIFICATE.

Sched. (*A*) *No.* 2, *Sects.* 4, 5, 8, 10, 11, 12, 13.

I, the undersigned,_____
being a (*a*) _____
and being in actual practice as a (*b*)_____
hereby certify, that I, on the _____day of
_____18   at (*c*) *Here insert the street,*
and number of house (*if any*) _____
in the County of_____separately
from any other Medical Practitioner, personally
examined_____of (*d*) (*State*
address and occupation, if any)_____
and that the said_____is a (*e*)_____
and a proper Person to be taken charge of and
detained under care and treatment, and that I
have formed this opinion upon the following
grounds ; viz. :—

1. Facts indicating Insanity observed by
myself (*f*) (*Some definite fact or facts must be*
specified)

_____
_____
_____

2. Other facts (if any) indicating Insanity
communicated to me by others (*g*) (*State the*
name of the person giving the information)

_____
_____
_____

(*Signed*)   *Name*_____
    *Place of Abode*_____

Dated this   day of   One
Thousand Eight Hundred and

(*a*) Here set forth the qualification entitling the person certifying to practise as a physician,
surgeon, or apothecary, ex. gra. :
—*Fellow of the Royal College of*
Physicians in London.
  (*b*) Physician, surgeon, *or* apothecary, *as the case may be.*
  (*c*) Here insert the street and
number of the house (if any), or
other like particulars.
  (*d*) A. B. of —— insert residence and profession, or occupation (if any).
  (*e*) Lunatic, *or* an idiot, *or* a
person of unsound mind.

(*f*) Here insert the facts. Some
definite fact or facts must be
specified.

  Please to write the facts legibly,
and on the lines.

(*g*) Here state the information,
and from whom received.

CHAPTER X.

LIABILITIES INCURRED BY THOSE CONCERNED IN THE CONFINE-
MENT OF PERSONS ALLEGED TO BE INSANE.

IGNORANCE of the law cannot be pleaded as an excuse for
its violation. It is the duty of all persons who undertake the responsibility of dealing with lunatics to make
themselves acquainted with the law relating to the confinement of the insane.

The plea usually set up in defence of an action
for infringement of the Lunacy Law is ignorance of the
statute.

Liabilities of Proprietors and Medical Superintendents.

Liabilities
of proprie-
tors and
medical
superin-
tendents.

A proprietor or medical superintendent renders himself liable to an action for :—

1st. Receiving a patient without an order and medical certificates.

2nd. Admitting a patient into an asylum on an
order dated by a person who has not seen the patient
within one month from the date of his signing.

3rd. Receiving a patient on a medical certificate in
which the examination of the patient was made more
than seven days prior to the admission.

The Commissioners in Lunacy are constantly impres-
sing upon the mind of proprietors of licensed houses
and asylums the great importance of carefully examining the various medical certificates and orders for admission before receiving the patient.

Infringement of the Law by receiving a Patient without an Order, Statement, and Certificates.

* The Commissioners were informed by the relieving officer of the Taunton Union that two persons of unsound mind were taken care of for profit by a certain Mr. D. at Langaller, near Taunton.

Action for taking care of a person of unsound mind without the legal documents.

An order was received from the Lord Chancellor,† and two members of the Board of Commissioners went to Taunton, and, accompanied by the relieving officer, entered the house of Mr. D.

One of the patients was found to be of weak mind, but not sufficiently insane to necessitate being placed under medical certificate.

The other patient was undoubtedly of unsound mind, suffering from chronic dementia and delusions.

The state of this patient's mind was quite apparent, and nobody in the house attempted to dispute or disguise this point. Upon further enquiry it was discovered that he had been residing with his daughter up to August 1869, but on finding that she could no longer manage him she applied to Mr. D., who agreed to take charge of him.

The room in which he slept was found, with the exception of a tin pan for water, quite destitute of furniture.

The Commissioners reported that Mr. D., having taken charge of a lunatic gentleman for profit, without the order, statement, and certificates, as required by law, had rendered himself liable to prosecution under the Lunacy Acts, and they desired very strongly to express their opinion that it was a case in which proceedings ought to be taken.

Two medical men made a special examination of the

* Commissioners' 25th Report, 1871.
† 8 and 9 Vict. c. 100, ss. 112, 113,

patient, and in their evidence before Baron Martin both described the case as one of chronic dementia of some months' duration.

The case was proved both by the witnesses for the defence and prosecution.

The defendant having withdrawn his plea of Not Guilty, said "the Act had no doubt been infringed," and threw himself on the mercy of the Court.

Baron Martin, addressing the defendant, said that he had no doubt that the patient was a lunatic, but there was no evidence to show that Mr. L. was not well treated by him or his servants, and that it would, in his opinion, be carrying the law to an extreme length if he were punished.

The defendant was fined 20*l*., to appear and receive judgment if called upon.

The Judge said that this lenient verdict was given in consequence of the defendant having taken charge of the patient "openly and publicly and by consent of the clergyman, and having treated him as one of his own family," adding that "he saw no reason to suppose the defendant knew anything about the Act of Parliament."

The Commissioners conclude the description of the case as follows :—

"The result of this trial was not anticipated by us, and was, in our judgment, much to be regretted; we thought it calculated to exercise a prejudicial effect by encouraging not only the idea that ignorance of the law is sufficient excuse for its violation, but that unless ill-treatment be proved the law may be violated with impunity. It was not without full consideration that we instituted these proceedings, and we remain strongly of opinion, on which we shall always act, that ill-treatment not being a necessary element in a case of prosecution for reception of an insane patient without a statutory order and certificate, the absence of proof of ill-treatment forms no ground for exempting the offender from punishment."

Liabilities of Persons who sign the " Order for Admission."

In an action brought by a patient against the proprietor, superintendent, or other persons in his employ concerned in the removal of a patient to an asylum, the order and medical certificates may be pleaded as a justification for so acting, and the action cannot be proceeded with, but the person who signs the order is not included in this section, or the medical men who have signed the certificates. It occasionally happens that the person who signs the order is threatened by the patient after his discharge with an action for, as he supposes, illegal confinement in an asylum.*

The order, statement, and med'cal certificates will be sufficient authority for the reception of a patient. The persons who sign the order and medical certificates are not so protected.

The action cannot be stayed, and the person signing the order remains subject to liabilities at common law.

In an action † brought by the plaintiff, Miss Nottidge, against her brother and brother-in-law to recover compensation for the incarceration of herself in a lunatic asylum, under the pretence that she was of unsound mind, the defendants, in answer to the charge, put the following pleas upon the record :—

Action brought against the person who signed the order.

1st. Not guilty.

2nd. That the plaintiff was of unsound mind, and that it was unsafe for herself and for others that she should be at large.

The plaintiff was placed in an asylum in November 1846, and detained there till January 1848.

She was at this time in possession of property to the amount of 6,000*l.*

In 1846 the plaintiff was living with her mother in Suffolk. In the autumn of that year she went on a visit

---

* 8 and 9 Vict. c. 100, s. 99.

† Nottidge *v.* Ripley, 1849.

to her three married sisters, who resided at Weymouth. She eventually travelled with them to Somersetshire.

Her sisters' husbands had adopted peculiar views and notions with regard to their religious services.

Miss Nottidge, together with two married sisters, joined a religious establishment called the "Agapemone," or " Abode of Love.'

The plaintiff was living in lodgings with one of the members of the community when the offence complained of was committed.

The plaintiff's brother-in-law, Mr. Ripley, in November 1848, went with two gentlemen to the cottage in which the plaintiff resided, and having entered the house by a back door, went into the room where she was, and, laying hold of her, forcibly removed her, notwithstanding her screams and struggles, into a carriage, without bonnet, shawl, or even shoes to her feet. She was brought up to London, and two medical certificates obtained, and she was placed in an asylum, where she was detained for seventeen months, when she managed to inform her friends of the place of her confinement. An application was immediately made to the Commissioners in Lunacy, who, having investigated the case, ordered the discharge of the plaintiff from the asylum.

The Lord Chief Baron directed a verdict of "Not Guilty" to be returned by the jury, in consequence of there not being sufficient evidence to prove that the defendants had been guilty of *some* of the acts entered against them. With regard to the plea of justification on the part of the defendants, that the plaintiff was "a person of unsound mind, and incapable of taking care of herself," the Lord Chief Baron said that if the jury were of opinion that the plaintiff was not in a condition dangerous to herself or to others, the verdict ought then to be for the plaintiff.

Verdict.   The verdict was given for the plaintiff, damages 40*l*., the jury adding to their verdict that in their opinion the defendants were not actuated by any unworthy motive.

In consequence of the opinion expressed during the trial by the Lord Chief Baron, that no person should be confined unless he could be proved to be dangerous to himself or to others, the Commissioners in Lunacy were induced to send a letter to the Lord Chancellor, in which they stated that the opinion as expressed by the Lord Chief Baron was not what was intended by the Lunacy Acts.

The Commissioners said, " The object of these Acts is not, as your Lordship is aware, so much to confine lunatics as to restore to a healthy state of mind such of them as are curable, and to afford comfort and protection to the rest.   Moreover, the difficulty of ascertaining whether one who is insane be dangerous or not is exceedingly great; and in some cases can only be determined after minute observation for a considerable time. It is of vital importance that no mistake or misconception should exist, and that every medical man who may be applied to for advice on the subject of lunacy, and every relative and friend of any lunatic, as well as every magistrate and parish officer (each of whom may be called upon to act in cases of this sort), should know and be well assured that, according to law, any person of unsound mind, whether he be pronounced dangerous or not, may legally and properly be placed in a county asylum, lunatic hospital, or licensed house, on the authority of the preliminary order and certificates prescribed by the Acts. "

Remarks made by Commissioners on the judgment

Liabilities of Medical Men who sign the Certificates.

By the Lunacy Act,* " any physician, surgeon, or apothecary who shall sign any certificate, or do any other act (not declared to be a misdemeanour) contrary to

---

* 16 and 17 Vict. c. 97, s. 122.

any of the provisions herein contained, shall for every such offence forfeit any sum not exceeding 20*l*., and any physician, surgeon, or apothecary who shall falsely state or certify anything in any certificate, under the Act, in which he shall be described as a physician, surgeon, or apothecary, not being a physician, surgeon, or apothecary respectively within the meaning of this Act, shall be guilty of a misdemeanour."

Mistakes made by medical men in signing a certificate which would lead to an action for misdemeanour.

The following may be mentioned as some of the chief mistakes made by medical men which might lead to a prosecution :—

1st. Stating facts not observed on the day of examining the patient. Thus, if a patient is examined on December the 5th, the facts only observed on that day must be stated, notwithstanding strong symptoms of insanity were observed on the 4th.

2nd. Examining the patient in the presence of another medical man is illegal.

3rd. Facts of insanity *falsely* stated.

4th. Facts falsely stated in the *first* part of the medical certificate—for example, a medical man stating that he is a physician, surgeon, or apothecary, or a registered practitioner, such not being the case.

Discharge of a Patient by the Commissioners in consequence of an Illegality in one of the Medical Certificates and Order.

Discharge of a patient, by Commissioners, who had been illegally admitted

A patient was admitted into an asylum on July 31, 1862, and on August 2, before any return had been made to the Commissioners' Office, the asylum in which the patient was confined was visited by two members of the Board, and on their examining the original certificates upon which the patient was admitted, they saw one of the certificates, dated July 29, was founded on a visit made by the medical man on June 13, six weeks previous to the admission, thus rendering the certificate illegal and invalid. The patient was immediately ordered to be discharged.

The certificate being invalid the patient had consequently been illegally detained.

The Commissioners considered the propriety of bringing an action against the medical man who had signed this certificate. He pleaded ignorance of the law respecting the dates of signing the certificate and the examination of the patient. He stated that he had in fact seen the patient several times subsequently to his examination, and once within three or four days before signing the certificate. The medical man was informed by the Commissioners in Lunacy that although he had been guilty of neglect in not making himself conversant with what was required by law, nevertheless, as it did not appear to them that he had wilfully acted in violating the law, no further proceedings would be taken against him.

The proprietor of the asylum pleaded inadvertency in omitting to observe the date of the examination of the patient.

The Commissioners in Lunacy addressed a letter to him, the following being an extract :—

" We are instructed by the Commissioners to say that, having fully considered your explanation, they cannot think it satisfactory. In their opinion there is no part of the duty of a proprietor of a licensed house which requires greater care than the examination of certificates. *Letter addressed to the proprietor who had received the patient.*

Your long experience ought to have rendered you familiar with the particulars, in regard to them which demand special attention. The Commissioners therefore consider your negligence on this occasion as a grave offence. They instruct us, however, to say that although they will at present forego any further proceedings, yet in the event of a similar occurrence they will without fail institute a prosecution against you."

Signing a Certificate of Lunacy without being a duly registered Medical Practitioner.

Action for falsification of facts in signing a medical certificate

A case occurred last year in which the defendant was indicted under 16 and 17 Vict. c. 96, s. 13, for illegally signing a certificate of lunacy.

The patient was undoubtedly of unsound mind, and one medical certificate having been signed by a duly registered practitioner, the defendant was called in to sign the second certificate, as required by the Act.

The defendant having filled up the certificate, signed "Alexander Ogilvie, R.N.," and the patient was forthwith removed to an asylum. The Commissioners in Lunacy having received copies of the certificates, in due course of time returned them for the signataries to more fully describe their qualifications. In the amended certificate Ogilvie described himself as being an M.D., St. Andrew's, but it was ascertained subsequently upon enquiry at the Admiralty that he was *not registered under the Medical Act*, nor connected with the medical department in the Navy, and that he did *not* possess the degree of M.D. from the University of St. Andrew's.

Pleas urged in defence.

The pleas set up in defence were, that he had been in practice for forty-two years; that he had signed the certificate at the *urgent* request of the patient's relatives; that he had testimonials of the highest character from surgeons and persons whom he had attended; that he had assisted his father and uncle, who had been surgeons in extensive practice, and that the act for which he was indicted had resulted in no pecuniary compensation to him.

Mr. Justice Lush observed that this was the first case in which the Court had been called upon to inflict punishment for a breach of the section of the Act referred to by the learned counsel for the prosecution. He had now, for the first time, to determine what was the proper punishment for such a violation of the Act as had been proved before him. The statute gave him no means of measuring the punishment, but merely classified the offence as one which might be dealt with by fine or imprisonment, or both. In short, there was nothing to guide him in the Act, or no precedent such as was furnished by former decisions. He had, therefore, to consider the mischief which the Act was intended to prevent; and, looking at the circumstances of this case, he did not doubt that the defendant's intentions were free from moral blame, and that he neither signed the certificate for any bad purpose of his own, nor with the intention of lending himself to any bad motives on the part of other people. The Act under which the defendant was indicted was intended for the good treatment of unhappy persons deprived of their mental powers, and as a bar to the machinations of evil-minded people, and, with that view, it required that, before any subject was deprived of his liberty, and shut up in a lunatic asylum, a request to that effect should come from a relative, and be accompanied by certificates from two medical men. He thought that, under all the circumstances, the justice of the case would be met by the imposition of a fine of 50l., and he should direct that the defendant be kept in custody until the fine was paid.

CHAPTER XI.

EPITOME OF SCOTCH LUNACY LAW, AND CONDITION OF LUNACY IN SCOTLAND.

IN order to place a patient in an asylum in Scotland a petition, accompanied by a statement and two medical certificates, has to be presented to the Sheriff.

Statement in Schedule C of 20 and 21 Vict. c. 71. Person who signs must state his relationship to the patient.

FORM OF STATEMENT TO BE LODGED WITH A PETITION TO THE SHERIFF FOR THE RECEPTION OF A LUNATIC.*

1. Christian Name and Surname of Patient at Length.
2. Sex and Age.
3. Married, single, or widowed.
4. Condition of Life, and previous Occupation (if any).
5. Religious Persuasion so far as known.
6. Previous Place of Abode.
7. Place where found and examined.
8. Length of Time insane.
9. Whether first Attack.
10. Age (if known) on first Attack.
11. When and where previously under Examination, and Treatment.
12. Duration of existing Attack.
13. Supposed Cause.
14. Whether subject to Epilepsy.
15. Whether suicidal.
16. Whether dangerous to others.
17. Parish or Union to which the Lunatic [*if a Pauper*] is chargeable.

---

* The person who presents this statement to the sheriff must state the degree of relationship or other capacity in which he stands to such lunatic.

18. Christian Name and Surname and Place of Abode of nearest known Relative of the Patient, and Degree of Relationship (*if known*), and whether any Member of his Family known to be or to have been insane.

19. Special Circumstances (*if any*) preventing the Insertion of any of the above Particulars.

I certify, That to the best of my Knowledge the above Particulars are correctly stated.

Dated this   day of   One thousand eight hundred and

[*To be signed by the Party applying.*]

FORM OF MEDICAL CERTIFICATE.

*I, the undersigned, [*set forth the Qualification entitling the person certifying to grant the Certificate, e.g.*, being a Member of the Royal College of Physicians in Edinburgh,] and being in actual Practice as a [Physician, Surgeon, *or otherwise, as the case may be*], do hereby certify on Soul and Conscience, That I have this Day at [*insert the Street and Number of the House (if any), or other like Particulars,*] in the County of   , separately from any other Medical Practitioner visited and personally examined *A.B.* [*insert Designation and Résidence, and if a Pauper state so*], and that the said *A.B.* is a Lunatic [*or an Insane Person, or an Idiot, or a Person of unsound Mind*], and a proper person to be detained under Care and Treatment, and that I have formed this Opinion upon the following Grounds, viz. :—

1. Facts indicating Insanity observed by myself [*state the Facts*].
2. Other Facts (*if any*) indicating Insanity communicated to me by others [*state the Information, and from whom*].

(Signed)   [*Name and Medical Designation and Place of Abode.*]

Dated this   day of   One thousand eight hundred and

The medical men who sign these certificates must have no immediate or pecuniary interest in the asylum in which the lunatic is to be placed ; but one of them may be the medical superintendent, consulting or as-

Medical certificate in Schedule D, 20 and 21 Vict. c. 71.

Persons authorised to sign the certificates.

---

* The law fixes no limit to the duration of the validity of the medical certificate.

sistant physician of such asylum, provided it is not a private asylum.

If the Sheriff is satisfied, he will grant an order for the reception of the lunatic into the asylum.

FORM OF ORDER TO BE GRANTED BY THE SHERIFF FOR THE RECEPTION OF A LUNATIC.

Schedule , 20 and 21 Vict. c. 71 Sheriff's order.

I, *G.H.*, Sheriff [*or* Sheriff Substitute, *or* Steward, *or* Steward Substitute] of the County [*or* Stewartry] of   , having had produced to me, with a Petition at the Instance of *I.K.* [*Name and Designation*], Certificates under the Hands of   , and   , being Two Medical Persons duly qualified in Terms of an Act [*specify this Act*], setting forth that they had separately visited and examined *A.B.* [*describe him, and if a Pauper state so*], and that the said *A.B.* is a Lunatic, [*or* an insane Person, *or* an Idiot, *or* a Person of unsound Mind,] and a proper Person to be detained and taken care of, do hereby authorise you to receive the said *A.B.* as a Patient into the Public [*or* Private] Asylum of   , and I authorise his Transmission to the said Asylum accordingly, and I transmit to you herewith the said Medical certificates and a statement regarding the said *A.B.* which accompanied the said Petition.

Dated this   day of   18

(Signed)   *G.H.*

To the Superintendent of the Public (*or* Private) Asylum.   [*Designation.*]

This order, signed by the Sheriff, must be dated within fourteen days prior to the reception of the lunatic, and no superintendent can detain a lunatic without such being the case. If the order is signed by the Sheriff of Orkney and Shetland, there must be an interval of twenty-one days between the date of the order of the Sheriff and the reception of the patient. But if one medical man certifies that the case is one of emergency, then the superintendent shall be justified in re-

Twenty-one days allowed for the alteration of defective certificates.

ceiving and detaining the patient for a period not exceeding three days. Twenty-one days are allowed for altering defective certificates; but no such amendment shall have any force without first receiving the sanction of the Board.

A copy of the order, medical certificates, petition, and statement must be sent to the Commissioners after the expiration of two clear days, and before the expiration of fourteen clear days, from the reception of the patient. *Documents to be sent to Commissioners within fourteen days from the admission*

A notice of the patient's admission must also be sent to the Board with these documents, and also a report signed by the medical attendant of the asylum into which the patient has been received.

NOTICE OF ADMISSION.

I hereby give Notice, that *A.B.* [*describe him*] was received into this House as a Private [*or* Pauper] Patient, on the day of , and I hereby transmit a Copy of the Order and Medical Certificates and Statement on which he was received. *Schedule F, 20 and 21 Vict. c. 71.*

Subjoined is a Report with respect to the mental and bodily condition of the above-named Patient.

(Signed) *E.F.*, Superintendent.

Dated at this day of One thousand eight hundred and

REPORT.

I have this day seen and personally examined *A.B.*, the Patient named in the above Notice, and hereby report and certify, with respect to his mental state, that [*insert Particulars*], and with respect to his bodily Health and Condition, that [*insert Particulars*].

(Signed) *L.M.*, Physician [*or* Surgeon].

Dated this day of One thousand eight hundred and

The Sheriff's clerk must, within seven days after the granting of the order, send a notice to the Board, stating who made the application, and to whom the order applied; also the names of the medical men who signed the certificates and the Sheriff who granted the order; and also the name of the asylum or house to which the order was addressed. *Sheriff's clerk must send notice to the Board, containing particulars relative to the patient's admission.*

Any Sheriff's clerk who fails to comply with such notice shall for every such neglect forfeit a sum not exceeding 10*l*.

Any person who *wilfully and falsely* grants a certificate to the effect that a person is a lunatic, the grantor of such certificate, according to the Act, is guilty of an offence, and liable for each offence to a fine not exceeding 300*l*., or to imprisonment for any period not exceeding twelve months.

The patient must be seen and carefully examined by the medical man who signs the certificate. If this is not complied with, the person signing is liable to a penalty not exceeding 50*l*.

All private houses and asylums must be licensed; and any person receiving lunatics into his house without first obtaining a licence is liable to a penalty not exceeding 100*l*., or to imprisonment for any space not exceeding twelve months.

This not only applies to the keeper of the asylum, but also to the person who sends the patient to the asylum or house, if he is aware that the same is not licensed.

Any person detaining or harbouring any lunatic in any asylum, whether public or private, or in any house, without proper order and certificates, is liable to a like penalty. This applies also to the person who sends the lunatic into the asylum or house without the legal order and certificates.

Resident Medical Officers.

All asylums licensed for one hundred patients, or more than this number, must have a medical man residing on the premises, as medical attendant thereof.

All asylums licensed for more than fifty and less than a hundred patients, having no medical man residing on the premises, must be daily visited by a medical man.

All asylums licensed for fifty or less than fifty

patients, and having no resident medical man on the premises, must be visited at least twice in every week by a medical man.

Asylums licensed for less than fifty patients are required to be visited twice during the week.

The Board have power to diminish or increase the number of visits, if they think proper ; and if they see sufficient cause, they may require a resident medical man to be appointed to any asylum licensed for more than fifty patients.

All asylums licensed for less than eleven patients may be visited by a medical man less frequently than twice in every week.

If licensed for less than eleven patients, the visits can be made less frequently than twice during the week.

This entirely rests with the Board, who give their written authority for these visits.

Discharge of Patients.

A relative or friend of the patient is legally empowered to authorise his discharge from an asylum, having previously procured the certificates of two medical men approved of by the Sheriff. The person who placed the patient in the asylum requires no such order. These certificates must be to the effect that the patient has recovered, or can be liberated without risk to himself or to the public. An order from the Sheriff for the discharge is also obtained ; and this, together with the two medical certificates, will require the superintendent to discharge the patient.

Relative or friend can authorise the patient's discharge.

The Board also have power, on being satisfied with the certificates of two medical men whom they may consult as to the recovery of a patient, to order his liberation.

The Board have power to discharge the patient.

It is necessary, previous to the liberation of any such lunatic by order of the Board or Sheriff, to give eight days' notice in writing of such intended liberation to the person at whose request such lunatic was confined ; or, in his absence, to the nearest relative of such patient.

Notice required previous to discharge of a patient.

In the case of a pauper lunatic notice must be given to the person or parish at whose expense his maintenance was defrayed.

The superintendent of an asylum, upon the removal or liberation of any patient, is required to enter, or cause to be entered, into a register to be kept by such superintendent the particulars of the removal of such patient, the date thereof, the authority on which such removal was made ; and, in the case of a lunatic discharged as incurable, the facts of such discharge must be stated in the register of the asylum, also a specification of the place where the patient has gone, and the person under whose care such lunatic has been sent. A copy of these entries must be transmitted to the Board by the superintendent within two clear days from the date of the patient's removal.

The superintendent must enter into a register the particulars relating to a patient's removal.

Register of Lunatics to be kept in Asylums.

In all public, private, and district asylums there must be kept a register ; a copy of this must be transmitted to the Board as they shall direct ; and all superintendents failing to comply with this are liable to a fine not exceeding 20*l*.

Register of lunatics required to be kept in all asylums.

REGISTER OF LUNATICS.

Number in order of Admission	Date of Admission	Christian and Surname at full length	Private per M.F.	M.F. (Pan)	Age	Married	Single	Widowed	Condition of Life and previous Occupation	Previous Place of Abode	County or Parish to which chargeable	By whose authority sent	Dates of Medical Certificates, and by whom signed	Bodily condition	Name of Disorder (if any)	Form of Mental Disorder	Supposed cause of Insanity	Epileptics	Congenital Idiots	Years	Months	Weeks	Number of previous Attacks	Age on first Attack	Date of Discharge, Removal, or Death	Recovered	Relieved	Not improved	Died	Observations
1	1850. Jan. 3	William Turner	–	–	23	–	1	–	Carpenter	–	–	–	–	–	–	Melancholia	–	–	–	–	4	–	–	17	1850. Sept. 1	1	–	–	–	–
2																														
3																														
4	1852. June 9	Henry North	–	–	25	–	1	–	–	–	–	–	–	–	–	Melancholia	–	–	–	–	–	3	–	3	1852. Dec. 2	–	–	–	1	–
5																														
6																														
7	1856. May 6	William Smith	–	–	29	–	1	–	–	–	–	–	–	–	–	–	–	–	–	–	1	–	–	4	1857. June 8	–	–	–	–	–
8																														

N

Death of Patients

In the event of the death of a patient confined in a public, private, district asylum, or private house, a statement must be prepared and signed by the medical man who attended the lunatic during his last illness or at the time of death. This statement, containing the following particulars—the time and cause of the death, and the duration of the disease from which the patient died—must be sent by the superintendent of the asylum within three days from the death to the Board, also to the person or parish by whom the expense of the lunatic's maintenance is defrayed, and to the person on whose application the lunatic was confined; and any medical man or superintendent failing to transmit this is liable to a penalty not exceeding 50*l.*

A " register of deaths " similar to the one given must be kept at all asylums.

REGISTER OF DEATHS.

Date of Death	Date of Last Admission	Duration of Disease	Christian and Surname at full Length	Sex and Class				Assigned Cause of Death	Age at Death		Observations
				Private		Pauper					
				M.	F.	M.	F.		M.	F.	
1850: Sept. 1	1850: Jan. 2	—	William Johnson	—	—	1	—	-	23	—	
1852: Dec. 2	1852: June 9	—	John Brown	1	—	—	—	-	25	—	
1856: June 8	1855: May 6	—	William Smith	—	—	1	—	Phthisis	27	—	

Boarders in Asylums.

Boarders
can be re-
ceived into
asylums,
having
previously
It is lawful for the superintendent of any asylum to receive as a boarder in an asylum any person who is desirous of submitting himself to treatment, having pre-

viously obtained the consent, in writing, of one of the
Commissioners.

The boarder must make written application to the
Commissioners to be admitted, and the mental condition
of the boarder must not be such as to render it legal for
certificates of insanity to be granted.

The Commissioners in Lunacy at the time of their
visit must examine every boarder.

Boarders have power to leave the asylum after having given three days' notice, unless medical certificates,
together with an order from the Sheriff, have been procured; but in this case neither of these certificates shall
be signed by any medical man connected with the asylum, or who has any immediate or pecuniary interest in
it. In the event of a boarder being received into an
asylum, or on the discharge or death of any such, notice
must be forwarded to the Commissioners as in the case
of a patient confined under certificate.

A boarder
can leave
the asylum
on three
days' notice.

Notice for-
warded to
the Com-
missioners
on the dis-
charge or
death of a
boarder.

Single Patients in Private Houses.

No person can receive a lunatic into his house for
profit without an order from the Sheriff, or the sanction
of the Board. Any person receiving a lunatic into his
house must, within fourteen clear days from the date of
his reception, make an application for such order or
sanction.

It is illegal
for a patient
to be de-
tained in a
house as a
single
patient
without the
legal docu-
ments.

If the lunatic is a pauper, the application must then
be made by the inspector of the poor, and in such a case it
is lawful for the Sheriff to grant his order on one medical
certificate.

All patients confined in private houses are visited by
a medical man as often as the Board shall regulate, and
he must enter in a book kept in the house the date of
each visit, the mental and bodily health of the lunatics
at the time of the visit; "and every medical man who
shall make an entry without visiting the patient within

seven days of making such entry, or who shall wilfully make any false entry in the book, is liable to a penalty not exceeding 20*l*."

The Board are empowered to order inspection and visitation of every private house, from time to time, as they may think proper.

Any person detaining, or aiding in detaining, any-one who upon enquiry is found to be of unsound mind, without an order or sanction of the Board, is liable to a penalty not exceeding 20*l*.

This does not apply to patients who have been sent under certificate of a medical man on temporary leave of absence for a period not exceeding six months.

The Board can authorise the transfer of any single patient. The Board, if they think proper, in consequence of ill-treatment or otherwise, may order the transfer of a patient to any other private house, or to any public, private, or district asylum, as they may deem expedient. The expense of the maintenance is chargeable on the property of the lunatic, if he possesses any, or on the person or parish legally bound for his maintenance.

Single Patients residing in Private Houses without Profit to the Occupier.

No person can detain in his house an insane relative beyond a year without permission from the Sheriff or Board. No proprietor or inmate of any private house can receive or detain therein a lunatic, although not for profit, notwithstanding the patient is one of the family and a relative of the inmate or proprietor, beyond the period of a year, the malady being such as to require seclusion, restraint, or coercion of any kind, without an order from the Sheriff or the sanction of the Board.

The proprietor or occupier must give the particulars of the case to the Board, stating the reasons which render it desirable that the patient should remain under private care. " If the Board have reason to believe that Section referring to the deten- any person of unsound mind, and whose case has been thus intimated to them, or of whose case no such intimation has been made, has been subjected to compulsory confinement in the house, or to restraint or coercion of any kind at any period beyond a year from the commencement of the insanity, or has been ill-treated, the Board, or one or more of its members, have power, having previously obtained the consent of one of Her Majesty's principal Secretaries of State, or Her Majesty's Advocate for Scotland, to visit and inspect such lunatic, and to make such enquiry concerning the treatment as such member or members shall deem fit; and if it appears that the patient has been detained for a space exceeding a year, and that seclusion, restraint, or coercion has been resorted to, or that the patient has been ill-treated, and that the circumstances are such as to render the removal of such patient to an asylum desirable, then it shall be lawful for the Board to make application to the Sheriff for transfer of such patient to any asylum or house."

Correspondence of Patients.

All letters written by patients in any asylum or house and addressed to the Board, or Secretary of the Commissioners, or to any one of them, must be forwarded unopened, and all letters from the Commissioners addressed to such patients, and marked "private," must be delivered to the patient unopened, and any person who shall intercept, detain, or open any such letters without the authority of the patient concerned, shall be liable to a penalty not exceeding 10*l.*

The Board have power to send a copy of such letter to the superintendent of the asylum if it appears necessary to acquaint him with its contents.

COMMISSIONERS IN LUNACY.

Chairman.—Sir JOHN DON WAUCHOPE, Bart.

Commissioners.—The Rt. Hon. GEORGE YOUNG, M.P., Lord Advocate for Scotland; GEORGE MONRO, Esq., Sheriff of Linlithgowshire; Sir JAMES CONE, M.D.; ARTHUR MITCHELL, Esq., M.D.

Deputy Commissioners.—G. A. PATERSON, Esq., M.D. ; J. SIBBALD, Esq., M.D.

Secretary.—WILLIAM FORBES, Esq.

Clerk to the Board.—W. J. BATT, Esq.

Clerks.—T. W. L. SPENCE, W. DENTON, and J. WILSON, Esqs.

Messenger.—W. LEAR.

Office : Post Office Buildings, Edinburgh.

The number and distribution of the insane in Scotland on January 1, 1871, exclusive of unreported lunatics maintained in private dwellings from private sources, were as follows :—

Mode of Distribution	Male	Female	Total	Private			Pauper		
				Male	Female	Total	Male	Female	Total
In Royal and District Asylums . .	2,243	2,281	4,524	488	464	952	1,755	1,817	3,572
„ Private do. .	130	208	338	103	158	261	27	50	77
„ Parochial do.	214	330	544	—	—	—	214	330	544
„ Lunatic Wards of Poorhouses	263	367	630	—	—	—	263	367	630
„ Central Prison . .	35	16	51	—	—	—	35	16	51
„ Training Schools for Imbeciles .	81	42	123	61	30	91	20	12	32
„ Private Dwellings . .	670	849	1,519	22	34	56	648	815	1,463
Totals .	3,636	4,093	7,729	674	686	1,360	2,962	3,407	6,369

Besides the number of insane given above, it is estimated that there were about 2,000 persons of unsound mind unreported, making the total number 9,729, the ratio per thousand of insane persons to the population being rather more than two.

Number of insane in Asylums
Jan. 1, 1871 . . . 5,406
Admitted during the year . 1,836 (excluding transfers)
Recovered 810
Died 539

The following table shows the distribution of the insane on January 1, 1858, and on January 1 from 1862 to 1871. This number does not include the inmates of idiot schools, who are not certified as lunatics :—

—	1858	1862	1863	1864	1865	1866	1867	1868	1869	1870	1871
In Royal and District Asylums .	2,380	2,820	2,822	2,919	3,125	3,207	3,519	3,874	4,041	4,461	4,524
In Private Asylums .	745	921	927	872	788	812	672	501	557	303	338
In Parochial Asylums and Lunatic Wards of Poorhouses .	839	838	878	910	925	1,008	998	1,007	1,024	1,127	1,174
In Lunatic department of Central Prison .	26	29	30	32	36	46	45	45	50	49	51
In Private Dwellings	1,804	1,762	1,700	1,658	1,630	1,589	1,573	1,549	1,535	1,518	1,519
Total .	5,794	6,370	6,357	6,391	6,504	6,662	6,807	6,976	7,207	7,458	7,606

From the following table it is seen that on an average of the ten years from 1862 to 1871, out of every 100 patients sent to asylums 25·8 were private and 74·2 pauper.

Years	Numbers placed in Establishments, excluding Transfers								
	Private			Pauper			General Total		
	Male	Female	Total	Male	Female	Total	Male	Female	Total
1862	192	192	384	449	541	990	641	733	1,374
1863	173	207	380	472	536	1,008	645	743	1,388
1864	181	169	350	513	558	1,071	694	727	1,421
1865	198	221	419	484	559	1,043	682	780	1,462
1866	235	210	445	538	585	1,123	773	795	1,568
1867	210	235	445	597	663	1,260	807	898	1,705
1868	182	215	397	628	691	1,319	810	906	1,716
1869	219	218	437	666	800	1,466	885	1,018	1,903
1870	208	223	431	607	750	1,357	815	973	1,788
1871	227	254	481	647	708	1,355	874	962	1,836
Average per year	202·5	214·4	416·9	560·1	639·1	1199·2	762·6	853·5	616·1

On the other hand, an analysis of the following table will show that in the same period out of every 100 patients discharged recovered 24·8 were private and 75·1 pauper; of those discharged not recovered 43·2 were private and 56·8 pauper; and of those who died, 17·9 were private and 82·1 pauper.

The ratio of recoveries among-private and pauper patients is very nearly according to the ratio of admissions. A large proportion of the private patients are discharged not recovered, and as a consequence the mortality of the private patients is in a lower ratio when compared with the admissions than that of paupers.

Years	Removed recovered		Removed not recovered		Deaths		Total Removals		
	Private	Pauper	Private	Pauper	Private	Pauper	Private	Pauper	Total
1862	137	439	148	144	76	362	361	945	1,306
1863	161	452	123	205	82	301	366	958	1,324
1864	155	429	101	172	63	335	319	936	1,255
1865	166	462	137	114	64	299	367	875	1,242
1866	191	482	106	159	91	342	388	983	1,371
1867	191	513	128	134	84	419	403	1,066	1,469
1868	169	584	127	142	103	349	399	1,075	1,474
1869	197	596	124	194	75	453	396	1,243	1,639
1870	196	646	117	173	92	449	405	1,268	1,673
1871	172	638	152	225	91	448	415	1,311	1,726
Totals	1,735	5,241	1,263	1,662	821	3,757	3,819	10,660	14,479

On the next page is given a table showing the causes of death in asylums during the year 1871.

Table showing the Causes of Death of Patients who Died in Public, Private, and Parochial Asylums, and Lunatic Wards of Poorhouses, in 1871.

ASYLUMS	Average Number Resident		Average percentage of Deaths which took place within a year after admission		Cerebral and Spinal Disease										Thoracic Disease						Abdominal Disease						Fever, Erysipelas, Cancer, &c.		General Debility and Old Age		Suicides and Accidents		Cause unknown	
					Apoplexy and Paralysis		Epilepsy and Convulsions		General Paralysis		Maniacal and Melancholic Exhaustion		Organic Disease of Brain, Tumours, &c.		Consumption		Inflammation of Lungs and other forms of Pulmonary Disease		Disease of the Heart, Aneurism, &c.		Inflammation of Stomach, Intestines, or Peritoneum		Disease of Liver, Kidneys, &c.		Dysentery and Diarrhoea									
	M.	F.	M.	F.	M.	F.	M.	F.	M.	F.	M.	F.	M.	F.	M.	F.	M.	F.	M.	F.	M.	F.	M.	F.	M.	F.	M.	F.	M.	F.	M.	F.	M.	F.
Royal and District Asylums	2246·0	2286·5	42·7	40·8	12	19	12	11	33	11	8	8	22	26	26	34	27	16	6	10	7	6	4	6	1	5	1	10	22	28	5	8	·	·
Private Asylums	130·5	215·5	80·0	66·7	2	··	··	··	4	··	1	3	··	··	1	··	4	3	1	··	··	··	··	··	1	1	··	··	3	2	1	··	··	··
Parochial Asylums	217·5	335·0	38·5	35·9	5	1	3	··	3	··	3	··	··	··	3	11	4	5	··	4	··	2	··	2	1	1	··	··	··	3	··	··	··	··
Lunatic Wards of Poorhouses	267·0	356·0	37·0	20·6	2	3	··	1	··	··	··	··	6	··	4	6	3	4	1	3	1	··	1	··	3	3	··	1	3	8	··	··	1	··
Totals	2861·0	3193·0	··	··	21	23	17	13	43	14	9	14	30	34	34	51	38	28	8	17	8	8	6	8	6	9	1	12	31	40	8	8	1	1

Private Asylums.

There are nine private licensed houses in Scotland.
The subjoined table shows the distribution of the
patients in private asylums on January 1, 1871, and
January 1, 1872 :

Town	Name of Asylum	On Jan. 1, 1871			On Jan. 1, 1872			Proprietor
		Male	Female	Total	Male	Female	Total	
Glasgow .	Garngad House .	16	9	25	13	..	13	Dr. Hill.
Edinburgh	Gilmer House .	11	12	23	10	11	21	Mrs. Saidleir.
Edinburgh	Hallcross House .	29	52	81	24	47	71	{ P. Mackenzie, Esq.
Bothwell .	Kirklands . .	19	23	42	37	34	71	Dr. Fairless.
Edinburgh	Melville House .	12	8	20	7	15	22	{ A. Chalmers, Esq.
Edinburgh	Newbigging House	2	30	32	2	30	32	Mrs. Moffat.
Edinburgh	Saughton Hall .	29	36	65	28	38	66	{ Drs. Smith & Lowe.
Dumbarton	Westermains . .	..	3	3	..	13	13	J. Laurie, Esq.
Inveresk .	Whitehouse . .	12	35	47	12	37	49	Mrs. Hackings.
	Totals . .	130	208	338	133	225	358	

Before concluding this chapter it might be as well
to mention that, in a case of emergency, a patient can be
admitted into an asylum on one medical certificate and
without an order from the Sheriff; but he can only be
detained for a period not exceeding three days. After
this period the order from the Sheriff and two medical
certificates must be obtained.

Table giving Particulars relative to Private Asylums during the Year.

Names of Asylums	Average Number Resident		Admissions		Recoveries		Discharges not Recovered		Deaths		Proportion of Recoveries per cent. on Admissions		Proportion of Deaths per cent. on Number Resident	
	Male	Female	Male	Female	Male	Female	Male	Female	Male	Female	Male	Female	Male	Female
1. Garngad	14·5	4·5	12	14	5	4	16	19	·1	...	26·3	28·6	6·9	...
2. Gilmer	10·5	11·5	1	5	...	1	1	5	1	...	...	20·0	9·5	...
3. Hallcross	26·0	48·5	17	33	4	8	12	19	6	7	23·5	24·2	23·1	14·4
4. Kirklands	28·0	28·5	34	28	4	7	8	9	4	1	11·8	25·0	14·3	3·5
5. Melville	9·0	11·0	6	9	2	...	4	3	5	...	33·3	...	55·6	...
6. Newbigging	2·0	30·0	...	11	...	4	...	6	...	...	...	36·4	...	...
7. Saughton Hall	28·5	37·5	10	11	4	2	5	4	2	1	40·0	18·2	7·0	2·7
8. Westermains	...	8·0	...	10	...	...	...	1	...	...	...	...	...	...
9. Whitehouse	12·0	36·0	1	11	...	5	...	1	1	...	...	45·5	8·3	...
General Results	130·5	215·5	88	132	19	31	46	67	20	9	21·6	23·5	15·3	4·2

District and Chartered Asylums.

County	Asylum	Superintending Physician or Surgeon	Visiting Physician or Surgeon	No. of Patients
				Abt.
Aberdeen .	Aberdeen Royal Asylum.	Dr. Jamieson. Assts., Drs. J. H. Smith and Yeates.	Dr. Macrobin	400
Argyle .	Argyle and Bute District Asylum.	Dr. James Rutherford	. . .	300
Ayr . .	Ayrshire District Asylum.	Dr. C. Skae . .	. . .	220
Banff . .	Banff District Asylum.	Dr. Mausen . .	. . .	90
Dumfries .	Crichton Institution, Dumfries; Southern Counties Asylum,Dumfries.	Dr. Gilchrist. Assts., Drs. Malan and Anderson.	Drs. Borthwick and Scott.	450
Edinburgh.	Edinburgh Royal Asylum.	Dr. Clouston. Assts., Drs. Haigh, Wright, and Sheaf.	. . .	700
Elgin .	Elgin Pauper Asylum.	Dr. Ross . . .	. . .	80
Fife . .	District Asylum .	Dr. Tuke. Asst., W. F. Morrison.	. . .	250
Forfar .	Dundee Royal Asylum.	Dr. Rorie . . .	Dr. Cocks.	200
,,	Montrose Royal Asylum.	Dr. Howden. Asst., Dr. Balfour.	Dr. Johnston	400
Haddington	District Asylum .	Dr. Howden . .	. . .	90
Inverness .	District Asylum .	Dr. T. Aitken. Asst., Dr. McDowal.	—	—
Lanark .	Glasgow Royal Asylum.	Dr. A. Mackintosh. Assts., Drs. Hay and Blair.	Dr. Fleming	600
Perth .	Murray's Royal Institution.	Dr. Lindsay . .	. . .	80
,,	District Asylum .	Dr. C. McIntosh. Asst., Dr. Wilson.	. . .	250
Roxburgh, Berwick, & Selkirk.	Millholme House, Musselburgh.	Dr. Grierson . .	. . .	120
Stirling .	Stirling District Asylum.	Dr. F. Skae . .	. . .	250

Poorhouses Licensed for Pauper Lunatics.

County	Poorhouse.	Governor
Aberdeen .	St. Nicholas, Aberdeen	W. Dalgleish.
,,	Buchan Combination Poorhouse .	Arthur Ramsay.
,,	Old Machar ditto	M. McLeod.
Ayr . .	Cunningham Combination, Irvine	A. M. R. Findlay.
Dumbarton	Dumbarton Combination . .	J. McLean.
Edinburgh	Edinburgh City	Daniel Kemp.
,,	South Leith	J. Cowan.
Forfar .	Dundee	D. Gunn.
,,	Liff and Benvie	S. Stewart.
Kincardine	Kincardine	J. Christison.
Lanark .	City Poorhouse, Glasgow . .	J. Robertson.
,,	Barnhill ditto	J. M. Mackay.
,,	Govan, Glasgow	J. McCulloch.
,,	Hamilton	G. Edwards.
Linlithgow	Poorhouse, Linlithgow . . .	D. B. Buglass.
Perth . .	Perth	J. Reddie.
Renfrew .	Abbey Poorhouse, Paisley . .	C. W. Laing.
,,	Burgh ditto, ditto	W. Mackenzie.
,,	Greenock ditto, Greenock . .	Archd. Blair.
Wigton .	Wigton	D. Moreland.

TRAINING INSTITUTIONS FOR IMBECILES.

Forfar—Baldovan, Dundee . Dr. Greig, Visiting Physician.
Mid Lothian—Columbia Lodge. Dr. Brodie, Physician and Professor
Stirling—Larbert . . . Dr. Ireland, Physician.

CHAPTER XII.

EPITOME OF THE IRISH LUNACY LAW AND CONDITION OF LUNACY IN IRELAND.

Licences.

IT is illegal for any person to receive two, or more than two lunatics into his house without first obtaining a licence from the justices, given on certificates from the Inspectors.

Fourteen days' notice of the application for licence must be given to the clerk of the peace for the county previous to the meeting of the justices of the quarter sessions.

The application must contain certain particulars relating to the number and sex of patients proposed to be received, description of the house and grounds, name and previous occupation of the proprietor, and, if the proprietor does not intend to reside on the premises, the application should contain the name of the proposed resident superintendent.

Statement and order.

No person can be received into a licensed house without an order and two medical certificates.

The order may be signed by a relative or friend of the patient.

On the next page is given a form of the order which is required previous to the admission of a patient into an asylum.

STATEMENT AND ORDER TO BE ANNEXED TO THE MEDICAL CERTIFICATES AUTHORISING THE RECEPTION OF AN INSANE PERSON.

The Patient's true Christian and Surname at full length . . . . _____

The Patient's Age . . . . . . _____

Married or Single . . . . . . _____

The Patient's previous Occupation (if any) . . _____

The Patient's previous Place of Abode . . . _____

The licensed House or other Place (if any) in which the Patient was before confined . . . _____

Whether found lunatic by Inquisition, and Date of Commission . . . . . . _____

Special Circumstances which shall prevent the Patient being separately examined by Two Medical Practitioners . . . . _____

Special Circumstances which exist to prevent the Insertion of any of the above Particulars . . _____

SIR,

Upon the Authority of the above Statement, and the annexed Medical Certificates, I request you will receive the said _____ as a Patient into your House.

I am, Sir,

Your obedient Servant,

Name . . . . _____

Occupation (if any) . . . . . _____

Place of Abode . . . . . . _____

Degree of Relationship (if any) to the Insane Person . . . . . _____

To Mr. _____

Proprietor of _____

The medical certificates are required to be properly filled up and signed by two medical men, who must not be in partnership with each other, and who are required to separately visit and personally examine the alleged lunatic within seven clear days previous to the admission. *Particulars relative to the signing the medical certificates.*

The certificates *must* be signed and dated on the day the patient is examined. If only one certificate can be obtained, the special circumstances which have prevented the patient from being examined by two medical men must be clearly stated in the certificate. If a patient has been admitted upon one medical certificate, it is necessary for another one to be obtained, signed by a medical man, within fourteen days from the signing of the first. The medical certificates cannot be signed by anyone who is wholly or partly the proprietor or regular professional attendant of the asylum, or whose father, son, brother, or partner is wholly or in part proprietor, or the regular professional attendant of such asylum. I give below a form of the medical certificate.

FORM OF MEDICAL CERTIFICATE.

I.

I, the undersigned, hereby certify, That I separately visited and personally examined _____ the person named in the annexed Statement and Order, on the _____ Day of _____ One thousand eight hundred and _____ and that the said _____ is of unsound Mind, and a proper Person to be confined.

(Signed) Name .   .   .   .   .   _____
Physician, Surgeon, or Apothecary . _____
Place of Abode   .   .   .   .   _____

II.

I, the undersigned, hereby certify, That I separately visited and personally examined _____ the person named in the annexed Statement and Order, on the _____ Day of _____ __ One thousand eight hundred and _____ and that the said _____ is of unsound Mind, and a proper Person to be confined.

(Signed) Name .   .   .   .   .   _____
Physician, Surgeon, or Apothecary . _____
Place of Abode   .   .   .   .   _____

Documents to be sent to the Inspectors of Asylums.

The proprietor, or medical superintendent, is required to send a copy of the order and medical certificates to the Inspectors of Asylums within two clear days from the admission of the patient. Subjoined is the form required to be sent in :—

NOTICE.

Sir,

I am to acquaint you, That _____ was received into my House on the _____ Day of _____ and I herewith transmit a Copy of the Order and Medical Certificates.

(Signed) _____

To the Inspectors of
Lunatic Asylums in Ireland.

The Inspectors of Asylums preserve copies of orders and certificates, and enter in a register, within five clear days, according to the following form:

FORM OF BOOK OF ENTRY OF PATIENTS TO BE KEPT IN THE LICENSED HOUSES, AND OF REGISTER TO BE KEPT BY THE INSPECTORS.

Surname and Christian Names, Sex and Age of Patient, and whether married or single	Occupation or Profession	Place of Residence	Date of Admission of Patient, and by whose Authority sent	Date of Medical Certificates, and by whom signed	Whether found Lunatic by Inquisition	When Discharged	Cured, not cured, or incurable	Death

Registers kept in licensed houses.

The Inspectors of Lunatic Asylums in Ireland are required to transmit to the registrar a copy of all medical certificates within two days from receiving the same, and in the event of a patient having been admitted into an asylum upon the warrant of a justice, a copy of the certificates upon which such warrant was issued must be sent within two days from the signing of this warrant

Documents forwarded to the registrar.

to the registrar; this must be sent either by the justice
or his clerk.

Book kept
by medical
superin-
tendent.

The medical superintendent is required to enter in
a book kept for the purpose, within three clear days
from the reception of a patient, particulars relating to
the following facts :—Name of the patient, Christian,
surname, occupation, place of abode of the person by
whose authority the patient was sent.

Return to
be made by
medical
superin-
tendent.

The resident medical superintendent or manager of
any district, county, or other public asylum, proprietors
of asylums, and all persons receiving lunatics into their
houses are required to transmit by post to the registrar,
within one week from the reception of the patient, a
notice or return stating his own name, description, and
residence, the name, last known residence, and description of the person upon whose authority the patient had
been received, the names of the medical men certifying
to the insanity, the age, nature of the lunacy, and property of the patient, together with all such other circumstances as the Lord Chancellor may require information
upon. Notice of the patient's discharge must also be
transmitted to the registrar.

Escape, Removal, or Death of a Patient.

Escape of
patients.

The proprietor or superintendent must transmit,
within two clear days, to the Inspectors of Asylums
notice of escape, removal, or death of a patient; and, in
the event of an escape, the circumstances connected with
it, and the mental condition of the patient at the time.
The patient can be recaptured and brought back to the
asylum upon the original certificates. Notice of this
recapture must also be sent, within two days, to the
Inspectors of Asylums.

FORM OF NOTICE ON DISCHARGE, REMOVAL, OR DEATH OF PATIENT.

I _____ of _____ hereby give you Notice, That _____ of _____ a Patient in the licensed House situate in _____ was removed therefrom by _____ of _____ [*or* Death] on the _____ Day of _____ One thousand eight hundred and _____ [*here describe the State of Mind on Removal*].

Dated this _____ Day of _____ One thousand eight hundred and _____

(Signed) _____

To the Inspectors of
Lunatic Asylums, Ireland.

If the patient has been removed, the notice must state by whose authority, to what place, and the mental condition at the time of removal.

All licensed houses which are not kept by a medical man are required to be visited by a medical man once a fortnight. He is required to make entries in a book kept at the asylum, and these are to be placed before the visiting Inspectors at the time of their visitation.

If a house is licensed for less than eleven patients, the Inspectors are empowered to order it to be visited once every four weeks.

All licensed houses are visited at least every six months by one of the Inspectors, who may be accompanied by a medical man, if the Inspector wishes it, and paid by him out of funds placed at his disposal. At this visit full enquiries are made into everything connected with the asylum and the patients confined therein; and it is required that a "Visiting Inspectors' Book" and a "Patients' Book" must be kept in all licensed houses; and entries in both of these made by the visiting Inspector at the time of his visit.

The Inspectors of Asylums must carefully examine

and consider the cases to which their attention has been specially drawn with reference to the sanity; and after two visits, fourteen days having intervened between them, the Inspectors have legal power to discharge the patient. In these visits the Inspector may have the services of a medical officer connected with the nearest district asylum.*

Single Patients Confined in Unlicensed Houses.

Single patients in private houses.

No person (except he be a guardian or relative who derives no profit from the charge, or a committee appointed by the Lord Chancellor, or a person with whom such lunatic has been placed by the committee) shall receive into his house a person of unsound mind without first obtaining an order and two medical certificates, as are required previous to the admission of an insane person into a licensed house.

It is required for the person who receives the patient to send a copy of the documents upon which he has been received within three months of such reception to the Inspectors of Asylums; and on January 1 in every year, or within seven days from that time, a certificate must be sent to the Inspectors, signed by two medical men, describing the mental condition of the patient.

In case of any action, the order and medical certificates upon which the patient has been received may be pleaded by the proprietor of the asylum as sufficient justification for receiving and detaining the patient. Any person receiving a person of unsound mind into his house without conforming to the law is liable to an action for misdemeanour.

Commissions in Lunacy.

Proceedings prior to Commission in Lunacy.

The Lord Chancellor, upon receiving a petition supported by evidence and affidavits for enquiry into the

* This does not apply to persons found lunatic by Inquisition.

capability of a person to manage his affairs, directs such inquiry to be held.

The alleged lunatic, if within the jurisdiction of the Chancellor, must have notice of the presentation of the petition for enquiry ; and may, by a notice signed by him and attested by his solicitor, and filed with the registrar within seven days after such notice, demand an enquiry before a jury ; but before the Lord Chancellor orders the enquiry to be so held he may examine the alleged lunatic as to his being mentally competent to form and express a wish for such enquiry. *Inquisition with jury.*

When a jury is not demanded, or when the Lord Chancellor by personal examination is convinced of the inability of the alleged lunatic to form an opinion, the Lord Chancellor is required to hear the case ; and having taken evidence upon oath and otherwise, and called for such information as he may think desirable, he declares whether the alleged lunatic is or is not of unsound mind and incapable of managing himself and his affairs. The Lord Chancellor, when the case is to be heard by a jury, may order it to be tried before one of the Superior Courts of Common Law in Dublin. *Inquisition without jury.*

The order of the Lord Chancellor and certificate of the judge are to be deemed as an inquisition. If the lunatic is not within the jurisdiction of the Lord Chancellor, the enquiry is held before a jury, and the alleged lunatic receives no notice of it.

All affidavits made in connection with Commissions in Lunacy must be divided into paragraphs, numbered consecutively, and expressed in the first person of the deponent. *Affidavits connected with Commission.*

The person having been pronounced to be of unsound mind, a committee of the person and estate is duly appointed, who will protect the interests and well-being of the patient. *Appointment of committees*

OFFICE OF INSPECTORS IN LUNACY.—DUBLIN CASTLE.

Inspectors of Lunatic Asylums.—JOHN NUGENT, B.A., M.D.,
L.R.C.S.I., Rutland Square, Dublin; G. W. HATCHELL, M.D., L.K.,
Q.C.P., F.R.C.S.I.

Clerks.—W. J. CORBET, Esq.; J. LOWNDES, Esq.; W. C. MOORE,
Esq.

The following is the usual summary, showing the
number of insane on December 31, 1872, and where
located, contrasted with the previous year's statement:—

	1871	1872
In Public Asylums	6,992	7,140
In Private do.	652	648
In Gaols	2	—
In Poorhouses	2,914	2,966
In Lucan, supported by Government . . .	35	30
In Central Asylum for Criminal Lunatics . .	172	175
Total number of registered Lunatics . .	10,767	10,959
Lunatics at large	7,560	7,219
Total number of insane in Ireland . . .	18,327	18,178

Number of insane persons in asylums, Jan. 1, 1873   . 7,999
Admitted during 1872 2,468
Recovered 1,098
Died 670

Table showing the Number of Patients in Private Asylums on December 31, 1871, and their Ages.

Asylums	Curable			Incurable			Idiots			Epileptics			Totals			Under 20 Years			20 to 40 Years			40 to 60 Years			Over 60 Years			Totals			Proprietor	Visiting Physician
	M	F	T	M	F	T	M	F	T	M	F	T	M	F	T	M	F	T	M	F	T	M	F	T	M	F	T	M	F	T		
Armagh Retreat, County Armagh	11	9	20	11	5	16					1	1	23	14	37	1	1	1	8	1		11	7	18	10	5	10	23	14	37	Mr. Allen	Dr. Leeper
Bellevue, Finglas, County Dublin	3			18	6	24							21	6	27				6			5	4	9	10	2	12	21	6	27	Mr. Telford Jones	{ Dr. W.S. Duckett
Bloomfield Retreat, do.	4	7	11	7	17	24		1	1	2	1	2	13	26	39				2	3		6	12	18	16	11	11	13	26	39	Dr. Bull	
Citadella, County Cork	8	7	15	7	3	10		1	1				15	10	25	4	6		10	6	4	8	4	12	3	3	3	15	10	25	Dr. Bull	Dr. Greig.
Cookstown House, Piltown, County Kilkenny				3	4	7							3	4	7					3		2	4	6	1	1	1	3	4	7	Dr. Peppard.	
Gorse Lodge, Co. Armagh	6	6			4	4								10	10							4	4	4					10	10	Mr. Orr	Dr. Riggs.
Esker House, County Dublin	2				4	4					1	1		6	6					2		3	3		1	1	1		6	6	{ Mrs. Mary Ann McDowal }	{ Dr. Gordon, assistant.
Farnham House, do.	5	4	9	20	11	31				1		1	25	16	41	8	5		13	5	8	12	7	19	9	5	9	25	16	41	Dr. Duncan.	
Hampstead House, do.	4			27	1	28				2		2	33	1	34	1			10		10	15		15	8	7	8	33	1	34	{ Drs. John and Marcus Eustace	

Table showing the Number of Patients in Private Asylums on December 31, 1871, and their Ages—CONTINUED.

Asylums	Curable			Incurable			Idiots			Epileptics			Totals			Under 20 Years			20 to 40 Years			40 to 60 Years			Over 60 Years			Totals			Proprietor	Visiting Physician
	M	F	T	M	F	T	M	F	T	M	F	T	M	F	T	M	F	T	M	F	T	M	F	T	M	F	T	M	F	T		
Hartfield House, Co. Dublin	11	..	11	19	..	19	..	..	..	2	..	2	32	..	32	..	..	..	15	..	15	14	..	14	3	..	3	32	..	32	Dr. Lynch.	
Highfield House, do.	1	1	1	10	11	11	..	..	..	..	..	..	..	12	12	..	..	..	..	3	3	6	6	6	..	3	3	..	12	12	Drs. John and Marcus Eustace.	
Lindville, County Cork	9	10	19	10	5	15	..	..	..	1	..	1	20	15	35	3	..	3	7	4	..	7	..	11	5	5	10	20	15	35	Dr. John Osborne.	
Lisle House, Co. Dublin	..	2	2	..	3	3	..	..	..	..	..	..	..	5	5	..	..	..	..	2	2	1	1	1	..	2	2	..	5	5	William Hayes	Dr. Leech.
Lucan Spa, do.	..	7	7	17	24	41	14	27	41	3	3	6	47	41	88	26	15	41	7	6	13	7	13	21	8	5	13	47	41	88		
Midland Retreat, Queen's County	3	4	7	3	..	3	..	2	2	..	..	..	8	4	12	3	..	3	2	1	..	4	2	5	3	..	3	8	4	12	Dr. D. Jacob	
Orchardstown House County Dublin.	1	1	1	3	5	8	..	..	..	1	..	1	4	6	10	..	..	..	..	2	..	4	2	2	..	2	2	4	6	10	Mrs. Stanley	Dr. Croly.
St. Patrick's (Swift's), Dublin City.	2	4	6	61	56	117	1	3	4	1	2	1	65	63	128	18	19	..	37	44	..	28	21	49	19	23	42	65	63	128		
Verville, Co. Dublin	4	4	4	..	10	10	..	..	..	..	2	2	..	16	16	..	..	..	7	7	7	6	6	6	..	3	3	..	16	16	Dr. Lynch.	
St. Vincent's, do.	46	46	46	..	40	40	..	..	..	..	..	..	..	86	86	..	..	..	..	44	44	32	32	32	..	9	9	..	86	86		
Woodville, County Wexford	..	..	..	1	1	2	..	..	..	..	..	..	1	1	2	..	1	1	..	1	2	..	..	..	..	..	..	1	1	2	Dr. H. Minchin.	
Totals	60	107	167	207	210	417	31	18	49	12	7	19	310	342	652	27	14	41	85	110	195	117	136	253	81	79	160	310	342	652		

District	Counties comprising District	Res. Phys. Superint.	Consult. and Vis. Phys. and Surg.	Apothecary
Armagh	Armagh	Robt. McKinstry, M.D.	Dr. Thos. Cuming	
Ballinasloe	{Galway, Roscommon}	Rich. Eaton, M.D.	Dr. Thos. Dillon	Jas. Moore
Belfast	Antrim	Dr. Robt. Stewart	Dr. H. McCormac	P. J. Cullen
Carlow	{Carlow, Kildare}	Dr. M. P. Howlett	Dr. Thos. O'Meara	
Castlebar	Mayo	Dr. J. Edmundson	Dr. M. J. Jordan	
Clonmel	Tipperary	Dr. W. H. Garner / Asst., Dr. R. P. Gelston	Dr. W. J. Hemphill	Richd. Graham
Cork	Cork	Dr. Thos. Power / Asst., Dr. A. S. Merrick	Dr. W. C. Townshend	
Downpatrick	Clare	Dr. G. St. G. Tyner	Dr. J. K. Maconchy.	W. Stamer, M.D.
Ennis	Wexford	W. Daxon, M.D.	P. M. Cullinan.	P. M. Cooke
Enniscorthy	Kerry	T. W. Shiell, M.B.	T. Drapes, M.B.	O'C. M'Dermot
Killarney	Kilkenny	W. Murphy, M.D.	L. T. Griffin, M.D.	J. B. Fitzsimons
Kilkenny	Donegal	Dr. Barry Delany	Dr. L. C. Kinchela	W. Dunlop
Letterkenny	Limerick	Dr. J. A. Eames	Dr. J. Ashe	S. Hunt
Limerick	Derry	Dr. Robt. Fitzgerald	Dr. Robt. Gelston	W. J. Eames
Londonderry		Dr. E. Smith	Dr. E. White	
Maryborough	{Queen's Co., King's Co.}	Dr. J. H. Hatchell	Dr. D. Jacob	J. B. Macnamara
Monaghan	{Monaghan, Cavan}	Dr. J. C. Robertson	Dr. A. K. Young	J. Whitla
Mullingar	{Meath, West Meath, Longford}	Dr. H. Berkeley	Dr. Jos. Ferguson	Wm. Middleton, M.D.
Omagh	{Tyrone, Fermanagh}	Dr. Francis J. West	Dr. H. Thompson	Francis Trenor
Richmond	{Dublin, Louth}	Dr. Joseph Lalor, / Asst., Dr. A. W. H. Leney	{Dr. R. Tuohill / Dr. J. Banks / John Hughes (Surg.)}	T. E. Hayes
Sligo	{Sligo, Leitrim}	Dr. John McMunn	Dr. W. S. Little	J. Lougheed
Waterford	{Wicklow, Waterford}	Dr. R. V. Fletcher	Dr. Pierce R. Conolly	J. Mackesy

Asylums Maintained Wholly or in Part from Charitable Resources.

Asylum	Superintendent	Visiting Physician	Apothecary
Bloomfield Retreat .	. . .	Dr. Wharton.	——
St. Vincent's Hospital	. . .	Dr. T. Fitzpatrick.	——
Swift's Hospital .	Dr. E. Lawless	Drs. J. Hamilton and Freke . . .	J. Nicholls.
Lucan Spa . .	Dr. F. Pim .	Dr. H. Stewart.	——

Further Duties of Inspectors.

The Inspectors are also Commissioners of Control with the two Commissioners of Public Works in Ireland. In them, as trustees, are vested *all* the public asylums in Ireland, lands, furniture, &c. They have, under the Lord-Lieutenant in Council, full power to erect new asylums, enlarge others, take or purchase more land, divide districts, &c.

CHAPTER XIII.

LUNACY IN FRANCE.

ALL Departments in France must provide a public institution to receive and treat insane persons belonging to that Department; or else make an agreement, having previously obtained the sanction of the Minister of the Interior, with a public or private asylum, in the same or adjoining Department, to receive their insane pauper patients. Department in France to contain an asylum.

It is, however, lawful to appropriate a separate division in civil hospitals for persons of unsound mind, if there is sufficient accommodation for not less than fifty patients.

Lunatic asylums are now under the immediate direction of the Préfet of the Department, the President of the Tribunal, the Judge of the Peace, Mayor of the Commune, and the local Procureur Impérial. It is the duty of the Procureur of the Arrondissement to visit every asylum once every six months, in addition to other visits made by the Préfet, accompanied by other official persons chosen by himself or by the Minister of the Interior. Asylums under the direction of the Préfet.

Before an asylum can be opened for the reception of lunatics, it is necessary to place before the Minister of the Interior the rules intended to be made use of in the management of that asylum. Regulations respecting asylums.

No person can superintend or organise a private asylum in France without having previously obtained the approval and sanction of the Government.

Asylums in France must be used exclusively for the treatment of the insane.

The Procureur of the Arrondissement is required to visit the private asylums in his district every three months, or more frequently if he thinks necessary. The Minister of the Interior, Préfet of the Department, and five members appointed by the Préfet and acting as Commissioners, have the direction and administration of all public asylums.

Appoint-
ment of
medical
officers of
asylums.

The Minister of the Interior has the nomination and appointment of the superintendent of such asylum, and also of the physicians attached to it; but if a vacancy afterwards occur in any of these appointments, the Minister selects from a list of three candidates proposed by the Préfet. The Minister has power to revoke the appointment of the superintendent and physicians, should he think fit to do so, upon the report of the Préfet, and he determines the stipend of all officers connected with public asylums. The principal medical officer connected with the asylum must reside on the premises, unless special permission is obtained from the Minister to reside elsewhere. If this permission is granted, he is required to visit every day all the patients confided to his care; or, if he is prevented from doing this, then a daily visitation must be made by a resident physician.

Licences.

Licences for
asylums.

All persons desirous of obtaining a licence to open a private asylum must petition the Préfet of the Department in which the proposed asylum is situated. It must be satisfactorily proved that the petitioner has attained the age of twenty-one years, is in the enjoyment of all his civil rights, that his conduct and morals have been good during the three previous years, and, lastly, that he has graduated as a Doctor of Medicine.

When the petitioner does not possess that qualifi- Residence of
medical
officer. cation, he may produce a certificate from some physician who undertakes to reside in the asylum, and to discharge the medical duties. The certificate that is produced must obtain the approval of the Préfet, who has power to revoke such nomination should he think fit to do so.

Besides the official persons before mentioned, there Visitation of
asylums. are two Inspector-Generals and one *adjoint* Inspector, whose special duty it is to visit all lunatic asylums, and report to the Minister of the Interior with regard to the condition and management of the insane.

There are at present two classes of patients in French asylums—1st, *voluntary* ; 2nd, those designated *d'office*.

1. *Voluntary Patients.*

Before a patient can be received into an asylum in Prelimina-
ries prior to
admission of
a patient
into an
asylum France, it is necessary for a petition to be presented to the authorities by some near relative of the alleged lunatic. Accompanying this document there must be a certificate of a legally qualified medical man, who will state that the patient is insane and requires confinement in an asylum.

The chief symptoms and characteristic features of the mental condition of the patient must be mentioned in the certificate.

The medical man who signs the certificate must have seen the patient within fifteen days from the day of signing the document, and must not be related to the patient or connected with the establishment to which the patient is to be sent. This preliminary step may, however, be dispensed with in very urgent cases, where the patient's safety or that of the public is in danger, but it must be remedied by subsequent proceedings. After the admission of the patient into the house, all documents respecting the case must be transmitted to the Préfet of the Department within twenty-four hours.

2. D'Office, or Judicial Lunatics.

The Préfet and certain public officers have power to order the admission into an asylum of any interdicted or non-interdicted persons considered as actually insane, in order to receive proper treatment; it is also in their power to confine any person whose mental condition is such as to endanger the public safety or to compromise public order.

Dangerous lunatics.

The Commissary of Police or the Mayor of the Arrondissement are empowered to place dangerous lunatics under restraint, provided an authorised medical man certifies such to be the case.

In these cases it is necessary to report to the proper officials, who, if they think it necessary, will make additional enquiries, and act accordingly.

Alleged Lunatics.

Alleged cases of insanity.

When a person in the middle or upper classes of society is supposed to labour under mental disorder, it is customary to assemble a *conseil de famille*, who, after having examined the alleged lunatic and investigated thoroughly the whole case, will draw up a *procès verbal* of the facts to be placed before the Procureur Impérial.

The Procureur will now order two medical men to visit the patient separately, take evidence, and afterwards forward to him their opinion of the case. Upon the written opinions of these physicians the Procureur gives his judgment, and the patient is sent to an asylum or otherwise treated as he may decide.

Special provision for dealing with alleged cases of insanity.

Though this is the usual way of dealing with alleged lunatics, there is a special provision relative to the management of sudden cases of insanity. If a legally qualified medical man believes that a patient under his care has become *suddenly* insane, so as to render himself dangerous to others or to himself, he may at once convey the patient to a *maison de santé*, and there leave him, with one certificate of insanity, in which certificate is embodied the full particulars of the case. The proprietor of thé asylum to which the patient has been taken must forward immediately a statement of every fact therewith connected to the Inspector-General of Lunatics, who shortly afterwards will send two physicians to examine the patient separately, and to report every fact connected with the case. Upon these facts the Inspector-General will make his decision.

I will give one case, taken from Dr. Webster's interesting paper upon the Lunacy Laws of France, published in Dr. Forbes Winslow's *Psychological Journal*, as an illustration.

An English nobleman consulted a medical man residing in Paris concerning his health, and having described certain symptoms which led the physician to suspect that his patient was of unsound mind—exhibited chiefly by his great excitement, and by the patient producing from his pocket a bowie-knife with which he threatened to kill a certain person—the physician, after some conversation with the patient, induced his lordship to take a drive, as if for recreation ; the patient was forthwith taken to a *maison de santé*, and there safely lodged, with one medical certificate. The Inspector-General, having been speedily informed of this occurrence, ordered two sub-inspectors to investigate the case and report their opinions thereon. Every legal formality being thus readily complied with, and as the patient was found to be unmistakably insane, he remained there under treatment until discharged convalescent.

By this rapid way of procedure, public scandal and

unnecessary violence, frequently accompanying acute
cases of insanity, may be avoided.

Statistics of Insanity in France.

On January 1, 1870, there were 38,036 lunatics, exclusive of idiots, residing in French asylums.   On
January 1, 1871, the number was 38,100 ; on January 1,
1872, the number of lunatics registered was 37,323.

Dr. Lunier, in a paper read before the Académie de
Médecine upon the question of the influence of the
events of 1870–71 on insanity in France, discusses the
subject as to whether political and social commotion
occurring in the country contributed to increase the
number of the insane.   We see by comparing the above
statistics that the number of the insane in France on
January 1, 1871, was 64 less than at the same time the
previous year ; and that on January 1, 1872, it was 713
less than in 1870.

Condition of
insanity
during the
late war.
Dr. Lunier, in his interesting paper, mentions the
fact that the number of patients admitted into the asylums of France from July 1, 1869, to July 1, 1870, was
11,655 ; and that in the following year—that is, during
the Franco-German war and the reign of the Commune
—the number decreased to 10,243, or 12 per cent. less
than the previous year.

During the last six months of 1871 the number of
patients admitted into French asylums was higher than
during the corresponding six months of 1869 ; but nevertheless the number remained notably below what it
would have been had the increase been followed by the
smallest decrease of the preceding years.   Out of the
10,243 patients received into French asylums from July
1, 1870, to July 1, 1871, 13 per cent. became insane in
consequence of the events of 1870–71.   Out of this
number, viz., 1,322, 15 per cent. were men and 9 per
cent. women.   During the last six months of 1871, 400

patients were admitted into French asylums who had
become insane in consequence of the events of 1870-71,
8 per cent. being men and nearly 6 per cent. women.

Dr. Lunier states the following facts :—The events
of 1870-71 have therefore produced two apparent con-
tradictory results: they have caused the outbreak of
from 1,700 to 1,800 cases of insanity, and yet they have
led to a decrease of more than 3,000 in the number of
the insane.

Dr. Lunier's
remarks
upon the
condition of
insanity
during the
war.

The principal causes for this decrease seem to be the
disturbance caused by the invasion in the organisation
regarding the insane ; the diversion produced by these
events in the minds of a certain number of persons predisposed to insanity, in certain parts of the country ; the
momentary decrease of excessive drinking of alcohol ;
and lastly, the rapid termination by death, or, much
more often, by recovery, of the insanity caused by the
events of the war.

Insanity in France.

The population taken at the last census was
37,988,905.

Number and Distribution of the Insane.

	Insane	Idiots	Totals
In asylums	31,992	3,980	35,972
At home	18,734	35,973	54,707
Totals . . .	50,726	39,953	90,679

	Males	Females	Totals
Insane	24,190	26,537	50,726
Idiots	22,736	17,217	39,953

By this it is seen that there was one insane person

P

in every seven hundred and forty-seven of the population, and one idiot in every nine hundred and fifty.

According to the official records the chief assigned causes for insanity in France were, epilepsy and convulsions, intemperance, destitution and misery, loss of fortune, and hereditary predisposition.

*List of Asylums in France.**

Where situated		Names of Directors
Department	Commune	
Ain	Bourg	{ Berger { Bourgarel
Aisne	Prémontré	Viret
Allier	Ste. Catherine, commune of Yzeure	Chasseloup of Châtillon
Ardèche	Privas	Nier
Ariége	St. Lizier	Sisteray
Aude	Limoux	Joly
Aveyron	Rhodez	Faucher
Bouches-du-Rh.	{ Marseilles	{ Guignard { Dubiau, Hildoubrand, Abram
	Aix 2.	Pontier
Calvados	Caen 1.	{ Lallier { Vatel, Faucon, Caron
Cantal	Aurillac	Meynial
Charente	Breuty, near Angoulême	Binet
Charente-Inférieure	Lafond, commune of Cognehors	Arnozan
Cher	Bourges	{ Renault of the Motey { Lhomme, Brunet
Corrèze	La Cellette 1.	Burin
Côte-d'Or	La Chartreuse, near Dijon	Fougères, Max Simon
Côtes-du-Nord	{ Lehon, near Dinan 1. { St. Brieuc 2.	N . . . Grosvallet
Eure	Evreux	Védie
Eure-et-Loir	Bonneval	Broc
Finistère	{ Morlaix (female) 2. { St. Athanase, near { Quimper (male)	Barazier-Lannurien Baume

1. Asylum not connected with a Hospital.   2. Connected with a Hospital.

* This list is taken from the Medical Directory of France, published in 1872.

*List of Asylums in France—*continued.

Where situated		Names of Directors
Department	Commune	
Garonne (Haute-)	Toulouse	Marchand
Gers	Auch	Bouteille
Gironde	Bordeaux (female)	{ Bigot { Bulard
	Cadillac (male)	{ Icard { Péon
Hérault	Montpellier 2.	Cavalier
Ille-et-Vilaine	St. Méen (Rennes)	Laffitte
Indre-et-Loire	Tours 2.	Danner
Isère	St. Robert, commune of St. Egrève	{ Pinot { Cortil
Jura	Dole	Rousseau
Loire (Haute-)	Le Puy 1.	Ramadier
Loire-Inférieure	Nantes 2.	Petit
Loiret	Orléans 2.	Payen
Loir-et-Cher	Blois	{ Lagarosse { Tardieu
Lot	Leyme 1.	Bonnefous
Lozère	St. Alban	Campan
Maine-et-Loire	Ste. Gemmes, near Angers	Combes
Manche	Pontorson	Sizaret
Marne	Châlons	Renault du Motey
Marne (Haute-)	St. Dizier	Lapointe
Mayenne	Laroche-Gandon, com. of Mayenne.	Bonnet (H.)
Meurthe	Maréville, near Nancy	{ Giraud { Bécoulet Petrucci
Meuse	Fains, near Bar-le-Duc	{ De Brouilly { Dauby
Morbihan	Vannes 2.	Pelé de Queral
Nièvre	La Charité	Brunet
Nord	Armentières (male)	{ Delair { Mérier, Dufour
	Bailleul (female)	{ Leblond { Espiau de Lamestre
Oise	Clermont 1.	{ Labitte { Pain
Orne	Alençon	Belloc
Pas-de-Calais	St. Venant	{ Giraut { Florimond

1. Asylum not connected with a Hospital.   2. Connected with a Hospital.

List of Asylums in France—continued.

Where situated		Names of Directors
Department	Commune	
Puy-de-Dome	Clermont 1.	Hospital
Pyrénées (Bas.)	Pau	{ Auzouy / Lièvre
Rhône	Lyon(Antiquaille) 2.	Arthaud Lacour
Sarthe	Le Mans	{ Barthélemy / Etoc-Demazy
Savoie	Bassens	Fusier
Seine	Asile Ste. Anne (clinical asylum)	{ Bayeux / Pr. Lucas / Dagonet / Bouchereau / Magnan
	Bicêtre (male) 2.	{ Berthier, J. Falret, Legrand of the Saulle
	Salpêtrière(female)2.	{ Delasiauve, Moreau, Trélat, Voisin
Seine-et-Oise	{ Asylum of Ville-Evrard / Asylum of Vaucluse	Dagron / Billod
Seine-Inférieure	{ Rouen, Quatre-Mares (male)	{ Dumesnil / Maret
	Rouen, St. Yon (female)	{ De Lagonde / Morel de Gany / Delaporte
Sèvres (Deux-)	Niort 2.	Lagardelle
Tarn	Alby 1.	Cassan
Tarn-et-Gar	Montauban 2.	Darnis
Vaucluse	Avignon	{ Cottard / Campagne
Vendée	Napoléon-Vendée	Guérinau
Vienne	Poitiers 1.	Solaville
Vienne (Haute-)	Limoges	N ...
Yonne	Auxerre	{ Teilleux / Poret junior

1. Asylum not connected with a Hospital.   2. Connected with a Hospital.

Private Asylums in Paris and its Vicinity.

Paris.—303 Rue du Faubourg St.-Antoine. Founded 1769. The first entry is 12th June, 1769. *Proprietary and Medical Officer,* Dr. Brierre de Boismont.

Near Paris.—106 Grande Rue de Saint-Mandé (environs of Paris). This Asylum is exclusively for ladies mentally afflicted. *Proprietress,* Madame Rivet, née Brierre de Boismont. *Resident Medical Officer,* Dr. Correggere. *Consulting Visiting Physician,* Dr. Brierre de Boismont.

Paris.—161, 163 Rue de Charonne. *Directors,* Dr. Mesnet, Physician of the Hôpital St.-Antoine, Dr. Motet, both residing.

Paris.—10 Rue Picpus (Asylum of Marcel Sainte-Colombe). *Director,* M. Conderc, assisted by Dr. Dassonneville.

Environs of Paris.—59 Grande Rue (St.-Mandé); 19 Avenue de l'Étang.

Maison de Convalescence.—Madame Albert Brierre de Boismont. *Visiting Physician,* Dr. Brierre de Boismont.

Paris.—90 Rue Picpus (Asylum of Reboul Richebraques). *Director,* Dr. Rota. *Consulting Physician,* Dr. Tardieu, 364 Rue St.-Honoré.

Vanves, near Paris.—This Asylum was opened in 1822. *Proprietor,* Dr. Voisin (since dead) and Dr. Jules Fabret; however, the Asylum is always under the name Voisin and Fabret; also 114 Rue du Bac. Jules Fabret is alone connected with the Hospital of Bicêtre.

Ivry-sur-Seine.—(Asylum of Santé-Esquirol), 7 Rue de Seine. *Directors,* Dr. Baillarger, 15 Quai Malaquais, Paris. Dr. Moreau de Tours, 17 Rue Bonaparte, Paris; Dr. Luys residing. These three physicians are consulted at 8 Rue de l'Université, and they are connected with the Hospital of Salpêtrière.

Paris.—17 Rue Berton, Quai de Passy. *Director,* Dr. Meuriot, ancien interne des Hôpitaux do Paris. *Consulting Physician,* Dr. Blanche.

Sceaux, near Paris.—(Villa Penthièvre, Asylum and Convalescent Hospital for patients of both sexes). *Director and Proprietor,* M. Reddon. *Resident Medical Officer,* Dr. C. Du Souchay.

Neuilly, near Paris.—Asylum of C. Pimel, to the Castle of Saint-James, Avenue de Madrid.   *Medical Director*, Dr. Semelaigne.

Commissioners in Lunacy (Inspecteurs généraux).

Dr. Constans, Rue du Bac, Passage Ste.-Marie, 11 bis.
Dr. Lunier, 52 Rue Jacob.
Dr. Dumesnil, 75 Rue de Vaugirard.

CHAPTER XIV.

LUNACY IN BELGIUM.

Licences.

No person is allowed to open or superintend an asylum without obtaining permission from the Government. Licences required before receiving patients.

All houses in which one or more lunatics are living are considered as asylums, except when a person is taken care of by a curator, relative, tutor, or provincial administrator.

Before a licence is granted certain facts have to be clearly established :— Particulars relative to the licence.

1. The situation of the proposed asylum must be a healthy one, the interior of the house properly arranged, and the grounds attached to the asylum tolerably extensive.

2. The male and female patients must be separated, and a proper classification adopted.

3. Medical men must be connected with the institution. The permanent deputation appointed for the nomination of the medical officers must renew every three years their approval of the professional attendants.

Admission into an Asylum.

In order to place a patient in an asylum in Belgium, a medical certificate describing his mental state must be obtained; this has to be signed not later than fifteen days previous to the admission, but cannot be signed by Preliminaries to be followed prior to the reception into an asylum.

the medical man who is connected with the asylum to which it is proposed to send the patient.

Medical certificates. Medical certificates contain an accurate description of the nature, duration, and characteristic symptoms of the insanity, stating when the attack commenced, and whether any previous treatment has been adopted.

A sealed statement by the medical man certifying is drawn up, containing the following particulars: the cause of the insanity, and whether any member of the patient's family has been similarly affected.

Certificates connected with pauper patients are granted gratuitously by the medical officer of the poor.

Special circumstances under which certificates are dispensed with. In urgent cases of insanity this certificate is dispensed with at the time of admission, but it is *absolutely necessary* for one to be obtained within twenty-four hours from the time of the patient's admission.

Notice of admission. Notice of the patient's admission must be sent within twenty-four hours to the following persons:—

1. The Provincial Governor.
2. The King's Procureur of the Arrondissement.
3. The Cantonal Judge of the Peace.
4. The Burgomaster of the Commune.
5. The Committee of Inspection.
6. The Secretary of the Permanent Commission.

Visitation of patients. Within three days from the reception of the notice sent to the permanent commission, two members of the commission who are in the medical profession are required to visit the patient and examine into his mental condition.

These visits must be repeated every two months during the first half-year of the patient's residence in the asylum, but during the second half-year the patient is only required to be visited once.

The results of these visits must be entered in a register kept at the asylum, and a copy sent to the secretary of the commission.

Eight days after the admission of a patient into a public or private asylum, a new certificate, containing the various symptoms and the frequency of the acute ones, must be sent by the medical officer of the establishment to the secretary of the permanent commission.

The Procureur of the Arrondissement must be informed where the patient formerly resided, so that he is enabled, through the local officer, to inform the patient's friends of the circumstance.

All asylums are visited by persons delegated by the Government, as follows :

1. Every year by the Burgomaster of the Commune.

2. Every three months by the Procureur of the Arrondissement.

3. Every year by the Provincial Governor, or a member of the Provincial Council nominated by the Governor.

Patients in Private Houses.

No person of unsound mind can be "*sequestrated*" in his own house, or in that of a relative, without two medical certificates first being obtained. One of the medical men who certify is appointed by the patient's family, and the other by the cantonal judge.

Lunatics in unlicensed houses must be under certificate.

The cantonal judge is required, by personal examination, to satisfy himself as to the insanity, and to visit the patient every month.

A certificate once every quarter has to be sent to the judge by the family physician, describing the progress of the case.

Discharge.

Notice of discharge must be sent to the same persons to whom notice of admission was required to be sent, within twenty-four hours from the discharge.

Discharge of patients.

The notice contains the patient's name, the asylum

in which he had been confined, his mental state at the time of discharge, and the name of the house in which he is going to reside.

Classification of Lunatics in Asylums.

According to the regulations existing, all asylums containing fifty patients of each sex must·be divided into two separate divisions, viz., Excited and Quiet lunatics.

If the number of each sex is more than fifty, four divisions of the patients are requisite, namely: 1. Quiet; 2. Excited and noisy; 3. Idiots and dirty patients; 4. Convalescent patients.

In asylums containing more than 100 patients of each sex, the clean and orderly patients must be separated from the dirty.

Medical Officers of Asylums.

Every asylum is required to have one or more medical men connected with it, and the patients have to be visited daily.

One attendant is required for every ten patients. No person can open an asylum, or make important alterations in any asylum, without first obtaining the sanction of the Government.

The special visitation of all asylums is confided in each Arrondissement to a committee of five, seven, or nine members, including the district commissary, who sits ex officio. These officials are required to visit annually all asylums situated within their immediate jurisdiction. Besides these local visitors, three Government Commissioners have officially to visit every year, and draw up a report containing a detailed statement of all asylums and everything pertaining to lunacy in Belgium, and this is published.

There are fifty-nine asylums in Belgium, three-fourths

of which are situated in towns or in their immediate vicinity, and one-fourth in the rural communes.

Asylums in Belgium are usually small, containing *Asylums in Belgium are small.* from ten to thirty patients, and chiefly situated at Ghent and Bruges, or in the immediate vicinity of these towns; but these institutions are not well adapted for the treatment of lunatics, in consequence of the small space occupied by them.

LIST OF ASYLUMS IN BELGIUM.

Province of Antwerp.

1. Antwerp. Hospital for patients of both sexes.
2. Antwerp. Asylum occupied by *les frères cellites*.
3. Malines. Asylum occupied by *les frères cellites* for male pensioners.
4. Duffel. Asylum for female pensioners.
5. Gheel. Large establishment for both sexes.

Province of Brabant.

1. Brussels. Asylum connected with the Hospital of Saint-Jean.
2. Brussels. Asylum at Uccle for pensioners of both sexes.
3. Schaerbeek. Asylum for pensioners of both sexes.
4. Erps Querbs. Asylum for female pensioners and poor patients.
5. Louvain. Hospital for male pensioners and poor patients.
6. Louvain. Hospital for female pensioners and poor patients.
7. Tirlemont. Hospital for male pensioners and poor patients.
8. Diest. Hospital for male pensioners.
9. Diest. Hospital for female pensioners.
10. Berthem. Hospital for female poor patients.

There is no public asylum in Brussels, only a small provisional depôt attached to the hospice of St. John. This is more like a prison than an insane receptacle. In this place lunatics are temporarily confined, previously to being transferred to other establishments.

There are some first-class private asylums in the neighbourhood of Brussels. Two large asylums are situated at Evère, one containing about fifty-six patients and the other about eighty.

Province of West Flanders.

1. Bruges. Hospital of Saint-Julien, for pensioners and poor patients of both sexes.
2. Bruges. Hospital of Saint-Dominique, for pensioners and poor patients of both sexes.
3. Bruges. Asylum of Saint-Michel, for male pensioners.
4. Courtrai. Hospital of Sainte-Anne, for pensioners and poor patients of both sexes.
5. Menin. Hospital for female pensioners.
6. Ypres. Hospital for pensioners and pauper patients of both sexes.
7. Thielt. Hospital for poor patients of both sexes.

The hospital of Saint-Julien is one of the most ancient asylums in Belgium. It is situated near the railway station, close to the Porta Santa, one of the gates of Bruges. Insane persons were received within its precincts about A.D. 1500. It contains about 400 patients, an equal number of both sexes. The best class of patients pay from 20*l.* to 90*l.* per annum. The pauper patients are received at the rate of 11*l.* per annum ; this includes food, clothing, and lodging.

St. Julien charges for patients.

The asylum is far too crowded, and the grounds too small for the use of the patients ; there are three medical officers attached to it, one of whom is required to visit the asylum every day, or oftener if necessary.

A convalescent home has been erected in the neighbourhood of the hospital, capable of receiving 450 patients. The erection of this appendage is a great benefit to the lunatics who are admitted into it ; they are enabled to breathe the pure air of the country instead of being shut up in a confined place.

With regard to the hospital itself, which is confined to the medical treatment of the patients, a great many improvements have recently taken place.

Asylum of Saint-Dominique.

This asylum was formerly an ancient convent, but has for many years been used as an asylum. There are five proprietors connected with it, who, in consequence of the accommodation for the patients being insufficient, have taken a château called Saint-Michel.

This château is about two miles' distance from Bruges, and has attached to it a garden, and farm of about 100 acres. About 70 to 80 patients are received in this building.

About 200 of each sex are confined at Saint-Dominique asylum.

The patients are classified as follows :—

Classification of patients at St. Dominique.

1. Convalescent patients.
2. Quiet patients.
3. Excited patients.
4. Noisy patients.
5. Idiots and dirty patients.

The asylum is managed by three physicians and one surgeon, who appear to do everything for the care and amusement of their patients.

Patients who are willing and able assist at the various employments to be obtained in the asylum.

This asylum has lately undergone complete reorganisation, both as regards new buildings and general management.

Province of East Flanders.

1. Ghent. Hospital of Guislain, for male pensioners and pauper patients.
2. Ghent. Hospital for female pensioners and pauper patients.
3. Ghent. Asylum situated in the Street d'Assaut, for female pensioners.
4. Ghent. Asylum of Strop, for male pensioners.
5. Ghent. Hospital of Grand Béguinage, for female pauper patients.
6. Ghent. Hospital of Saint-Jean-de-Dieu, for male pensioners.

7. Ghent. Hospital of Selzaete, for male pensioners and pauper patients.

8. Saint-Nicolas. Hospital for male pensioners and poor patients.

9. Saint-Nicolas. Hospital of Ziekhuifs, for female pensioners and pauper patients.

10. Alost. Asylum for male pensioners.

11. Velsique-Ruddershove. Hospital for female pensioners.

12. Lede. Asylum for female pensioners and pauper patients.

13. Ninove. Hospital for poor patients of both sexes.

14. Nevele. Hospital for poor patients of both sexes.

15. Sleydinge. Hospital for poor patients of both sexes.

A new hospital has been opened at Selzaete, at Ghent, capable of receiving when completed 250 patients.

The asylum of Saint-Jean-de-Dieu, at Ghent, has been rebuilt and arranged in a manner more suitable to its situation. The yard has been converted into a garden containing a fountain, and domestic animals are kept in the garden, and these serve to occupy the attention of and amuse the patients.

The number of patients residing at Ghent or in its immediate neighbourhood amounts to 700, the majority of whom are female.

The Province of Hainault.

1. Mons. Asylum for female pensioners and pauper patients.

2. Froidmont. Asylum for male pensioners and pauper patients.

3. Tournai. Asylum for female pensioners and pauper patients.

4. Wez-vel-vain. Asylum for female pensioners.

5. Chièvres. Asylum for female pensioners.

The asylum at Froidmont ranks among some of the first in Belgium. The pensioners and poor patients occupy separate and distinct apartments. The division of the asylum appropriated to the pensioners consists of two wards, one reserved for the quiet and one for the noisy patients; and two new wards are in course of construction for the dirty and excitable patients.

The part of the asylum occupied by the pauper

patients is divided into five distinct wards, for quiet, half-quiet (*semi-paisibles*), excited, rather noisy (*semi-agités*), and idiots.

The two divisions occupied by the pensioners and pauper patients are separated by a large and beautiful gallery, in which the pensioners are allowed to walk, and which serves as an easy communication between the various parts of the house.

There is a large public hall and refractory ward in each of these divisions; large dormitories, properly lighted and well ventilated, are situated on the various floors.

In the part of the asylum occupied by the noisy and idiotic patients the dormitories are on the ground-floor.

The grounds in which the patients take their exercise contain a number of trees and flowers, over which are situated covered galleries, and these enable the patients to be protected in case of rain. A great improvement existing at the present time is that the various exercising grounds are separated by hedges, and not by walls, this helps to remove all idea of seclusion, and allows a free current of air to pass. There is accommodation in this establishment for 500 lunatics.

The medical superintendent and his assistant are nominated by Government.

Province of Liége.

1. Liége. Hospital for male pauper patients.
2. Liége. Hospital for female pauper patients.
8. Ans-et-Glain. Asylum for pensioners of both sexes.
4. Faubourg Sainte-Marguerite. Asylum for pensioners of both sexes.

Province of Limbourg.

There are two establishments situated at Saint-Trond, one for male pensioners and pauper patients, the other for female.

Insane Colony at Gheel.

Gheel was formerly occupied by the Texandrians, mentioned in Cæsar's "Commentaries," and, according to tradition, has for a long time been a refuge for lunatics. There is a legend respecting the origin of the supposed power possessed by Gheel for the cure of insanity.

Origin of Gheel. In the sixth century, Dymphna, a daughter of an Irish king, was converted to Christianity through the agency of an anchorite named Jerebert.

The father was very much enraged at the conversion of his daughter, and threatened vengeance.

Legend connected with it. Dymphna and her companion fled across the sea to avoid the vengeance of her father, who eventually, upon discovering her retreat, insisted upon her again changing her religion. Upon her not consenting to this, her father drew his sword and cut off the head of Jerebert, and also that of his daughter.

Some lunatics who were said to be present at this massacre were very much terrified, and the legend reports that they were immediately cured. This faith having spread abroad, lunatics were brought to Gheel from far and near, to be cured through St. Dymphna's intercession.

Gheel founded 1200. About A.D. 1200 a church was erected on the spot where the murder was perpetrated, in which the bones of the murdered Dymphna were deposited. In the church there are several paintings of groups of insane people chained down, and also oak carvings representing the circumstances connected with the murder of Dymphna.

There is a small house attached to the principal church tower, in which lunatics were deposited by their friends for nine days consecutively. This was the period considered essential for their recovery.

Nine young virgins, hired for that purpose, made a daily procession round the church aisles, passing nine times on their bended knees under St. Dymphna's tomb ; during this time prayer was offered up for the lunatic's recovery. A priest at the same time recited prayers appointed for such occasions.

Gheel contains a population of about 4,000 ; but that contained by the whole commune is 9,000. Formerly 1,000 persons of unsound mind were distributed in, or in the neighbourhood of, Gheel. The number is now increased to 1,230. These patients are distributed in about 89 houses; 30 of these are cottages and farmhouses situated in the country, and the remainder in Gheel itself. The district through which these patients are distributed occupies a circumference of thirty miles, and is divided into four divisions. Each of these divisions is under the superintendence of a physician. *Population of Gheel.*

All householders of the commune who are authorised to receive lunatics are divided into two classes : 1. Hosts; 2. Nourriciers.

The first of these classes receive patients who pay at least 25 francs per annum more than indigent lunatics. The second class, or nourriciers, receive patients at the minimum rate of payment.

The householders who receive lunatics have their names inscribed upon a register, and the distribution of the patients is effected according to rotation, though the friends of the patients have power to select any registered person they may think fit to place their friends under. *Hosts and nourriciers receiving patients have their names registered.*

Except under certain circumstances only three lunatics are permitted to reside in one house; but special sanction can be granted by the permanent committee to receive a larger number, after they have received a report from the divisional and inspecting physicians.

Rules are laid down respecting the food and clothing provided for the patients, and no patient is allowed to work unless he is in a fit state to be employed.

Q

The hours in which patients are permitted to leave their domiciles are, in summer, between 6 A.M. and 8 P.M., and in winter, 8 A.M. to 4 P.M.

Very stringent police regulations respecting these lunatics are in force. If one escapes, the person in whose house he is at the time will have to pay three-fourths of the expenses incurred in his recapture.

They are permitted to wander about within the limits of their district, unless any symptoms of violence or a desire to escape are exhibited.

Prelimina-
ries respect-
ing the
admission of
patients into
Gheel. The patients are first received into the infirmary, where their symptoms are carefully watched for a time, before they are entrusted to the care of a nourricier or host. Those in the infirmary receive proper medical treatment, and remain there as long as their condition renders it necessary for them to be under immediate medical supervision. The medical superintendent has the power to direct, as he may determine, the removal of a patient from the infirmary to the care of a nourricier or host, whose duty it is to provide occupation for them. The patients occupy their time in various ways : some in agricultural pursuits, others in music or painting. In the event of a severe bodily illness occurring, they are transferred to the infirmary to undergo the requisite medical treatment.

Payments usually made at Gheel.

Charges for
patients
at Gheel. There are four different classes of payment.

In the 1st class, about 49 patients pay from 16*l.* to 60*l.* per annum.

In the 2nd class, about 147 pay at the rate of 15*l.* per annum.

In the 3rd class, about 266 patients pay at the rate of 13*l.* 5*s.* per annum.

In the 4th class, about 312 patients pay at the rate of 11*l.* 12*s.* 6*d.* per annum.*

* These reside with the nourriciers.

These payments include lodging, food, clothing, &c. All patients who are able to work are employed on the farms and fields, or as ordinary servants. Most of the quiet patients reside in Gheel, and the noisy and more excitable ones in the country. About fourteen patients in every hundred recover, and about fifteen per cent. die.

We rarely hear of the perpetration of any violence ; suicides are very rare ; and morality is less outraged than in more protected classes.

The '*Médecin Inspecteur*' is Dr. Bulckens, who has kindly sent me full particulars relating to Gheel. He has it in his power to visit at any hour a patient confined, and, if necessary, order his removal. The system adopted here has been generally attended with favourable results, though much objection has been raised against it.

Regulations affecting the Colony at Gheel.

Gheel is affected by the same laws applicable to asylums throughout Belgium, being under the inspection of the Permanent Commission charged with the supervision of all lunatics. Besides this, a committee of eight members superintend the whole establishment. Visitation and inspection of patients at Gheel.

Four of these members are appointed annually by the special Commission from their own body, or from persons resident in the commune of Gheel. The Minister of Justice appoints four more members, from a list given to him by the council of the commune.

The Burgomaster or one of the sheriffs presides over this committee. These officials manage everything, receive all moneys paid, and are responsible for all payments; visit the houses in which the lunatics are confined, and look after their welfare.

On January 1, 1873, according to statistics kindly forwarded to me by Dr. Bulckens, there were 1,230 persons of unsound mind residing in Gheel and its immediate vicinity.

Classification of Patients at Gheel on January 1, 1873.

	Male	Female	Total
Natives . . . {	572	658	1.230
	492	575	1,067
Foreigners, *i.e.* not Belgians	80	83	163
Pensioners	97	43	140
Poor patients . . .	475	615	1,090
Curables	97	43	140
Incurables	475	615	1,090

Admissions during the year 1872, 310 patients.

	Male	Female	Total
Curable.	32	53	85
Incurable	116	109	225
Total	148	162	310
Pensioners	23	12	35
Pauper patients	126	149	275
Total	149	161	310
Discharges during } Pensioners .	8	5	13
1872 . . ʃ Paupers . .	94	91	185
Total	102	96	198
Recoveries	31	30	61
Deaths	35	42	77
Discharged	20	5	25
Removed by friends . . .	6	13	19
Escaped	10	6	16
Total	102	96	198

The average rate of mortality during the last eighteen years was seven per cent., but during the year 1872 the proportion was five per cent. out of 1,428 cases under treatment during the year.

The recoveries form but a very small proportion, because the asylum receives a large proportion of the infirm and incurable patients from other institutions, so that the incurable patients form seven-tenths of the total inmates.

Gheel contains 85 *hosts* (hôtes) and 806 *nourriciers*, making in all 891 families in which patients are received and treated like members of the family of the proprietor.

Gheel is situated about thirty-two miles from Antwerp; the most direct route is by rail to Herenthals. This occupies about one hour, and from thence by omnibus or private conveyance in an hour and a half.

Condition of Lunacy in Belgium.

The last census, taken in 1868, contains the following particulars relating to the insane :—

1. The number and the sex of insane persons in Belgium.
2. Their antecedents, and where they were born.
3. Their age.
4. The age at which they became mentally afflicted.
5. Their condition in society, and amount of education.
6. Their profession.
7. The number and age of lunatics detained in each establishment.
8. The province in which they were born.
9. The province in which they lived.

At the last census, the number of insane persons in Belgium was found to be 8,240, distributed as follows :—

	In Asylums			Living at home			General Totals	
	Male	Female	Total	Male	Female	Total	Male	Female
Free . . .	—	—	—	1,280	850	2,130	4,287	3,953
Deprived of their liberty	2,972	3,060	6,032	35	43	78		
Totals .	2,972	3,060	6,032	1,315	893	2,208	8,240	

The population in Belgium is 4,897,794, there being one insane person in every 594 of the population. If this is compared with the census taken in the four previous times, it will be found that the increase of insanity is unmistakable.

Years	Population according to the Census	One Insane Person in every
1835	4,165,953	816
1842	4,172,706	924
1853	4,516,361	920
1858	4,623,300	714
1868	4,897,794	594

I have drawn up a statistical table of the admissions and discharges from the year 1866 to 1870 inclusive.

The Commission of Enquiry of 1842 visited 37 asylums; in 1852 there existed 59; and on December 1, 1871, this number was reduced to 47. The following table will show the various changes that have taken place during this period :—

Number of Asylums in Belgium.

Provinces	Visited in 1842	In existence 1852	Remaining Jan. 1, 1871	Licensed	Closed by public authority	Built since 1852	Asylums closed
Antwerp	6	6	5	5	—	—	1
Brabant	8	13	10	10	1	1	3
Flanders, West . .	6	7	7	7	—	—	—
Flanders, East . .	7	21	15	15	4	5	7
Hainault. · . . .	4	5	5	5	—	—	—
Liége	4	5	4	3	—	—	1
Limbourg . . .	2	2	2	2	—	—	—
Total . . .	37	59	48	47	5	6	12

During the first four years which followed the reorganisation of asylums the population remained nearly stationary, but in 1856 it increased in a notable proportion, as will be perceived by the following table, which shows the number of lunatics living in asylums on December 31 each year from 1852 to 1871 inclusive:—

Lunatics residing in Asylums on Dec. 31	Pensioners			Pauper Patients			Total		Total general
	Male	Female	Total	Male	Female	Total	Male	Female	
1852	454	444	898	1,521	1,422	2,943	1,975	1,866	3,841
1853	493	532	1,025	1,527	1,502	3,029	2,020	2,034	4,054
1854	614	606	1,220	1,418	1,456	2,874	2,032	2,062	4,094
1855	608	628	1,236	1,390	1,448	2,838	1,998	2,076	4,074
1856	636	600	1,236	1,501	1,541	3,042	2,137	2,141	4,278
1857	626	666	1,292	1,574	1,565	3,139	2,200	2,231	4,431
1858	622	691	1,313	1,618	1,877	3,195	2,240	2,268	4,508
1859	627	750	1,377	1,678	1,622	3,300	2,305	2,372	4,677
1860	647	762	1,409	1,840	1,633	3,473	2,487	2,395	4,882
1861	646	801	1,447	1,835	1,751	3,586	2,481	2,552	5,033
1862	681	782	1,463	1,951	1,756	3,707	2,632	2,538	5,170
1863	725	792	1,517	1,972	1,877	3,849	2,697	2,669	5,366
1864	701	859	1,560	1,939	1,942	3,881	2,640	2,801	5,441
1865	724	861	1,585	1,950	1,887	3,846	2,683	2,748	5,431
1866	724	896	1,620	2,032	1,960	3,992	2,756	2,856	5,612
1867	779	858	1,637	2,085	2,069	4,154	2,864	2,927	5,791
1868	769	889	1,658	2,214	2,155	4,369	2,983	3,044	6,027
1869	761	935	1,696	2,349	2,234	4,583	3,110	3,169	6,279
1870	772	924	1,696	2,423	2,343	4,766	3,195	3,267	6,462
1871	745	898	1,643	2,446	2,392	4,838	3,191	3,290	6,481

Statistical Table from 1866 *to* 1870.

Year	Number of insane persons		Discharges during the year				Ratios per cent. upon the			
	On Jan. 1	Admitted during the year	Recovered	Relieved	Not improved	Deaths	Recoveries	Relieved	Not improved	Deaths
1866	5,404	1,912	642	172	288	592	8·78	2·35	3·94	8·09
1867	5,612	1,865	627	140	263	656	8·39	1·87	3·52	8·77
1868	5,790	2,008	626	178	410	557	8·03	2·28	5·26	7·14
1869	6,027	2,268	593	220	519	684	7·15	2·65	6·26	8·25
1870	6,279	2,127	596	182	415	749	7·09	2·17	4·94	8·91

CHAPTER XV.

ABSTRACT OF THE LAW RELATING TO PRIVATE ASYLUMS IN GERMANY.

A LICENCE granted by the Minister of Police is re- No Asylum can be opened without a Licence.
quired by all proprietors of private asylums. In order
for a patient to be admitted into a private asylum, a
medical certificate must be obtained and produced before the Minister of Police, or any person whom he may
authorise to act for him, and if it is satisfactory and
conclusive as to the patient's mental condition, permission is granted to the proprietor to receive the patient
into his asylum. All proprietors of private asylums are
obliged to keep a "day journal" according to a prescribed form, and to draw up a special statement concerning each patient, and forward to the proper authorities an annual report describing the condition of their
asylum.

*Lunatic Asylums belonging to the German Confederation.**

Name of Town	Description	Patients on Jan 1, 1864	Admitted during the Year
Aix-la-Chapelle	Annunciated Institution	87	56
,,	Alexianer Convent (incurables) . . .	47	10
Allenberg .	Provincial Institution	260	83
Bamberg . .	Local Hospital, St. Getreu . . .	36	6
Bayreuth . .	St. Georgen Hospital	67	10
,, .	For patients of the Jewish persuasion . .	8	2
Bendorf . .	Private asylum of Dr. Brosius . . .	21	15
Coblenz . .	,, ,, Dr. Erlenmeyer . . .	74	36
Berlin .	City Lunatic Asylum, connected with } Charity Hospital . . . . }	56	182

* Report of Dr. Laehr on German Asylums.

German Confederation—continued.

Name of Town	Description	Patients on Jan. 1, 1864	Admitted during the Year.
Berlin . .	City Hospital for Insane	340	356
,, . .	Private asylum for females	20	2
,, . .	Dr. Klinsman's private asylum for both sexes	47	19
Bernau . .	Private asylum for females	15	1
Blankenburg .	Connected with Convent	90	13
Blankenhain .	Karl Friedrich's Hospital for Insane . .	86	7
Bonn . .	Albers Institution	11	8
,, . .	Private asylum	21	17
Brake . .	Public ,, ...	98	34
Braunschweig.	Provincial asylum (for curables) . . .	65	25
Bremen . .	Department connected with the hospital .	76	38
Breslau . .	,, ,,	50	89
Brieg . .	Provincial institution	173	5
Brünn . .	Moravian ,, ...	208	229
Bunslau . .	Provincial ,, ...	227	143
Burgdorf. .	,, ,, (for quiet patients) .	—	—
Canstatt . .	Private asylum of Dr. Rühle's . . .	12	4
Carlsfeld . .	Private asylum opened by Dr. Niemeyer .	15	25
Charlottenburg	Private asylum for females	21	10
Coblenz . .	,, ,, . . .	9	2
Coburg . .	Provincial hospital	—	—
Cologne . .	Citizens' ,, ...	63	12
Colditz . .	Provincial institute for males . . .	615	83
Dessau . .	Ducal institution	49	19
Dömitz {	Instituted for incurable and dangerous patients, connected with the fortress . }	126	10
Düsseldorf .	Public asylum for incurables . . .	433	164
Eichberg . .	,, ,, ,, . . .	268	54
Eitorf . .	Private asylum receiving from 20 to 30 patients	—	—
Elberfeld . .	Public asylum for incurables . . .	38	64
Endenich . .	Private asylum	33	27
Erlangen . .	District ,, ...	205	78
Eupen . .	Private ,, ...	21	10
Frankfurt .	Public ,, for insane and epileptics .	101	73
Gesecke . .	Provincial institution for incurables . .	—	26
Near Bayreuth.	Private asylum of St. Gilgenberg . . .	9	7
Gladbach . {	Institution connected with the Alexianer Convent . . . . . }	—	—
Gmünd . .	Private asylum of St. Vincenz . . .	—	—
Göppingen {	Private asylum, to which is attached 120 acres of land, and farm house. It forms an insane colony . . . . . }	226	91
Görlitz . .	Private asylum	33	33
Göttingen .	New institution for 200 patients . . .	—	—
Gotha . {	Institution for the insane ; contains about 18 patients . . . . . }	—	—
Graetz . {	Provincial institution for the insane of Steiermark . . . . . }	165	78
Greifswald .	Public asylum	33	49
Grimma . .	Private asylum of Villa Bochlen . . .	16	6
Haina . {	Institution for the insane, formerly a convent of monks . . . . . }	399	42
Hall . .	Provincial institution	114	45
Halle . .	Institution for province of Saxony . .	488	113
Hamburg .	Friedrichsberg institution at Barmbeck . .	—	—
Helmstädt .	Private asylum	3	14
Hermannstadt.	Provincial institution		

German Confederation—continued.

Name of Town	Description	Patients on Jan. 1, 1864	Admitted during the Year.
Hildesheim	Horticultural Colony and Institution for the Insane	810	179
Hofheim . .	Provincial hospital	428	88
Hornheim .	Private asylum at Kiel	—	—
Hubertusburg .	Insane hospital for women and children .	722	112
Jena . .	Institution for the insane . . .	74	53
Illenau .	„ „ formerly at Heidelberg	439	345
Ilten . .	Private asylum	—	—
Irsee . .	Institution for insane	—	76
Kaiserwerth .	Lutheran Institution for female patients .	29	22
Kennenburg .	Institution for the insane	20	19
Kessenich .	Private asylum	2	11
Klagenfurt .	Branch connected with the general hospital	—	—
Klingenmünster	Institution for the insane	326	123
Königslutter .	„ „	—	—
Kowanowko .	Private asylum	27	25
Laibach .	Provincial institution connected with general hospital	—	—
Laichingen .	Private provincial institution . . .	—	—
Leipzig .	House of St. George, is also used as a House of Correction	16	76
Lemberg .	Connected with the general hospital .	189	250
Lengerich	Institution for the insane . . .	—	—
Leubus .	Provincial institution (public) These are connected and under same supervision	110	256
„ „	„ „ (pensionnat)	36	15
Lindenburg .	Private asylum	296	101
Lindenhof .	„ „	15	37
Linz . .	Connected with the Provincial Hospital	—	96
Linz-on-Rhine	Institution for Catholic women, under supervision of Sisters of Charity . .	—	—
Lübeck .	Public institution	53	15
Luxemburg	Connected with a convent, under supervision of Sisters of Charity . . .	—	—
Marsberg .	Public provincial institution . . .	469	144
Merkhausen .	Institution for females (chronic) . . .	200	11
Munich . .	Royal District Institution	265	104
Münster .	Connected with Clemens Hospital . . .	11	5
Neu-Ruppin .	Provincial institution	157	87
Neuss .	„ „ in Alexianer Convent .	—	—
„ „	Connected with St. Joseph's Hospital .	—	—
Neu-Eberswalde	New institution	—	—
„	Private asylum	—	—
Osnabrück .	Institution for 200 patients just opened .	—	—
Owinsk, Posen	Provincial hospital for 100 patients .	—	—
Pforzheim .	Institution for Grand Duchy of Baden .	499	93
Pfullingen .	Private asylum for 10 to 20 patients .	—	—
Pirna . .	Private asylum	16	12
Popelwitz .	Private asylum	32	25
Posen . .	Connected with the City Hospital . .	25	17
Prag . .	Provincial institution	744	386
Roekwinkel .	Private asylum	—	—
Regenburg .	Institution near Regenburg (Carthaus Prüll)	201	84
Roda . .	Institution for curables	139	54

German Confederation—continued.

Name of Town	Description	Patients on Jan. 1, 1864	Admitted during the Year
Rostock . .	Institution for about 80 patients . . .	—	—
Rudoestadt .	Institution for the insane	42	8
Rügenwalde .	Provincial institution	116	5
Sachsenberg .	Institution for the insane	233	91
Salzburg . .	Provincial institution	89	29
„ . {	Institution for harmless lunatics (Leprosen-hans) . . . . }	—	—
Scheibe . {	Connected with a convent, 30 patients being received . . . . . . }	—	—
Schleswig .	Institution for the insane	639	109
„ .	Private asylum	8	1
Schmiedeberg .	„ „	20	5
Schweizerhof .	„ „ near Berlin for female patients	46	36
Schwetz . .	Provincial institution	—	—
Sieburg . .	„ „ for curable patients .	207	282
Sigmaringen {	Public institution connected with Prince Charles's Hospital . . . . }	40	16
Sonnenstein .	Royal Lunatic Hospital	369	212
Sorau . .	Lower Lusatian Institution for the insane .	243	69
Stralsund .	Institution for the insane	—	—
Strelitz . {	Lunatic asylum, workhouse, and house of correction combined . . . . }	59	—
Telgte . .	St. Rochus's Hospital for female patients .	31	17
St. Thomas .	Institution for the insane . . .	197	35
Thonberg .	Private asylum	44	26
Trier . {	Hospital, workhouse, and insane department combined . . . . . }	—	—
Trieste . .	Royal State Provincial Institution . .	136	—
„ . .	Connected with hospital	30	—
Troppau . .	Provincial institution	51	—
Waiblingen .	Royal Curative Institution (Winnenthal) .	134	97
Waigolshausen	Castle Werneck	—	—
Wehlnen . .	Institution for the insane . . .	77	54
Wesel . .	City institution ("Hohehaus") . .	—	—
Wien . .	Provincial institution	807	789
„ . .	Private asylum	54	41
„ . .	„ „	43	34
„ . .	„ „	30	—
„ . .	„ „	40	—
Wittstock .	Department connected with almshouse .	143	49
Würsburg .	„ „ Julius Hospital .	82	111
Ybbs . {	Lower Austrian Provincial Institution for the insane . . . . . }	363	59
Zwiefalten .	Royal Curative Institution (Würtemberg) .	168	4

Public Asylums in Berlin.

The public asylums at Berlin are :—

1st. The lunacy division of the royal " Charité."

2nd. The City of Berlin Lunatic Asylum.

The lunacy division of the " Charité " receives

curable patients, and is limited to the city of Berlin.
In consequence of the insufficient accommodation for
lunatics in Berlin, the Government are contemplating
building a large public asylum. In the " Charité " the
clinical lectures are given to the students of Berlin.
The director of the hospital is Dr. Westphal, professor
of psychological medicine at the University at Berlin.
His assistants are Dr. Fastowitz and Dr. Obermeier.

The City of Berlin Lunatic Asylum was originally a
division of the city workhouse, but is now unconnected
with it, though the financial administration of the two is
the same, and they are both superintended by the
same person. The asylum is composed of two divisions :
one for male, and the other for female patients. These
two divisions are not only overcrowded, but they do not
even contain the requirements which should now be
found in all asylums.

The food is inadequate for the patients, and comes
from the kitchen of the workhouse. There is no classification of the patients.

The terms are 29s. per month.

The medical superintendent of the asylum is Dr.
Idler, but it is in contemplation shortly to appoint an
assistant.

Before a patient can be received into this asylum the
permission of the Guardians of the Poor must first be
obtained, but in very urgent cases this permission can
be granted by a magistrate.

Private Asylums in Berlin.

Private asylums are divided,

1st. Into those which receive only incurable cases.

2nd. Into those which receive both curable and incurable patients.

A special licence for each of these is required.

There is only one private asylum situated in Berlin

kept by a medical man, the other asylums are kept by non-medical persons.

Dr. Filter (Waldemar Strasse, 59) is the physician who keeps the asylum above mentioned, and resides on the premises. The institution is only for female patients, and is conducted on the non-restraint system entirely. It contains from twenty to thirty patients, nearly all being incurable. The terms for patients are from 6*l.* to 7*l.* 10*s.* per month, but a reduction is made for those who stay for a longer period.

Mrs. Schneider's Asylum, 9 Schönhausen Allee (formerly known as Klinsman's).

This asylum contains about fourteen male and twenty-four female patients, chiefly incurables.

Dr. Lander, the medical officer attached to it, does not reside in the asylum, but visits it daily. The terms vary from 3*l.* 15*s.* to 9*l.* 15*s.* a month.

Mrs. Gierasch's Asylum, 133 Schönhausen Allee.

This asylum is only for incurable female patients. The number received is about ten. Dr. Becker is the medical visitor. The terms are 2*l.* 5*s.*, 3*l.* to 4*l.* 10*s.* a month.

Mr. and Mrs. Rupp's Asylum, 98 Schönhausen Allee.

This asylum receives a few incurable patients of both sexes; it is under the control of the " President of Police." The medical visitor is Dr. Mendel. The terms are (15, 20 to 25 thalers) 2*l.* 5*s.*, 3*l.* to 3*l.* 15*s.* a month.

Professor Boesch's Asylum, 135 Schönhausen Allee.

This asylum is chiefly for idiots; the number received is about 50.

Dr. Lohde is the medical visitor. The terms for lunatics are 3*l.* 15*s.*, 5*l.* to 6*l.* 5*s.* a month, for idiots 2*l.* 10*s.* a month.

Private Asylums and Hospitals in the neighbourhood of Berlin.

Dr. Lewinstein's asylum, situated at Schoenberg, near Berlin, 12 Botanische Garten Strasse.
This is a very large institution, under the immediate direction of the Government at Potsdam. It is divided into two separate divisions.

1st. The division for invalids.

2nd. The division for lunatics.

The first of these divisions is very highly recommended as a residence for invalids desiring a warmer climate, for the autumn and winter months. It contains large bath, fountains, and whey-establishments. The terms are from 9*l.* to 18*l.* 5*s.* a month, but a reduction is made when two persons occupy the same room. Payment is made in advance every month, and before leaving it is necessary to give fifteen days' notice. The accommodation is very superior, and "full boarding, attendance, light, fuel, whey, fountains, baths, and use of the electrical apparatus, medicines, and cold water cures" are all included in the payment.

In the division for lunatics, before a patient can be received, a certificate from the doctor who has treated the case, containing a full report, must be submitted to the proprietor, besides the ordinary Government certificate.

This division contains both male and female patients. The terms are—for curable cases, one room, 15*l.* a month; for two rooms, 22*l.* 10*s.* a month; for incurable cases, 7*l.* 10*s.* a month.

Payment is made in advance every month, and thirty days' notice before leaving is required. The director of this large institution is assisted by a resident medical man, and other physicians may be called in to consultation as the patients or their friends desire.

Dr. Laehr's asylum, "Schweizerhof," near Zehlendorf (about half an hour by rail from Berlin).

This private asylum is for female patients, chiefly curable cases.

It was founded in 1854, and is under the direction of the Government at Potsdam. Beautiful grounds of about 300 German acres are attached to it, and in these grounds are separate pavilions for patients. The number received is 70. A few of the patients whose mental state will permit of it, are boarded with families in the immediate neighbourhood. Dr. Laehr, assisted by two or three assistants, superintends the medical treatment of the inmates.

Everything is done with a view to effect a cure. Lectures upon instructive and scientific subjects are given, and patients are placed under judicious medical treatment. The terms are, according to the accommodation afforded, from 5*l*. 19*s*. to 10*l*. 4*s*. a month for separate rooms. The rooms in the pavilions situated in the garden are more expensive, 12*l*. 15*s*. a month.

Before, or immediately after, a patient has been received, a full report, drawn up by a medical man, is required, stating the origin and course of the disease.

The asylum contains 67 patients, of which number eight are residing with families in the immediate vicinity of the asylum.

Asylum of Pankow.

(Five English miles from Berlin.)

This asylum was opened about three years ago, and is under the control of the Government at Potsdam.

It is under the direction of Dr. Mendel.

It contains about twenty-two male and seven female patients, curable cases. The terms are 7*l*. 10*s*. per month.

Dr. Edel's Asylum at Charlottenburg.

(Five English miles from Berlin.)

This asylum was opened in 1870, and is under the control of the president of police. Male patients only are received, and the charges for curable cases are 6l. 9s. per month, and in chronic cases 4l. 10s. per month. Upon the admission of a patient, besides the medical certificates required by Government in all cases, a full and detailed report of the history of the case must also be sent with the patient.

Mrs. Prillowitz's Asylum at Charlottenburg.

This asylum is under the control of the president of police, and receives only female patients. No medical man resides on the premises, but Dr. Lieber visits it. From thirty to forty, mostly incurable, patients are received, and the lowest terms are 3l. 15s. per month.

Mrs. Becker's Asylum at Charlottenburg.

This asylum is under the control of the president of police, a few incurable female patients only being received. The terms are 2l. 5s. per month.

Mrs. Feyh's Asylum at Pankow.

This asylum was opened August 3, 1862, and receives about twenty-five female patients.

Miss Welzer's Asylum at Pankow.

This asylum was opened in 1865, and contains about twenty-five female patients.

Mr. Reyher's Asylum at Pankow.

This asylum was opened in 1866 for male patients. The number received is about forty.

The last three asylums are under the control of the

R

Government at Potsdam, and receive only patients whose incurability is certified by medical reports.

The terms commence at 3*l.* per month.

Condition of Insanity in Germany.

No reliable statistics of insanity have been published since the Franco-German war, and consequently I am unable to give the condition of insanity that existed in Germany before the annexation of Alsace and Lorraine.

Out of a population of 13,747,637 there were 10,595 persons of unsound mind, making a proportion of one insane person in every 1,267 of the population.

The chief causes for insanity in Germany were hereditary predisposition and intemperance.

CHAPTER XVI.

INSANITY IN THE UNITED STATES OF AMERICA.

Population . . . 38,555,983.

	Insane	Idiots
White	35,560	21,324
Black	1,605	2,743
Mulatto	169	443
Chinese	35	5
Indian	13	10
Total	37,382	24,527

Total of Insane and Idiots, 61,909.
Proportion of Insane to the Population.—1 in 623, or
1·06 per 1,000.
Principal Causes of Insanity.—Intemperance, grief,
physical disease, religious excitement, epilepsy.
Chief Causes of Death.—Exhaustion, epilepsy, general
paralysis, consumption.

It is not my intention to epitomise the lunacy law
of America, as each State has its own law, and to do
this would occupy a larger amount of space than I can
now afford.

ASYLUMS IN THE UNITED STATES OF AMERICA.

States	Towns	Character	When opened	Number of Patients	Charges	Superintendents
Alabama	Tuscaloosa	State	1861	279	3$ 50 c.	Peter Bryce
California	Stockton	Corporate	1852	1,090		J. A. Shurtleff
Connecticut	Hartford	State	1821	157		J. S. Butler
"	Middletown	State	1868	230		A. M. Shew
"	Litchfield	Private		12		H. W. Buel
Georgia	Milledgeville	State	1842	220		T. F. Green
Illinois	Jacksonville	"	1851	460	Paid by the State	H. F. Carriel
Indiana	Indianapolis	"	1848	500		O. Everts
Iowa	Mount Pleasant	"	1861	438	Paid by Counties	M. Ranney
Kansas	Ossawatamie	"	1866	41		G. O. Gause
Kentucky	Lexington	"	1824	525	4$ to 10$	J. W. Whitney
"	Hopkinsville	"	1854	325	Half paid by the State	J. Rodman
Louisiana	Jackson	"	1848	166		
Maine	Augusta	"	1840	345	4$ to 7$	H. M. Harlow
Maryland	Baltimore	"	1834	125	6$	R. F. Stewart
"	Mount Hope Retreat	Corporate	1867	193		W. H. Stokes
"	Catonsville	State				
Massachusetts	Worcester	"	1833	425	3$ 80 c. to 10$	M. Bemis
"	Taunton	"	1854	403	3$ 50 c. to 5$	W. W. Godding
"	Northampton	"	1858	420		P. Earle
"	Tewkesbury			291		
"	Boston	City	1839	230	15$ to 50$	C. A. Walker
"	Somerville	Corporate	1818	190	5$ 8 c.	G. F. Jelly
Michigan	Kalamazoo	State	1859	305		G. H. Van Densen
Minnesota	St. Peter	"	1866	206		
Mississippi	Jackson	"	1855	160		
Missouri	Fulton	County and City	1851	288	3$ 50 c.	W. M. Compton
"	St. Louis	"	1869	211	Paid by County	C. H. Hughes
"	St. Vincent	Corporate	1858	250	5$ to 25$	C. W. Stephen
New Hampshire	Concord	State	1842	253	5$ to 10$	J. B. Bancroft

State	Location	Type	Year	No.	Charge	Superintendent
New Jersey	Trenton	,,	1849	648	4$ to 6$	H. A. Buttolph
New York	Utica	,,	1843	658		J. P. Gray
,,	Poughkeepsie	,,	1858		Paid by the State	J. M. Cleaveland
,,	Auburn	State criminal	1869	62		J. W. Wilkie
,,	Ovid	State	1821	243		J. B. Chapin
,,	Bloomingdale	Corporate	1861	165		T. Brown
,,	Blackwell's Island	City	1846	1,300		R. L. Parsons
,,	Flushing	Private	1855	40		J. A. Barstow
,,	Flatbush	County	1855	602		E. R. Chapin
,,	Canandaigua	Private	1859	73		G. Cook
,,	Troy	Corporate & City	1861	109		J. D. Lomax
,,	New York	Immigrant	1856		8$ to 25$	G. Ford
North Carolina	Raleigh	State	1859	230		E. Grissom
Ohio	Columbus	,,	1839	330		W. L. Peck
,,	Newburg	,,	1859	559		J. M. Lewis
,,	Dayton	County	1855	571		R. Gundry
Oregon	Longview	State	1853	122	Paid by the State	O. N. Langdon
Pennsylvania	Portland	Corporate	1841	360		J. C. Hawthorne
,,	Philadelphia	,,	1817	62		T. G. Kirkbride
,,	Frankford	State	1851	430	8$ 50 c. to 30$.	J. H. Worthington
,,	Harrisburg	,,	1856	401	County patients	J. Curwen
,,	Dixmont					J. A. Reed
,,	Danville					S. S. Schultz
Rhode Island	Philadelphia	City	1849	750		D. D. Richardson
South Carolina	Providence	Corporate	1822	160	5$ to 35$	J. S. Sawyer
Tennessee	Columbia	State	1840	250	2$ to 3$ 50 c.	J. F. Ensor
Texas	Nashville	,,	1861	356		J. H. Callender
Vermont	Austin	,,	1837	48		W. H. Rockwell
Virginia	Brattleboro	Corporate	1773	518	3$ to 4$	D. R. Brower
,,	Williamsburg	State	1828	203		F. T. Stubbing
,,	Staunton	,,	1870	324		D. H. Conrad
West Virginia	Howard Grove	,,	1866	150		R. Hills
Wisconsin	Weston	,,	1854	207		A. M. Dill
,,	Madison	,,		360		
District Columbia	Washington	Government	1855	541		C. C. Nichols

Table illustrating the gradual Increase in Insanity.

UNITED STATES OF AMERICA, TWENTY YEARS.

Year	Population	Number of Insane & Idiots	Ratio per 1000 to population	Proportion to population
1850	23,191,876	31,397	1·35	1 in 738
1860	31,443,322	42,864	1·36	1 ,, 733
1870	38,555,983	61,909	1·60	1 ,, 623

ENGLAND, TEN YEARS.

1862	20,336,467	41,129	2·02	1 in 494
1865	20,990,946	45,950	2·18	1 ,, 456
1868	21,649,377	51,000	2·35	1 ,, 424
1871	22,704,108	56,755	2·49	1 ,, 400

SCOTLAND, TEN YEARS.

1862	3,083,989	6,341	2·05	1 in 486
1865	3,136,057	6,468	2·06	1 ,, 484
1868	3,188,125	6,931	2·17	1 ,, 459
1871	3,358,613	7,808	2·32	1 ,, 430

IRELAND, NINETEEN YEARS.

1851	6,552,385	15,098	2·03	1 in 434
1856	6,164,171	14,141	2·29	1 ,, 435
1861	5,798,967	16,749	2·88	1 ,, 346
1870	5,195,236	17,194	3·39	1 ,, 303

FRANCE, FIFTEEN YEARS.

1851	35,783,170	44,970	1·25	1 in 795
1866	37,988,905	90,679	2·38	1 ,, 418

CHAPTER XVII.

LUNACY IN RUSSIA.

THERE are no public records printed in Russia, containing information with reference to the state of lunacy in that country. Each government public asylum issues its own report, and these are difficult to procure. Through the courtesy and kindness of Dr. Seifert, Conseiller d'État, one of the physicians of the Imperial Asylum at St. Petersburg, I have obtained the following information. Each city has its own public asylum for the admission of private as well as pauper patients. There are two classes—1st, *Placement volontaire*, these are called private patients. 2nd, Public or government patients. The first class or private patients are admitted on the order of a relative and one medical certificate. The second class or government patients are sent by the police, no medical certificate on admission being necessary. The police require the patient to be examined by their own medical man previously to his being sent to the asylum, but this certificate is not presented at the asylum when he is admitted. After the reception of the patient, the medical officers of the asylum write to the police authorities for the details of the case, and for the certificate drawn up by their own medical officer. A return is made relative to the mental state of the patient to the chief governor of St. Petersburg. In the course of the second, third, or sixth week the governor issues a command for the patient to be brought before him, in order that he may be examined by a medical man appointed by himself. If owing to illness or any other cause, this command cannot be complied with, the governor, accompanied by his own medical adviser, visits the asylum and examines the patient. When restored to health the patient returns to his relatives. Nothing is paid for the maintenance of pauper patients in an asylum, everything, including clothes and linen, are provided gratuitously for them. In the high class private asylums of Russia the expense of maintenance ranges from 20*l.* per month to a higher sum. There are three private asylums in St. Petersburg, the Imperial Asylum of that city contains 400 patients, and has four resident medical officers—viz., Dr. Lawrence, the chief physician, Dr. Herzog, Dr. Sheman, and Dr. Seifert. These physicians have separate suites of rooms allotted to them, but no private residences. They have fixed salaries, and, with the exception of lodgings, lights, and firing, they have to provide for themselves. As compared to what the English resident medical officers receive, the pay of the Russian physician is very small, but they are not like the English medical men, who are the resident medical officers of public asylums, debarred from practice. The usual fee in cases of lunacy is never less than three guineas, sometimes much higher fees are received.

CHAPTER XVIII.

RECENT LUNACY STATISTICS AND INSTRUCTIONS.

SINCE the preceding portion of the volume has been sent to press, the Annual Report of the Commissioners in Lunacy for 1873 has been issued; and, with a view of placing before the reader the most recent information relative to the subject of lunacy, I append the following particulars:—

Statistics of Insanity, Jan. 1, 1873.

The following summary shows generally the classification and distribution of the patients registered on Jan. 1, 1873:—

	Private			Pauper			Total		
	M.	F.	T.	M.	F.	T.	M.	F.	T.
In County and Borough Asylums	183	196	379	13,799	16,295	30,094	13,982	16,491	30,473
In Registered Hospitals . . .	1,213	1,084	2,297	191	160	351	1,404	1,244	2,648
In Licensed Houses	1,734	1,516	3,250	405	838	1,243	2,139	2,354	4,493
In Naval and Military Hospitals, and Royal India Asylum . .	323	15	338	—	—	—	323	15	338
In State Criminal Asylum . .	272	64	336	134	38	172	406	102	508
Private Single Patients . .	170	253	423	—	—	—	170	253	423
In Workhouses .	—	—	—	6,209	8,134	14,343	6,209	8,134	14,343
Out-door Paupers	—	—	—	2,839	4,231	7,070	2,839	4,231	7,070
Total . .	3,895	3,128	7,023	23,577	29,696	53,273	27,472	32,824	60,296

These numbers do not include 188 persons found

lunatics by inquisition. There is an increase of 1,656 upon the number returned on January 1, 1872.

Year	Population	Lunatics on Jan. 1, 1873	Ratio per 1,000 to Population
1873	23,356,414	60,296	2·58

New Asylum for Middlesex.

A new asylum, in conformity with the suggestions of the Commissioners in Lunacy, for the county of Middlesex is to be opened at Banstead, in the county of Surrey.

An estate of about one hundred acres has been purchased at a cost of 10,000*l.*

The Asylum will probably be fit for occupation at the end of 1875.

There are at present 725 patients belonging to the county of Middlesex for whom no provision has been made by the county.

THIRD ASYLUM FOR MIDDLESEX.*

Instructions to Architect, issued by the Committee of Justices.

1. The general plan of the Metropolitan District Asylum at Leavesden is to be followed.

2. Provision is to be made for 580 male patients, of whom 100 are to be in an infirmary, consisting of 3 dormitories for 30 beds each, with 10 single rooms, and the remaining 480 in 3 blocks. Each block to consist of a day-room on the ground floor, 14 feet high, and 2 dormitories on the first and second floors, each containing 70 beds, with 20 single rooms. Store rooms, sculleries, padded rooms, and attendants' rooms to be provided in each block.

3. Provision is to be made for 1,020 females, of

* Appendix E, Commissioners' Report, 1873.

whom 100 are to be in an infirmary, 800 in 5 ordinary blocks, and 120 in a block of like construction, but connected with the laundry. Single rooms, sculleries, padded rooms, and attendants' rooms to be provided as on the male side.

4. Provision will have to be made for the following staff:—

Two medical superintendents, who will be married men, and must be provided with separate houses and all necessary offices, but connected with the main buildings, one with the male side, and the other with the female side.

Two assistant medical men, and for whom apartments without offices will be sufficient.

One matron in apartments, with accommodation for a servant, kitchen, &c., in connection with the female side.

One steward, a married man, who will require a separate house.

One workmistress, who will require a separate sitting-room and bedroom.

One laundry matron, the like.

The superior male attendants, one sitting-room in common, and a bedroom apiece.

Two female ditto the like.

Thirty-two male attendants, of whom 6 must sleep in the infirmary, 4 in each block, and the rest where they can be most conveniently placed.

Fifty-eight female attendants, of whom 6 must sleep in the infirmary, 10 in the laundry ward, 4 in each block on the female side, and the remaining 22 where they can be most conveniently placed.

Defective Certificates. Instructions by Commissioners.

The Commissioners, in their Report, draw special attention to the various defects in medical certificates in consequence of carelessness on the part of those signing. Last year, out of 12,176 notices of admission sent to the office, 2,314 were returned for amendment. The Commissioners, with the view of assisting the proper filling-up of the statutory forms, have drawn up a paper of instructions in Appendix P of their Report just issued.

LUNACY.*

PRIVATE PATIENTS.

Private patients Instructions.

In order to justify the charge or detention of a lunatic (which expression includes an idiot and a person of unsound mind) as a private (*i.e.*, not pauper) patient in a county or borough asylum, hospital, or licensed house, or as a single patient † elsewhere (except where no payment is made for, or profit derived from, the charge, or where a committee has been appointed by the Lord Chancellor), the law requires,—

1. An *order of reception*, signed by some person, requesting the superintendent or proprietor of the asylum, hospital, or house, or the person who is to take charge, to receive the patient.

2. Two *certificates*, each signed by a registered medical practitioner, stating that he has separately examined the patient, and on such examination found him to be of unsound mind.

INSTRUCTIONS AS TO ORDER AND CERTIFICATES.

It being unlawful to receive or take charge of a lunatic, except as above, without these documents, it follows that both the order and the certificates must be signed *before* the reception takes place, and must bear

---

* Appendix P. Report, 1873.

† No *licence* is necessary where merely one insane patient at a time is received. Such one patient is called a "single patient."

date either on or before, *but not after*, the day of such reception or of first taking charge. The order may be signed before or after the certificates, or either of them. Private patients.
Instruc-
tions.

Two blank forms (duplicates) of order and accompanying statement of particulars and certificates, if not sent herewith, must be procured.* These forms are statutory (Acts 16 & 17 Vict. c. 96, Schedules A. and C.; c. 97, Schedule F., Nos. 2, 3, 4), and must be strictly adhered to.

One of these forms must be completed as an original, by the person giving the order and by the two certifying medical men. On the reception of the patient, this original document is to be given to the proprietor, superintendent, or person receiving or taking the charge, and must be carefully preserved by him, being his sole authority for detaining the patient.

The second blank form is for the use of the proprietor, resident superintendent, or person taking charge, who is bound by law to make and transmit exact copies of the original order, statement, and certificates to the Commissioners in Lunacy.† He must fill up and sign the notice of admission, which is on the first page of the form, and, *within one clear day* from the day of reception, post the copies and notice, addressed—

THE SECRETARY,
 Office of the Commissioners in Lunacy,
  19, *Whitehall Place, London, S.W.*

---

* These forms, and others prescribed by the Lunacy Acts. are kept in stock by Messrs. Shaw and Sons, Fetter Lane, and Messrs. Knight and Co., 90 Fleet Street, London, E.C.

† From houses licensed by justices, copies and notice must go to the Clerk of the Visitors.

STATEMENT OF CONDITION.

After two clear days, and before the expiration of
seven clear days, from the day of reception, the patient
must again be examined, and a statement of his mental
and bodily health as observed at the time of examination must be transmitted to the Commissioners in
Lunacy.*

This document, which must be in the statutory form,
must be signed—

(*a*.) In the case of an asylum, hospital, or licensed
house, by the medical officer, medical superintendent,
proprietor, or attendant :

(*b*.) In the case of a "single patient," by the
"medical attendant" appointed by the friends of the
patient. He must be a registered medical practitioner,
*who did not sign either of the certificates of insanity, or
the order for reception*, and who derives no profit from
the *care* or *charge* of the patient, and who is not a
partner, father, son, or brother of any person deriving
profit from such care or charge.

AMENDMENT OF DEFECTIVE ORDERS AND CERTIFICATES.

If requiring and capable of amendment, the original
order or certificates may be amended, with the sanction
of the Commissioners, within fourteen days next after
the reception. In such a case instructions will be sent
as to the amendments required in the originals, and
the copies will be returned for precisely corresponding
alterations. No corrections or amendments in the
original order or certificates are to be made by anyone
except the person who signed the defective document,
and he should affix his initials opposite to each alteration.

* And to the Clerk of the Visitors, where the house is licensed
by Justices.

MEDICAL EXAMINATION.

The patient must not be medically examined in the house where he is to remain, nor on the premises. Should he have been living in the house previously to legalising the charge, the date of admission given in the notice of admission should be that of the day whereon he returns to the house after signature of the order, medical examinations, and signature of the certificates. *Private patients. Instructions.*

Should it become necessary to obtain fresh certificates the patient should, as above, be removed for examination. In this case, and where a fresh order has been required, a fresh notice of admission must be transmitted.

Certificates signed, or founded on medical examinations made, elsewhere than in England or Wales (the extent of the Commissioners' jurisdiction), are not accepted as a valid authority for the detention of a patient within that jurisdiction.

CAUTIONS.

1. No order is valid unless the person signing it has seen the patient within one month previous to the date of the order.

2. An order becomes invalid and useless if the reception does not take place within one month from the date of the order.

3. No certificate is valid if signed—

(*a.*) By a non-registered practitioner;

(*b.*) By the partner or assistant of the person signing the other certificate;

(*c.*) By the person who signs the order, or by his father, brother, son, partner, or assistant.

4. A certificate becomes invalid and useless if the reception does not take place *within seven clear days* from the date of the medical examination on which the certificate is grounded.

5. *For reception into a county or borough asylum* no certificate is valid which is signed by any medical officer of the asylum in question.

6. *For reception into a licensed house or hospital* no certificate is valid which is signed by—

(*a.*) A medical man, who is wholly or partly the proprietor of, or a regular professional attendant in, such licensed house or hospital; nor by

(*b.*) The father, brother, son, partner, or assistant of such last-mentioned persons, or of either of them.

7. *For reception into a licensed house* no certificate and no order is valid which is signed by—

(*a.*) Any person receiving any percentage on, or otherwise interested in, the payments on account of any patient received into the house in question;

(*b.*) Any medical man keeping, or in his medical capacity attending, such licensed house.

8. *For reception of a " single patient " into a private house* no certificate and no order is valid which is signed by the person who takes the charge, or who receives a percentage on, or is otherwise interested in, the payments for the patient.

N.B.—The person who is intended to act as the regular medical attendant will be precluded from so acting if he signs either order or certificate.

9. No medical man can receive a " single patient " into his house on a certificate signed by himself, or by his father, brother, son, partner, or assistant.

CHARLES SPENCER PERCEVAL, *Secretary.*

Office of the Commissioners in Lunacy.

Changes in the Commission.

Mr. John Forster, who has filled the office of one of the Visiting Commissioners in Lunacy for a period of five years, has, in consequence of ill health, resigned his post. His great experience and knowledge will still be available to the Board, as he will act as one of the Honorary Commissioners. Mr. Charles Palmer Phillips succeeded Mr. John Forster as Commissioner, and Mr. Charles Spéncer Perceval succeeded to the Secretary-ship of the Commission, vacated by Mr. Phillips. Mr. Lutwidge, who for many years was connected with the Commission, I regret to say, during a visit paid by him in conjunction with Mr. Wilkes a few months since to Fisherton House lunatic asylum, Salisbury, was murderously attacked by a patient, and killed. It is a matter of great regret that the Board has been deprived of the valuable services of one of its oldest members. Mr. Lutwidge was always ready and willing to say a kind word to all the patients during his official visitations, and his sympathy, consideration, and kindness were conspicuous. The Hon. Greville Howard has been appointed by the Lord Chancellor as a successor to Mr. Lutwidge. Col. Clifford retired from the Honorary Board of Commissioners during the year.

Patients in Asylums.

The asylums, hospitals, and licensed houses visited by the Commissioners during the year amounted to 182. The average daily number resident in asylums during the year is 30,302. The percentage of recoveries on the admission for the past year was 38·34—being more favourable than in any year since 1862. The percentage of deaths upon the number of insane persons treated was 7·53, the rate of mortality being lower than in any year since 1858.

The number of persons of unsound mind confined in county and borough asylums on January 1 was 30,473; out of which number only 2,476, or 8·12 per cent., were deemed as curable cases.

The number of patients admitted into asylums,

s

hospitals, and licensed houses during 1872 was 12,016.
Of this number 1,356 were transfers from other institutions. If this number is deducted from the total
number of admissions, the admissions will amount to
10,660, or 90 more than in 1871.

Private Asylums. Remarks by Commissioners.

Licensed
houses.

"In the houses licensed for the reception of the
insane we continue to observe a general improvement.
As may easily be understood, the houses themselves
vary in their style of building, in the character of their
management, and in the degree of accommodation which
they afford. However frequently the houses may be
inspected by ourselves or by the Visitors, the amount of
comfort enjoyed by the patients, and the provision for
the proper treatment of their malady, must still to a
great extent depend upon the special aptitude of the
resident licensee for his post, upon the ability and willingness of the proprietor to incur liberal outlay, and
upon the numerical strength and efficiency of the staff
of attendants employed by him.

"Thus, in the proprietary establishments of the best
class, where the scale of payment is high, a corresponding amount of comfort is enjoyed by the patients. In
some instances, individual patients occupy well-furnished
villas in the pleasure-grounds detached from the principal building. They are attended by their own servants,
make use of their own equipages, and, indeed, are
debarred from no enjoyments, however luxurious, which
are compatible with their own welfare and not liable to
endanger other persons. Others of less affluence jointly
occupy the main building. Usually, in houses of this
class, each person has his separate bedroom, and, where
his means justify it, his private sitting-room. But in
those establishments where the rate of payment is more
moderate, the patients, classified according to their

mental condition, occupy associated dormitories and Licensed houses.
day-rooms.

"For a long time both out-door exercises and in-door occupation have been encouraged more or less in all licensed houses. Such of the patients as can be trusted not to abuse these privileges enjoy a considerable amount of freedom, many being even permitted to extend their walks beyond the grounds unattended. The airing-courts, formerly bare gravel yards, are now changed for pleasant gardens, containing conservatories for the supply of flowers for the decoration of the interior of the house.

"In the treatment of the insane, much depends on sufficient means of amusement and employment; and it is gratifying to us to be able to report that this fact appears at the present day to be freely admitted by the proprietors of licensed houses both in town and in the country. In most of them, daily gatherings of the patients take place at family prayers, at meal times, and for out-door games. The inmates are also periodically assembled for dramatic and musical entertainments.

"Our aim has always been, and still is, to take from these houses, as far as practicable, the appearance of mere receptacles for the insane, to do away with all unnecessary mechanical contrivances for security, and to assimilate their arrangements to those of a well-regulated boarding-house or family residence. To a certain extent we have been successful. The sexes are now in many licensed houses brought into more frequent association, to their mutual advantage. The patients' relatives are occasionally induced to become boarders for days, and even weeks, and so to alleviate the distress incident to compulsory residence within an asylum; lady companions are also provided to amuse female patients of the first class; and trips to the sea-side break the monotony of routine life. Reading, drawing, music, and needlework are among the amusements of the ladies, and for the gentlemen's recreation, books and newspapers, and billiard tables, continue to be supplied.

"In fact, licensed houses are at the present day very different institutions from what they were within the memory of many members of our Board, and the difference would, we believe, astonish those who only remember the old state of things, and have not watched the gradual alteration since this Commission was first appointed. The defects which remain are chiefly those inherent in establishments kept for profit; and it is therefore, we think, of the first importance that the selection of the licensees should be carefully considered. We fear that in some instances the grants of licences by the Courts of Quarter Sessions have been rather too much matters of course; but in that direction, also, we observe gradual amendment.

"There is yet, beyond question, great room for improvement in the description of attendants employed in licensed houses. They should always be selected from a very superior grade, and we frequently remind licensees that such can only be attracted by good wages. It must, however, be borne in mind, that patients are in some houses received at too low a scale of payment to admit of a high rate of remuneration for those who take personal charge of them, or, indeed, of much outlay in other directions."

Remarks of the Commissioners on Seclusion.

"Without questioning the utility of seclusion in certain cases of excitement, especially amongst epileptics, we think that in a remedial point of view its value has been much exaggerated, and that in many instances it is employed unnecessarily and to an injurious extent, and for periods which are quite unjustifiable.

"By patients themselves seclusion is no doubt

usually regarded as a punishment, and besides being most objectionable on this ground, it is too often resorted to in cases of temporary excitement, which might be readily subdued by treatment of a less repressive character. Upon the attendants themselves also its frequent use has a most injurious effect, by leading them improperly to seek through its means relief from the duties and responsibilities involved in a constant and vigilant supervision of those placed under their charge.

" The frequent resort to seclusion in the treatment of the insane we can only attribute in most cases to defective organisation or management of the asylums, more especially as regards an adequate staff of properly-trained and diligently-supervised attendants, and we think that in all such instances persevering efforts should be made by improved arrangements to diminish its employment, and keep it within the narrowest possible limits."

Single Patients. Remarks of Commissioners in Lunacy.

" The following tabular statement shows the num- Single bers of Single Private Patients subject to our jurisdiction patients. and visitation, as they existed at the commencement and termination, respectively, of the year 1872, and the changes in the same which took place during that year :—

—	Males	Females	Total
Numbers, January 1, 1872	168	252	420
Registered during the year	60	100	160
Discharged and removed .	47	87	134
" of whom recovered	8	10	18
Died .	11	12	23
Remaining January 1 last	170	253	423

" In accordance with the resolution referred to in

Single patients.

our Seventeenth Report, which had received the express approval of the Lord Chancellor, we have, ever since the passing of the 'Lunacy Regulation Act, 1862,' discontinued visiting single patients found lunatic by inquisition, as rendered quite unnecessary by the 20th section. Of the single patients on January 1 last, 118, viz., 55 of the male and 63 of the female sex, came within the class of lunatics under commission, leaving, as patients to be regularly visited by us, 305, viz., 115 of the male and 190 of the female sex.

"During the last ten years the single patients regularly visited by us have trebled in number. At the commencement of that period the total number of single patients was only 150, of whom very nearly one-third were found lunatic by inquisition.

"The accessions from time to time have no doubt been in great measure attributable to the prosecutions instituted by our Board for illegal reception of patients without certificates, to the wider promulgation of the law by these criminal proceedings, and to the circulars and papers of instructions published and generally disseminated by us with that view.

"In illustration of this statement we may refer specially to the fact, that towards the end of the year 1864, pending the prosecution (adverted to in our Nineteenth Report) of a medical man, as many as 16 notifications were received by us from parties having charge of uncertified patients, with requests to be furnished with such forms and papers as would then enable the applicants to comply with all the statutory requirements. After the conviction of this person, who was fined 50l., and before the end of the same year, a period of less than three months, no less than 37 fresh returns were made to this office.

"We continue to receive frequent voluntary communications from medical men and others, disclosing

their reception of insane persons, or persons of ques- Single
patients.
tionable sanity, placed under their charge by relatives.
In such cases generally, we are satisfied by immediate
and due compliance with the statutory requirements.

"The results of inquiry and correspondence, and the
information collected by us in the course of official
circuits, satisfy us that there are throughout the country
a considerable number of insane persons who are not,
but ought to be, placed under orders and medical certificates as single patients. In many instances, no
doubt, ignorance of the law applicable to such cases
might fairly be pleaded by non-professional persons, but
we cannot admit such a plea on the part of medical
men, who assuredly ought to be aware of the provisions
of the Acts relative to lunatics, idiots, and persons of
unsound mind.

"There are other reasons for concealment and
non-compliance with the law which, we have reason to
think, mainly actuate parties thereto. We refer, amongst
others, to a reluctance on the part of relatives, by disclosing the circumstances, to brand the family with the
taint of insanity. In this point of view, they object to
submitting the patients to our jurisdiction and visitation.
When influenced by such considerations, the parties are
possibly not aware, or fail to bear in mind, that every
one in this department is sworn to secrecy, and, consequently, that publicity through the medium of our
office is out of the question.

"Another actuating motive for evading the fulfilment of the provisions of the Lunacy Acts is, we cannot
doubt, a fear of inquiry into the sources, amount, and
administration of the patient's property and available
income, a subject which we invariably investigate.

"In our Fourteenth Report we stated at length our
general views on the subject of single patients, their
care and treatment, the payments made for them, the

question of management and application of their property, and the mental state of those who had come under our notice.

"In order that single patients may have all the benefit of medical care and treatment intended by the Legislature, we, as a rule, even where the patient is residing under the charge of a professional man (physician or surgeon), decline to sanction any dispensation of the statutory medical fortnightly visits, until the Board shall have received a report of a visit to the patient by one of their number.

"The visits which, as a rule, we make annually to patients of this class, now upwards of 300 in number, necessarily entail a great expenditure of time, money, and labour. These patients are scattered over all parts of England and Wales, and frequently reside in remote country districts, many miles distant from railway stations. In fact, the visit to one patient in some cases occupies an entire day, and, of course, involves proportionate travelling and personal expenses."

Regulations respecting Detention of the Insane in Workhouses.

"Local Government Board, Whitehall, S.W.,
"August 10, 1872.

"Sir,—The Local Government Board are informed by the Commissioners in Lunacy that, in the course of their periodical visits to workhouses, they have had occasion to notice that the provision in Section 20 of the Lunacy Amendment Act, 1862, 25 & 26 Vict. c. 111, so far as it imposes a duty on the medical officer, is very imperfectly observed.

"The former part of that section is as follows : ' No person shall be detained in any workhouse, being a lunatic or alleged lunatic, beyond the period of 14 days, unless, in the opinion given in writing of the medical officer of the union or parish to which the workhouse belongs, such person is a proper person to be kept in a workhouse, nor unless the accommodation in the workhouse is sufficient for his reception; and any person detained in a workhouse in contravention of this section, shall be deemed to be a proper person to be sent to an asylum within the meaning of Section 67 of the Lunacy Act, cap. 97.' (See 16 & 17 Vict. c. 97.)

Circular from Local Government Boar

" In order, therefore, to justify the detention in a workhouse, beyond the above-mentioned period of 14 days, of any lunatic or alleged lunatic, it is in strictness necessary that the medical officer of the workhouse should certify in writing that such person may properly be kept there. The statute, it will be seen, imposes the further condition, that the accommodation in the workhouse shall be sufficient for the reception of the lunatic or person of unsound mind.

" In the event of this important provision having been overlooked in your union, I am directed by the Board to request that the guardians will at once call the attention of the medical officer to the omission, in order that the law in this respect may be strictly complied with in future.

" The certificates given from time to time by the medical officer should be preserved by the master of the workhouse, and laid before the Visiting Commissioner in Lunacy, with the book or list of insane inmates required to be kept by Section 37 of the Act 25 & 26 Vict. c. 111, above referred to.

" I am, Sir, your obedient servant,
" H. FLEMING,
" *Secretary.*

" To the Clerk to the Guardians."

Statistics of Insanity in all Countries.

In arranging the Statistical Tables I have derived great assistance from the Report of Dr. Williams, Com missioner in Lunacy for California, published December 1871. It is a most valuable and interesting compilation of facts relating to the insane. The two following Tables, I have copied from his Report: they show the condition of the insane in various parts of the world.

Table I.

Countries	Census taken once in	Census of	Population	Males	Females	Total	Ratio to Population
Ireland . .	10 years	1861	5,798,967	3,500	3,565	7,065	1 in 821
England and Wales .	„ „	1861	20,066,224	11,249	13,096	24,345	„ 824
Newfound-land . .	„ „	1857	122,638	50	38	88	„ 1,394
Nova Scotia	„ „	1861	330,857	166	174	340	„ 973
Prince Ed-ward's Isld.	7	1861	80,857	.	.	148	„ 546
United States	10	1860	31,445,080	.	.	23,999	„ 1,310
France . .	5	1856	36,012,669	.	.	35,031	„ 1,028
Savoy . .	4	1861	542,535	143	167	310	„ 1,750
Belgium .	10	1856	4,529,560	2,019	1,998	4,017	„ 1,128
Holland .	„	1859	3,308,969	1,038	1,101	2,139	„ 1,547
Hanover .	3	1861	1,888,048	1,591	1,493	3,084	„ 612
Prussia . .	„	1858	17,739,913	.	.	.	.
Saxony . .	„	1861	2,225,240	.	.	1,559	„ 1,427
Bavaria .	„	1861	4,689,837	2,576	2,323	4,899	„ 957
Wurtemburg	„	1861	1,720,708	690	648	1,338	„ 1,286
Hesse Darm-stadt . .	„	1861	856,907	.	.	.	.
Oldenburg .	.	1855	287,163	446	508	954	„ 301
Denmark .	5	1860	2,605,024	2,543	2,592	5,135	„ 507
Sweden . .	„	1855	3,641,011	1,898	1,995	3,893	„ 935
Norway .	10	1855	1,490,047	619	710	1,329	„ 1,121
Piedmont .	10	1858	5,041,853	.	.	1,750	„ 2,881
Italy . .	.	1867	24,263,320	.	.	8,191	„ 2,962
Austria . .	.	1864	13,000,000	.	.	3,215	„ 4,043
New South Wales .	.	1867	447,620	.	.	1,156	„ 387
California .	.	1870	560,247	.	.	1,233	„ 1,454

Table II.

Countries	Year	Population	Number of Insane and Idiots		Total	Proportion of Insane and Idiots to Population
			Insane	Idiots		
United States .	1870	38,555,983	37,382	24,527	61,909	1 in 623
England . .	1870	22,090,163	. .	. .	54,713	,, 403
Scotland . .	1870	3,222,837	. .	. .	9,571	,, 336
Ireland . .	1860	5,195,236	11,122	6,072	17,194	,, 302
France . .	1866	37,988,905	50,726	39,953	90,679	,, 418
Prussia . .	1867	23,971,337	16,929	21,031	37,960	,, 631
Belgium . .	1865	4,984,451			7,431	,, 671
Total . .		136,008,912	—	—	279,457	1 in 486

CHAPTER XIX.

DEFINITIONS AND EXPLANATION OF TERMS GENERALLY USED TO DENOTE VARIOUS FORMS OF INSANITY.

I DO not propose to enter minutely into this subject. My object is, as far as practicable, to briefly define those types of mental derangement which medical men may be called upon to describe when certifying as to a patient's mental unsoundness prior to legal confinement, or when giving evidence in courts of law relative to cases of criminal insanity or disputed testamentary capacity.

The principal terms used to denote various forms of insanity are as follows :—

Varieties of insanity.

1. Mania ; acute, chronic, and recurrent.
2. Monomania.
3. Melancholia ; acute and chronic.
4. Dementia ; acute, and chronic.
5. Imbecility.
6. Idiocy.
7. Nymphomania.
8. Kleptomania.
9. Delusions ; hallucinations, and illusions.
10. Delirium.
11. Dipsomania.
12. Homicidal and moral insanity.
13. Puerperal insanity.
14. General paralysis of the insane.

ACUTE MANIA is usually defined to be an active disorder of the brain, affecting the propensities and all the operations of thought. It is generally associated with symptoms of bodily disease and indications of active mischief going on in the brain, such as congestion of the cerebral vessels or inflammation of the brain itself and its membranes (*meningitis* and *cerebritis*). In this form of insanity delusions of a painful character crop up; the conversation is generally wild and incoherent ; the patient is morbidly suspicious, often fancying that he has been or is about to be poisoned. Under the effect of these delusions he often becomes violent—furiously so—and occasionally tries either to injure himself or others. Sleeplessness (*insomnia*) and excessive garrulity are among the prominent and earliest symptoms of an attack of acute mania. The mind is in a state of intense morbid exaltation, the judgment, will, and in fact all the faculties of the mind are perverted, and the patient is in a constant state of physical restlessness, often unconscious of the calls of nature, and eventually becomes filthy in his habits and conversation. There are, in cases of acute mania, a great variety of symptoms ranging from extreme violence to milder manifestations of the disease.

In CHRONIC MANIA the symptoms are less acute, delusions, however, generally exist, the perceptions are disordered, and the conversation incoherent.

RECURRENT MANIA.—This is a variety of insanity often met with. The patient, after labouring under an attack of mania for a variable period, suddenly becomes for a certain time, apparently of sound mind and appears to be free from all delusions. He continues well for perhaps a month or even longer, and then will have another attack, which will pass off, to be followed again by apparent restoration of the mental faculties. The interval between the attacks of mania is

Characteristics of acute mania.

Recurrent mania.

called a *lucid interval.* Lord Coke describes a patient
who is suffering from recurrent insanity as " a lunatic
that hath sometimes his understanding and sometimes
not." "*Aliquando gaudet lucidis intervallis,* and therefore he is called *non compos mentis* so long as he hath not
understanding."

It is curious to observe a person who for one month
is quite insane, the next apparently recovered. Lucid
intervals occur in patients who have been insane for
many years.

Dr. Pritchard says " that no person should be convicted for a crime committed during a lucid interval,
because there is a probability that at the time of the
offence he might have been under the influence of that
degree of cerebral irritation that renders a man insane."

A will made by a patient during a lucid interval is
valid.*

MONOMANIA is a form of insanity associated with
some prominent delusion, often confined to one idea,
the patient being apparently sane on all other points.
It is a vexed question whether it is possible for the
mind to be deranged on one subject only. Cases of
pure monomania are certainly of rare occurrence, for
even in patients who appear to be monomaniacs the
mind, if carefully analysed, will be found to be under
the influence of several delusions. The principal morbid ideas met with in the " monomaniac " are as
follows :—

1. That a conspiracy exists against him.
2. That his food is poisoned.
3. That he has been guilty of some great crime, and
under this delusion he will often wish to deliver himself up to the police or public magistrate.

Marginal notes:
Dr. Pritchard on crime committed during a lucid interval.

Monomania.

Delusions frequently met with in monomania.

---

* Two forms of lucid interval are spoken of, one in which there
is an apparent suspension of the *disease,* and the other in which
there is a temporary suspension of its *manifestation.*

4. That he is addressed by strange and imaginary voices (auricular delirium); a most unfavourable form of monomania.

5. That he has committed the unpardonable sin, is forsaken of God, and out of the pale of salvation.

6. That he is Jesus Christ.

7. That he is a king, or some great person; under this delusion he will comport himself accordingly.

8. That he has at his command great wealth.

9. That he is ruined and on the eve of bankruptcy.

The monomaniac is unable to talk rationally upon the subject connected with his particular delusion, but in all other respects he appears perfectly sane. Beyond this no unsoundness of mind is perceived. Pritchard says that " the mind in monomania is unsound, not unsound in one point only and sound in other respects, but this unsoundness manifests itself principally with reference to some particular object or person."

Dr. Pritchard on monomania.

MELANCHOLIA, acute and chronic.—This affection is indicated by a state of profound mental depression, often associated with suicidal ideas and delusions on religious and other subjects. These patients often refuse their food, and are obliged to be fed by mechanical means. The mind is often occupied in the contemplation of one or more prominent delusions, and the unhappy man will sit for hours together moping and gloomy in the corner of the room, apparently unconscious of what is going on. This acute state of melancholia often lapses into CHRONIC MELANCHOLIA. In this form of mental disorder the symptoms are generally similar to the type previously described, but are less acutely manifested. It may be defined as a condition of mental depression generally associated with some delusion or hallucination. In some cases the physical health is but slightly deranged. The liver and digestive organs however are often found to be in a disordered state, hence the term

Characteristics of melancholia.

melancholia is derived from a Greek word signifying "black bile." * The delusions of these patients are often of a religious character, the patient believing that he has committed the unpardonable sin, sin against the Holy Ghost, or that he is doomed to eternal punishment, having no hope of salvation.

Varieties of Melancholia.

Melancholia assumes various forms, viz., melancholia *concentrica*, in which the fancies relate to the *internal* sensations of the patient ; and melancholia which is confined to *external* objects, and is called melancholia *peripherica*. There are also melancholia *religiosa*, *dæmonia*, and *attonita*. These acute forms of melancholia are often preceded by severe attacks of profound *hypochondriasis*. This latter state of mind is accurately described by the poet Burns, in a letter to his biographer, Mr. Cunningham, in which he says :—" Canst thou not minister to a mind diseased ? Canst thou not speak peace and rest to a soul tossed on a sea of troubles, without one friendly star to guide his course, and dreading that the next surge may overwhelm him ?' If thou canst not do the least of these, why should'st thou disturb me in my miseries with thy enquiries after me ? "   In another letter in which he refers to himself he says :—" I have been for some time pining under secret wretchedness. The pang of disappointment, the sting of pride, and some wandering stabs of remorse settle on my life like vultures, when my attention is not called away by the claims of society or the vagaries of the Muse. Even in the hour of social mirth my gaiety is the madness of an intoxicated criminal under the hands of an executioner. My constitution was blasted, *ab origine*, with a deep incurable taint of melancholy that poisoned my existence.'' How accurately has old Burton, in his " Anatomy of Melancholy," described the terrible sufferings of the hypochondriac. He says :—" They are soon tired with

* μέλανος χολή.

all things: they will now tarry, now begone; now in bed they will rise, now up then they go to bed; now pleased, and then displeased; now they are like, then dislike all. '*Sequitur nunc vivendi nunc moriendi, cupido,*' to quote Aurelianus. Discontented, disquieted upon every light occasion or no occasion; often tempted to make away with themselves; they cannot die, they will not live; they complain, weep, lament, and think they live a most miserable life; never was any man so bad. Jealousy and suspicion torment them; they are peevish, distrustful with their best friends." Charles Lamb poetically delineates these unhappy persons :—

> By myself walking,
> To myself talking,
> When I ruminate
> On my untoward fate
> Scarcely seem I
> Alone sufficiently.
> Black thoughts continually
> Crossing my privacy:
> They come unbidden,
> Like foes to a wedding;
> Thrusting their faces
> In better guests' places.
> Peevish and malcontent,
> Clownish, impertinent:
> So like the fashions,
> Dim cognitions
> Follow and haunt me,
> Striving to daunt me.
> Fierce anthropophagi,
> Spectra diaboli.
> What scared St. Anthony?
> Hobgoblins, Lemures,
> Dreams of antipodes,
> Night-riding incubi.

In acute attacks of melancholia, it is often useless to attempt to dissipate the morbid ideas that are so distressing the patient. He appears to take a pleasure in

T

hugging his imaginary sorrows, and steadily refuses to
be comforted. In the words of the poet, he exclaims:—

> "Go ! you may call it madness,—folly,
> You *shall not* chase my gloom away ;
> There's such a charm in melancholy,
> I would not, if I could, be gay."

Stages met
with in
dementia.

DEMENTIA (acute and chronic). This term is often
used synonymously with that of fatuity and idiocy, and
is divided into,

1. *Dementia naturalis.*
2. *Dementia adventitia.*

The first state is that of *idiocy*. The second refers
to persons who originally possessed reasoning power.
It may be described as a general enfeeblement of the
intellect, and in some cases an apparent abolition of all
mental power. This state of intellect may arise from
accidental injury to the head, or may result from long-
continued disease of the brain affecting the operation of
thought.

Dr. A.
Taylor's re-
marks on
dementia.

"Dementia, when confirmed," says Dr. A. S. Taylor
in his valuable work on Medical Jurisprudence, "is a
total absence of all reasoning power, an incapacity to
perceive the true relations of things ; the language is
incoherent, and the actions are inconsistent ; the patient
speaks without being conscious of the meaning of what
he is saying ; memory is lost, and sometimes the word
or phrase is repeated for many hours together ; words
are no longer connected in meaning, as they are in
mania and monomania. This state is often called *fatuity*;
it is not an unfrequent consequence of mania and monomania."

CHRONIC DEMENTIA is often the result of acute attacks
of insanity. All intelligence appears to be abolished, and
the unhappy patient is reduced to the lowest degree
of fatuity, being utterly unable to understand any question addressed to him. He ceases to obey the calls of

nature, is dirty in his habits, and is reduced almost to the level of the brute creation. Occasionally this state of mental prostration is accompanied by sudden paroxysms of violence; but as a general rule these patients are very tractable, and are easily controlled.

IMBECILITY may be either congenital or acquired. The mind is often able to understand simple propositions, and the memory occasionally retains its power. In this form of *mental impairment* the patient is susceptible of a certain degree of *improvement*, is facile to the bad influence of other persons, is easily led in consequence of an enfeeblement of volition. All the higher faculties of the mind are undeveloped, or but slightly manifested. In this type of insanity the patient is pronounced to be in legal phraseology "*non compos mentis*," or of unsound mind. Of course this term is applicable to *all* forms of disordered mind, unfitting the person for the management of himself or his affairs; but is more generally applied to chronic forms of imbecility or want of capacity, either the effect of congenital defect of the brain, or some mechanical injury to the head, or mental shock. This term, "unsound mind," originated with the late Lord Eldon, and was intended to convey the idea of a person not acutely insane, or altogether imbecile or fatuous, but in such a condition of intellect as clearly to unfit him for the management of himself or government of his affairs.

IDIOCY may generally be defined undeveloped or arrested intelligence, arising from malformation of the cranium and defective organisation of the brain. It may be a *congenital* or an *acquired* condition of intellect. It is often an *intra-uterine* state, and is generally manifested at birth. It is occasionally the effect of some form of disease of the brain, such as inflammation, acute softening, and hydrocephalus, or the result of mechanical injury to the head during parturition.

Imbecility either congenital or acquired.

Idiots as
defined by
Fitzherbert.

An idiot is defined by Fitzherbert to be "from birth a person who cannot count or number twenty pence, or tell who was his father or mother, nor how old he is." According to Lord Tenterden, an idiot, in strict legal phraseology, is "a man who cannot repeat the letters of the alphabet, nor read what is set before him. There are degrees of idiocy. Occasionally there are faint scintillations of intelligence, and often the affections are strongly manifested even in advanced cases of this type of mental weakness.

Dr. Ray on
idiocy.

"Idiocy is that condition of mind in which the reflective, and all or a part of the effective powers, are either entirely wanting, or are manifested to the slightest possible extent. The intellectual and moral faculties, in cases properly falling under this head, are almost null, the effect being in most instances congenital, and arising in all cases from want of development of the senses is almost equally defective. The power of speech does not exist, or exists only so far as to enable the patient to articulate a few unintelligible monosyllables. This incapacity depends sometimes on the imperfect conformation of the organs of speaking, sometimes upon those of hearing, but more frequently on a deficiency in or want of the powers of imitation; so that even when the hearing and the speech are both entirely mature, the patient remains unable to do more than in the one case to show his knowledge of the existence of sound, and in the other, to give utterance to noises not above, if equal to, those of the brute creation. Taste and smell are equally imperfect. In many cases there is an inability to perceive odours, and in most, nothing but the coarsest discrimination in the selection of articles of food. Wallowing in personal filth, devouring even excrement with apparent avidity, indisposition to eat at all unless food be placed directly before the eye, drinking urine with as little appearance of distaste as water, are inci-

dents one or more of which are to be found in almost
every case of idiocy. And the same low grade of
sensibility and of flexibility is found in the purely physical system. The nerves are almost torpid. Limbs
sometimes have been amputated without apparent pain,
and Esquirol even tells of labour having been undergone
without the patient being conscious of the fact or of its
meaning. The arms are frequently of unequal length,
and misshapen; and the limbs generally are crooked and
feeble. A careless and broken gait distinguishes them
in most cases. Even the eyes are defectively hung, and
seem incapable of poising themselves at a right level.
And in the lower class of cases there is sometimes so
great a defectiveness of vision as to prevent the patient
from perceiving the most obvious objects. And even
when the powers of vision and of motion exist, the
intellectual powers are sometimes so attenuated as to
make attempts to reach a desired point entirely abortive,
though there be entire muscular power for such a purpose."*

Idiots of the lowest class are mere organisms, masses
of flesh and bone in human shape, in which the brain
and nervous system have no command over the system
of voluntary muscles; and which consequently are
without power of locomotion, without speech, without
any manifestation of intellectual or affective faculties.

Fools are a higher class of idiots, in whom the brain
and nervous system are so far developed as to give
partial command of the voluntary muscles; who have
consequently considerable powers of locomotion and ani-
mal action; partial development of the intellectual and
affective faculties, but only the faintest glimmer of
reason, and very imperfect speech.

Simpletons are the highest class of idiots, in whom
the harmony between the nervous and muscular systems

* Dr. Ray.

is nearly perfect; who, consequently, have normal powers of locomotion, considerable activity of the perceptive and affective faculties, and reason enough for their simple individual guidance, but not enough for their social relations.*

Nympho-
mania,
probably a
disease of
cerebellum.

NYMPHOMANIA.—This insane condition of mind is supposed to arise from an irritation or an enlargement of the *nymphœ*. Hence its name. But the disease is generally *cerebral*, or in other words *reflex*, the effect of disease or disorder of the brain, probably the cerebellum. It may shortly be defined to be a morbid exaltation of the sexual appetite associated with lascivious desires and unnatural habits, not always, as is erroneously supposed, the effect of local irritation. This disease often attacks truly modest women, who heroically struggle to keep in check this terrible malady. This morbid affection is generally found to be associated with uterine disturbance and catamenial irregularity.

Distinction
between
kleptomania
and wilful
stealing.

KLEPTOMANIA.—In some forms of insanity patients are often irresistibly impelled to steal, and to carefully conceal what they pilfer from others. Within the precincts of most asylums these cases are met with. One lunatic will steal from another, or pilfer anything they can lay their hands upon in the house. But these cases are not made matters of public observation and inquiry. It is only when this morbid propensity exhibits itself in the higher or middle classes of society outside of a lunatic asylum that it comes under judicial notice, and is matter for legal investigation. It is sometimes difficult to distinguish *kleptomania* from ordinary acts of theft. The circumstances of the alleged crime or monomania are of course carefully to be considered. In numerous cases the unhappy patient (generally female) is in good circumstances at the time the imputed offence was committed, having at command the means

* In accordance with Dr. Howe's Classification of Idiocy.

of purchasing all the necessaries and even luxuries of life; and yet, with a purse full of money, she finds it impossible to restrain on certain occasions her "fingers from picking and stealing." Women of known honesty, truth, intelligence, and worth, in full possession of everything that can make life desirable, find it impossible, when suffering from this malady, to resist this insane propensity. It is often associated with physical disorder of the nervous system—uterine irritation—ovarian disease—general nervous debility and ill-health —hysteria, &c. It is occasionally an hereditary malady,* and is often seen to follow some shock, physical or mental. It frequently manifests itself during the period of *utero-gestation*, or shortly after childbirth, or an attack of puerperal mania. All these particulars have carefully to be weighed and considered before forming a *diagnosis*.

Kleptomania often hereditary.

"There are persons," says Dr. Rush, "who are moral to the highest degree as to certain duties, but who, nevertheless, live under the influence of some one vice. In one instance, a woman was exemplary in her obedience to every command of the moral law, except one, she could not refrain from stealing. What made this vice more remarkable was, that she was in easy circumstances, and not addicted to extravagance in anything. Such was the propensity to this vice, that when she could lay her hands on nothing more valu-

Remarks by Dr. Rush on kleptomania.

---

* Alluding to the hereditary character of crime, a writer says: —"I was present one day at a factory or barrack in New South Wales, where the convicts are kept until engaged by a master, when a gentleman came in, and seeing a youth whom he thought would suit him, said, 'Well, lad, what are you?' 'A London thief,' was the boy's reply, touching his hat. 'What can you do?' 'Thieve, sir.' 'No doubt of that; but how were you brought up?' 'To thieve, sir.' 'Nonsense; what was your father?' 'A thief, sir.' Upon further inquiry the gentleman ascertained that the boy had *five* brothers and *five* sisters, all of whom had been convicted thieves."

able, she would often, at the table of a friend, fill her pockets secretly with bread. She both confessed and lamented the crime." "Cases like this," says Dr. Ray, "are so common, that they must have come within the personal knowledge of every reader who has seen much of the world, so that it will be unnecessary to mention them more particularly. It would be difficult to prove directly that this propensity continuing as it does throughout a whole life, and in a state of apparently perfect health, is, notwithstanding, a consequence of diseased or abnormal action in the brain; but the presumptive evidence in favour of this explanation is certainly strong. First, it is very often observed in abnormal conformations of the head, and accompanied by an imbecile condition of the understanding. Gall and Spurzheim saw, in a prison of Berne, a boy twelve years old, who could never refrain from stealing. He is described as ill-organised and rickety. At Hainau they were shown an obstinate robber, whom no corporeal punishment could correct. He appeared about sixteen years of age, though he was in fact twenty-six; his head was round, and about the size of a child's one year old. He was also deaf and dumb, a common accompaniment of mental imbecility. An instructive case has been lately recorded, in which this propensity seemed to be the result of a rickety and scrofulous constitution. Secondly, this propensity to steal is not unfrequently observed in undoubted mania. Pinel says it is a matter of common observation, that some maniacs, who, in their lucid intervals, are justly considered models of probity, cannot refrain from stealing and cheating during the paroxysm. Gall mentions the case of two citizens of Vienna, who, becoming insane, were distinguished in the hospital for an extraordinary propensity to steal, though previously they had lived irreproachable lives. They wandered over the house

Dr. Ray on klepto-mania.

from morning to night, picking up whatever they could lay their hands upon, straw, rags, clothes, wood, &c., which they carefully concealed in their room." *

DELUSIONS, HALLUCINATIONS AND ILLUSIONS. — It is necessary to bear in mind the legal as well as medical definitions of these often-used technical terms. Lord Brougham defines *delusion* to be "a belief of things as realities which exist only in the imagination of the patient." Sir John Nicholl says a delusion is "a belief in a fact which no rational reason would have believed." Dr. Forbes Winslow thus defines the word delusion: "a belief in the existence of something extravagant which in reality has no existence except in the *diseased* imagination of the patient, the absurdity of which he cannot perceive and out of which he cannot be reasoned." † Dr. Winslow thus makes an important legal distinction between the *eccentric* conceptions of a *healthy* and the *morbid* creations of a *diseased* imagination and judgment.

HALLUCINATIONS are insane impressions made upon the mind by *external* objects. Such patients often fancy they see the apparition of persons long dead coming into the room, or believe that they have been transformed into various species of animals. Some fancy that they are pregnant, are dead, or are made of glass, butter, and wax. Others imagine that voices are addressing them, speaking through the panels of the room from or in the street, addressing them by name, accusing them of certain crimes, or urging them to commit suicide. The words, "Kill yourself, kill yourself!" are words which the unhappy patient fancies he hears addressed to him. The morbid phenomena of those who so suffer are of an *objective* character.

ILLUSIONS are the effects of a morbid state of the *perceptions* and are often combined with hallucinations.

Delusions defined.

Hallucinations.

Illusions.

* Ray " On Insanity."
† "Lettsomian Lectures on Insanity."

It is sometimes difficult to diagnose one state from the other. *Schümayer* defines *illusions* to be mistakes in the conception and interpretation of the perception of objects *actually present;* whilst in *hallucinations*, the perception which originates in a diseased action of the senses appears in the patient as if the sensation were produced by a real object acting upon the senses. Illusions are *subjective* phenomena. These false and disordered impressions arise from an *internal* cause. Chronic and organic disease of the stomach, liver, or bowels will often give rise in persons who become insane to the idea that they are satanically possessed and are undergoing the tortures of the damned; or that a snake, frog, or reptile has been swallowed, and is gnawing their vitals. In cases of profound dyspepsia, hepatic and intestinal derangement, the patient is often under the illusion that his food is poisoned, that the head on his shoulders does not belong to him,* and that everything he sees and touches is dirty or contaminated. Esquirol relates a typical case of the kind. A

Case related
by Esquirol.

---

* A person who became insane during the French Revolution imagined that he had, with numerous other persons, been guillotined, and that when Bonaparte was raised to power all the heads of the guillotined persons were given to their respective owners. In the scramble that then occurred to regain the lost heads, he had got the wrong one, and under this delusion he went about shouting in great misery, "This is not my head," "These are not my teeth," "These are not my eyes," "Give me my own head," "This head belongs to another person." Tom Moore thus alludes to this singular case in his "Fudge Family in Paris" :—

> "Went to the Madhouse—saw the man,
> Who thinks, poor wretch, that while the Fiend
> Of discord here full riot ran,
> *He*, like the rest, was guillotin'd ;
> But that when under Boney's reign
> (A more discreet, though quite as strong one)
> The heads were all restor'd again,
> He in the scramble got a *wrong one.*"

lunatic was for the greater part of his life under the delusion that he had a wolf inside him. After death it was discovered that he had for many years been afflicted with cancer of the stomach. Occasionally these patients imagine they are being pursued or watched by the police; and that they are to be tried for some imaginary crime.

When *in extremis*, and in certain forms of low fever, patients are often seen picking the sheets and blankets under the delusion that insects are crawling over the bedclothes.

DELIRIUM (*de, lira*) off the tract, or the mind off its balance. This is a temporary mental disorder, often caused by acute bodily disease, such as fever, typhoid, puerperal, and typhus, renal disease, abuse of stimulants causing *delirium tremens*.* The latter form of delirium is associated with delusions and hallucinations, especially of the senses, but they are usually not of a fixed and permanent character like those seen in actual insanity. The delusions in delirium are constantly changing and are transient in their manifestations. Delirium.

* " The experienced physician is not likely to confound delirium tremens, clearly the consequence of an excessive indulgence in, or the *effect* of a *sudden* abstraction of stimulants from the brain, with insanity. The acute accession of the delirium, remarkable insomnia which precedes its development, and continues through its course; peculiar muscular tremor; anxiety and distress of mind so characteristically marked in the physiognomy, the *fussy* and *busy* nature of the delirium, fumbling of the bedclothes, extreme loquacity of the patient, peculiar sensorial illusions and mental hallucinations, suffused face, injected conjunctivæ, soft and feeble pulse, moist and creamy tongue, wild look of suspicion, terror, and alarm, clammy state of the skin, accompanied by a peculiar cutaneous exhalation similar to that observed in rheumatism, and perfectly obvious to the sense of smell, great agitation of manner, and increasing restlessness, are all specific and peculiar diagnostic features of this type of cerebro-mental disorder, clearly distinguishing it from the ordinary and specific forms of insanity."— *Obscure Diseases of the Brain and Mind:* by Forbes Winslow, M.D., D.C.L., Oxon., 4th edition.

Great caution should be exercised before signing a certificate in a case of *delirium tremens* with the object of placing such patients in a lunatic asylum. In a few instances it is absolutely necessary to do so, but, as a general rule, if properly treated they recover at home. Personal or mechanical restraint, except in extreme cases, should always be avoided.

Distinction between delirium and insanity.

In forming a diagnosis between delirium, the result of active *bodily* disease, and the delirium of *insanity*, it should be borne in mind that the delusions in true delirium are often evanescent, and are generally accompanied by some acute form of bodily disorder, as *cerebritis* or *meningitis*, &c.

In insanity the delusions are more fixed and are often *apparently* independent of any acute bodily disease, though as a rule we find insanity associated with a bad state of physical health.

The brain functionally or organically affected in delirium.

In all forms of delirium and disordered mind the brain is either *functionally* or *organically* affected. No mental derangement can occur unless the brain, the seat of thought, is disordered (not necessarily structurally). The vessels may be congested, the blood poisoned, or the membranes of the brain may be undergoing changes, all of which often give rise to delirium. There may be extensive organic disease of the brain, tubercles, abscess, and even *ramollisement* or induration of the brain, without the mind being at all affected; but directly the *ceneritious* or cortical structure is involved, the mind and mental faculties are immediately implicated. No disorder of the *vesicular* neurine can take place without mental disturbance.

Dipsomania often confounded with ordinary drunkenness.

DIPSOMANIA—chronic alcoholism, as it is sometimes termed. It is often difficult to distinguish this form of mental disease from ordinary attacks of drunkenness. The attacks of dipsomania are generally paroxysmal, and associated with some form of brain disorder or mental or bodily ill-health. The patient has often regular *lucid intervals*—*id est*, he will abstain from stimulants for a considerable time—and then suddenly have a relapse, and indulge freely in their use. In numerous cases the patient is conscious of his infirmity, and bitterly laments his inability to control his morbid craving for intoxicating drinks. He will affirm that he has no real pleasure in this indulgence, but finds the habit irresistible and uncontrollable. He apparently struggles against the propensity, and for a time succeeds in mastering the passion; but in some cases the slightest smell or taste of alcoholic drinks induces a paroxysm of the disease, and he then drinks till he becomes brutally intoxicated. The true dipsomaniac bitterly deplores his unhappy condition, and begs that measures to restrain him may be adopted. Often these patients voluntarily place themselves under restraint in asylums; but when restored to sane sobriety it is difficult, in consequence of the absence of delusions, to retain them as patients. The Commissioners in Lunacy, however, in some chronic cases sanction the detention of these invalids, even after apparent recovery, provided they show signs of undoubted mental disorder, exhibiting itself in an insane desire for stimulants.[*]

The subjoined quotations in relation to this subject I extract with the permission of the author:—[†]

"In these cases the morbid craving for physical sti-   Dr. Forbes Winslow on dipsomania.

[*] When alluding to this subject the Commissioners observe :— "We have considered that a lunatic asylum is not a place for the permanent detention of persons who have recovered the use of their reason, and are not obnoxious to the charge of unsoundness of mind otherwise than on account of the liability to run into their former excesses when restored to liberty."

[†] "On Uncontrollable Drunkenness considered as a Form of Mental Disorder, with Suggestions for its Treatment, and the Organisation of Sanatoria for Dipsomaniacs." By Forbes Winslow, M.D., D.C.L. Oxon.

muli of all kinds is uninfluenced by any motives that can be addressed to the intellect, heart, or conscience. Self-interest, self-esteem, friendship, love, religion, morality, are appealed to in vain. The passion for intoxicating drinks paralyzes the will and obtains a complete mastery over the understanding and moral sense, making every other emotion of the soul subservient to its base and demoralizing influences.

" This disposition for stimulants is often associated with an intense horror of the practice. The invalid (for so he must be considered) is often painfully conscious of his infirmity, and bitterly laments his inability to conquer the disordered appetite.

" When speaking of this mental malady, Esquirol says : ' *Si l'abus de liqueurs alcooliques est un effet de l'abrutissement de l'esprit, des vices de l'éducation, des mauvais exemples, il y a quelquefois un entraînement maladif qui porte certains individus à abuser des boissons fermentées. Il est des cas dan lesquels l'ivresse est l'effet du trouble accidentel de la sensibilité physique et morale, qui ne laisse plus à l'homme sa liberté d'action.*'

Want of control exhibited by dipsomaniacs.

" So intensely developed in many cases is this yearning for intoxicating stimulants that the unhappy victim allows no sense of decency, no feeling of propriety, no regard for family or domestic ties, to stand for a single instant in the way of his sensual indulgence. As in other forms of disordered intellect and perverted instinct, the most remarkable cunning and ingenuity are frequently exhibited by the patient in his endeavours to obtain access to stupifying drink. I have, in my own experience, known both men and women (occupying high social positions) of decided genius, of wonderful attainments, and cultivated intellectual taste, fall a prey to this form of insanity, and become utterly wrecked in mind, body, and estate.

" It is difficult for those unprofessionally conversant

with these cases to appreciate the extent to which this vice prevails in all ranks of society, and the difficulties connected with its successful treatment. In the majority of instances, and in those too where the habit of intemperance has reduced the person almost to the level of the beast, the ordinary reasoning powers for a time appear to be intact, and the mind is apparently free from the influence of delusions, hallucinations, or any other form of mental alienation. The person, when not actually muddled by drink, talks rationally, consecutively, and often with great acuteness and sagacity. Hence the medical and legal difficulties that arise when asked what amount of *personal interference* can be imposed in such cases with the view of destroying the insane impulse to drink, and of saving the patient, if not from a horrible death, at least from irretrievable ruin. It is absurd, except in cases where the mind has become decidedly disordered or impaired, to talk about placing such patients as *lunatics* in public or private asylums. If it were thought desirable so to confine and treat them with a view of re-establishing the bodily health and restoring the lost, or I should say, *suspended* power of self-control, the law very properly would not permit it. It is only when the mental disorder from intemperance culminates in a commonly-recognised form of insanity that the law interferes to save the individual from himself, and to protect his relatives and friends, or the community.

Inability to deal legally with dipsomaniacs.

"During the whole of the nascent and maturing stages of the alienation, during the progressive degradation of the moral faculties of the individual, the medical man is compelled to look on, and witness the most heart-rending ruin of a family, often in soul individually as well as in worldly possessions, by one whose intemperance is the manifestation of a true insane impulse, hereditary or acquired. The control of friends or relatives, experience shows fails utterly, as a rule, to destroy the morbid propensity for drink."*

Homicidal insanity generally associated with melancholia. HOMICIDAL INSANITY.—In this form of lunacy there is often an absence of all impairment or aberration of the *intellectual* powers, but in numerous cases delusions are detected. Patients predisposed to this form of madness are liable to sudden paroxysms of murderous violence. Occasionally they appear to be influenced by the most trifling exciting cause, and in numerous cases the crime appears to be entirely motiveless. An intense desire to destroy the lives of those whom they most tenderly love overpowers the reason and will of the unhappy sufferer. In this type of insanity there is generally found symptoms of melancholia associated with strange erratic conduct. These patients are gloomy and morose, combining often with the ferocity, the cunning, of the tiger. This phase of mental disorder is frequently classed under the head of

Dr. Forbes Winslow on moral insanity. MORAL INSANITY. On this subject I cannot do better than quote the following passage, as it fully describes this form of lunacy :—

" Let me consider the subject of ' moral insanity,' or, as Pinel terms it, ' *emportement maniaque sans délire*,' not *pathologically* but *metaphysically*. All authorities agree in opinion, that the specific characteristics of this form of derangement are dependent upon a lesion of the

---

* Drunkenness cannot be pleaded in excuse for crime. The drunkard is, in the words of Lord Coke, " *Voluntarius dæmon*." His drunkenness aggravates his offence : " *omne crimen ebrietas et incendit et detegit*." (Coke on Litt. 274, *a*.). Baron Alderson told a jury that " if a man chooses to get drunk it is his own voluntary act : it is very different from madness, *which is not caused by any act of the person*." (This is not psychologically accurate). Baron Parke declared that " if a man makes himself voluntarily drunk it is no excuse for any crime he may commit whilst he is so." According then to the English law, drunkenness is no valid defence in a criminal case.

carefully investigate the cases quoted by Pinel, Esquirol,
and Prichard, and referred to as *types* of moral insanity,
we are irresistibly led to the conclusion, that the malady,
as described by these authorities, was not in *any one
case restricted to the affective or motive powers of the understanding*. The faculties of judgment, reason, and
comparison are represented in this form of insanity to
be healthy and *intact*. Apparently, upon a superficial
examination, they may be so; but do not the 'tyrant
passion'—predominant vice—overpowering emotion—
loss of self-respect—brutality of conduct—prostration of
all the more refined sensibilities of the mind—uncontrollable impulse—impetuous will—and the suicidal or
homicidal idea, during the crisis of the paroxysm, *and
contemporaneously with the commission of the act*, dethrone
reason, and paralyze the operations of the judgment?
Do not violent and ungovernable temper, impulsive
emotion, and unreasonable conduct, leading to overt acts
of what are termed moral insanity, suspend the exercise
of the will, and interfere with the healthy balance or
equilibrium of the *intellectual* faculties? In cases where
the faculty of volition appears to be suspended, and the
patient is unhappily the willing and facile slave of every
wicked, sensual appetite and vicious propensity, and is
guilty of most extravagant conduct—are, I repeat, the
powers of *judgment, reason*, and *comparison*, the more
exalted and intellectual functions of the mind, entirely
free, unclouded, unfettered, and in a healthy state of
activity? Is the 'moral maniac' capable of pursuing
an ordinary and healthy process of induction, and competent to exercise the powers of reason, comparison, and
reflection, *quoad* the specified features of his so-termed
'moral' disease? He may be apparently of sound understanding, able to solve with great rapidity a difficult
mathematical problem; have great capacity for the
ordinary business of life; may converse with ease upon

points of science, art, and philosophy ; and astonish the world by the tenacity of his memory, the vividness of his fancy, the playfulness of his satire, the brilliancy of his wit, and the majesty and sublimity of his eloquence —all these elevated states of mind are compatible with *latent delusive ideas and intellectual disorder.** Lord Brougham makes some pertinent remarks on this subject. When applying his able powers of philosophical analysis to this question, his Lordship observes : ' We cannot with any correctness of language speak of general or "partial" insanity ; but we may most accurately speak of the mind exerting itself in consciousness without cloud or imperfection, but being morbid when it fancies ; and so its owner may have a diseased imagination, or the imagination may be diseased, and yet the memory may be impaired, and the owner be said to have lost his memory. In these cases we do not mean that the mind has one faculty, as consciousness, sound, whilst another, as memory or imagination, is diseased ; but that the mind is sound when reflecting upon its own operations, and diseased when exercising the combination termed imagination, or casting the retrospect called reflection.' Then again, as to what is termed impulsive insanity, a form of disease generally considered to be unassociated with derangement of the ideas, I would ask, is it a fact that these cases are invariably unaccompanied by delusive impressions, or by a disturbance of

Dr. Forbes Winslow on moral insanity.

* "In many cases, designated as illustrations of moral insanity, I feel assured that undetected and unrecognised delusions often actually exist, influencing the conduct of the patient. I could narrate several instances of the kind. M. Marc mentions the case of a man, who for many years had been in the habit of licking the walls of the apartment with his tongue, until he had actually worn away the plaster. No one could imagine what was the cause of this perseverance in so painful and disgusting a habit, until one day in the author's presence he confessed that he tasted and smelt the most delicious fruit on the walls."

Moral in-
sanity.

the reasoning faculties? Admitting the existence of a morbid impulsive propensity, does it become absolutely irresistible and uncontrollable except during a crisis of delirium? It has been maintained, that at the moment of the impulsion an intellectual perturbation and positive derangement of ideas occurs. 'We believe,' says a French writer, 'that the doctrine of a temporary insanity, of a sudden eclipse of the reason at the time of the act, is a safer and more philosophical doctrine than the hypothesis of modern medical jurists, who assert that no monomania, whether homicidal, suicidal, or incendiary, can compel to the consummation of the act, without insanity in the ordinary acceptation of the term, or intellectual disturbance. We repeat that we cannot admit this theory or principle of monomania with irresistible desire, and without delirium during the act, because it appears to us to be dangerous, inasmuch as it suspends the course of free-will, is destructive of the morality of human actions, and tends to favour impunity of crimes. For if the impulse be irresistible, and is unaccompanied by delirium during the act, what becomes then of free-will? In our minds, the disturbance of the reason will always be more comprehensible and conformable to the common-sense of mankind than a perversion of the will without delirium.' " *

Puerperal
mania
generally
immediately
following
confine-
ment.

PUERPERAL MANIA may occasionally precede parturition, but, as a general rule, it follows delivery. The insanity in these cases is more of the character of delirium, especially in its early stage, than that of true mental derangement. The patient is often troubled with hallucinations and illusions instead of any fixed delusions, although these occasionally crop up. This form of lunacy is often associated with a desire to murder or injure the infant. In the acute stage the

* "Lettsomian Lectures on Insanity," by Forbes Winslow, M.D., D.C.L., Oxon.

patient and child require to be closely watched. These cases are generally curable, and ought not to be removed from home. In some chronic forms of the malady it is absolutely necessary to place the patient under surveillance with a view to efficient remedial treatment.

GENERAL PARALYSIS OF THE INSANE.—This mental affection is often caused by organic changes in the membranes or substance of the brain, and is associated with morbid conditions of the mind, muscular system, and speech. It is a most insidious malady, and it is most difficult to trace its origin. It is characterised by three distinct and well-marked stages. In the early stage the mind becomes affected by exalted or ambitious delusions; the patient, probably imagining that he is in possession of a large amount of property, will order various things for which he has no use, and at the same time no money to pay for; he will also draw cheques upon banks in which he has no effects, being under the delusion that he has vast resources at his command, and under the influence of these false impressions if not restrained he will beggar himself and his family. He may fancy that he has gigantic strength, and that it is in his power to accomplish anything he may attempt, or that he is a regal personage, and will consequently dress up in extravagant costumes. The patient is completely wrapped up in his own ideas of grandeur, and nothing can persuade him that he is labouring under false impressions. All these symptoms are characteristic of the first stage of general paralysis of the insane. We have in addition great loquacity, restlessness, and defective memory for recent events.

In the second stage of the disease paralysis becomes evident, the first indication showing itself in the speech, which is thick; he articulates with difficulty and speaks

General paralysis of the insane.

First stage.

Second stage.

with a muffled voice resembling very much the articulation of a drunken man, and as if the tongue were too large for the mouth. He is unable to give utterance to certain words, or pronounce particular letters of the alphabet. There is an uncertainty in his gait, and loss of power, especially in the lower extremities, is very apparent. The delusions existing in the first stage of the disease are also present, the memory and other faculties of the mind are much impaired, and there is an *entire* absence of all moral feeling.

Third stage.　　In the third stage of this disease the patient passes into a state of helpless dementia, he cannot recognise his immediate friends and relatives, he is completely paralysed, very dirty in his habits, and entirely lost as to what goes on about him. In this stage he remains until death terminates his unhappy existence.

Detection of feigned insanity.　　FEIGNED OR SIMULATED INSANITY.—Insanity is often feigned by the criminal to escape punishment, or by the soldier to obtain his discharge from the army. In these cases the pseudo-lunatic overacts his part, so that the experienced eye of the skilled physician ought not to be easily deceived. These cases, however, require to be under close observation for a time before the imposition can be detected. It is occasionally necessary to watch the person closely by day and night in order to discover the simulation. The tests are the physiognomy, the appearance of the eyes, the character of the voice, and feigned incoherence of the conversation, the absence of all bodily illness usually accompanying cases of insanity. It will be easy to distinguish the nonsensical gibberish of a person feigning insanity from the disjointed, rambling, incoherent conversation of a *bonâ fide* madman. It is not easy to describe the difference, but an expert will have no difficulty in detecting it. In all suspected cases it may be necessary to get the alleged lunatic to put in writing his ideas, to associate him with other lunatics, and then observe his conversation and conduct. Occasionally the mask is thrown off when it is proposed in the patient's presence to use some very painful local remedies with the view of curing his insanity, such as the actual cautery, shaving and applying blisters to the scalp. The dread of a prolonged shower bath has had the effect of discovering feigned insanity. Monomania *cannot be* easily simulated. The physician accustomed to observe these cases ought not to be baffled. When feigning incoherence the person generally talks a quantity of bosh from ignorance of the true characteristics of the disease which the skilled medical man has never heard a really insane person indulge in. This phenomenon is well pourtrayed by Sheridan in the *Critic*, where he makes Tilburina thus imitate the ravings of a lunatic :—

> " The wind whistles—the moon rises—see
> They have kill'd my squirrel in his cage !
> Is this a grasshopper?—Ha ! no ; it is my
> Whiskerandos—you shall not keep him—
> I know you have him in your pocket—
> An oyster may be cross'd in love !—Who says
> A whale's a bird ? Ha ! did you call, my love?—
> He's here ! he's there !—He's everywhere !
> Ah me ! he's nowhere ! "

In Sheridan's case of mimic madness the simulation is said to have been detected by the " mangled metre ! "

Contrast the gibberish uttered by Sheridan's mock madwoman with the truthful delineation of the insane ravings of Poor Tom, as pictured by the immortal bard :—" Who gives anything to poor Tom ? whom the foul fiend hath led through fire and through flame, through ford and whirlpool, over bog and quagmire ; that hath laid knives under his pillow, and halters in his pew ; set ratsbane by his porridge ; made him proud of heart, to ride on a bay trotting-horse over four-inch'd bridges, to course his own shadow for a traitor."

Again, compare the incoherence of Sheridan's poetic lunatic with the *ipsissima verba* of Dr. Rush's madman, and the difference between the conversation of an imaginary lunatic and the disjointed language of a person' really insane will at once be recognised :—"No man can serve two masters. I am King Philip of Macedonia, lawful son of Mary Queen of Scots, born in Philadelphia. I have been happy enough ever since I have seen General Washington with a silk handkerchief in High Street. Money commands sublunary things, and makes the mare go ; it will buy salt mackerel, made of tenpenny nails. Enjoyment is the happiness of virtue. Yesterday cannot be recalled. I can only walk in the night-time, when I can eat pudding enough. I shall be eight years old to-morrow. They say R. W. is in partnership with J. W. I believe they are about as good as people in common—not better, only on certain occasions, when, for instance, a man wants to buy chin-copins, and to import salt to feed pigs. Tanned leather was imported first by lawyers. Morality with virtue is like vice not corrected. L. B. came into your house and stole a coffee-pot in the twenty-fourth year of his majesty's reign. Plum-pudding and Irish potatoes make a very good dinner. Nothing in man is comprehensible to it. Born in Philadelphia. Our forefathers were better to us than our children, because they were chosen for their honesty, truth, virtue, and innocence. The Queen's broad R. originated from a British forty-two pounder, which makes too large a report for me. I have no more to say. I am thankful I am no worse this season, and that I am sound in mind and memory, and could steer a ship to sea, but am afraid of the tiller * * * * * * son of Mary Queen of Scots. Born in Philadelphia. King of Macedonia." *

Medical Evidence in Court.

The medical man, when called upon to give evidence, should abstain from the use of pedantic terms and technical phraseology. Duties of medical witness in Court.

The more simple, unaffected, and unadorned his statement, the greater will be its moral weight. He should carefully and scrupulously avoid all *positiveness*, *dogmatism*, and *partisanship*. His testimony ought to be accompanied with judicious qualifications, when relating to cases of difficulty, doubt, and obscurity, respecting which there may, even among scientific men, be great discrepancy of opinion. His evidence should impress the Court with the conviction that his opinion has not been hastily, indiscreetly, or rashly formed. It should appear as the result of a full, careful, and scientific consideration of the case.

Having a lucid conception of the nature of the evidence he is prepared to give, he should quietly and firmly maintain his position, and not allow himself to be confused or driven from his point by the cunning artifice of counsel, or thrown off his guard by the remarks of the court.

He should be careful not to lose his temper, or to indulge in witticisms or retorts upon the counsel.

Many witnesses seriously commit themselves by an undue *loquacity*. This fault, and it is a prevalent and a very serious one, cannot be too carefully guarded against.

The witness had far better keep to the text; answer the questions tersely and epigrammatically, and if called

* Dr. Rush on the Mind, pp. 242-3.

upon for a further explanation, it should be brief and to the point.

All attempts at a *definition* of insanity should be carefully avoided.

The counsel who knows the obscurity of the subject, and the difficulty with which the medical witness has to contend in giving an accurate definition of insanity, most unfairly endeavours to pin him down to one ; and then, by demonstrating the fallacy of his definition, to overthrow the whole moral effect of his testimony.

If the witness be asked to define insanity, it will be more judicious for him at once to candidly acknowledge his utter incapacity to do so—

> For to define true madness,
> What is't ? but to be nothing else but mad.*

-----

* Hamlet.

APPENDICES.

———◦⋄◦———

I.

ANNO OCTAVO & NONO VICTORIÆ REGINÆ.

CAP. 100.

An Act for the Regulation of the Care and Treatment of Lunatics.
August 4, 1845.

BE it enacted by the Queen's most excellent Majesty, by and with the advice and consent of the Lords Spiritual and Temporal, and Commons, in this present Parliament assembled, and by the authority of the same, That from and after the passing of this Act an Act passed in the Session of Parliament holden in the second and third years of the reign of his late Majesty King William the Fourth, intituled "An Act for regulating for three years, and from thence until the end of the then next Session of Parliament, the Care and Treatment of Insane Persons in England;" and an Act passed in the Session of Parliament holden in the third and fourth years of the reign of his said late Majesty, intituled, "An Act to amend an Act of the second and third year of his present Majesty, for regulating the Care and Treatment of Insane Persons in England;" and an Act passed in the Session of Parliament holden in the fifth and sixth years of the reign of his said late Majesty, intituled "An Act to continue for three years, and from thence to the end of the then next Session of Parliament, two Acts of the second and third year and the third and fourth year of his present Majesty, relating to the Care and Treatment of Insane Persons in England;" and an Act passed in the Session of Parliament holden in the first and second years of the reign of her present

The following Acts repealed, except as they repeal other Acts:

2 & 3 W. 4. c. 107.

3 & 4 W. 4. c. 64.

5 & 6 W. 4. c. 22.

1 & 2 Vict. c. 73.

Majesty, intituled "An Act to continue for three years, and from thence to the end of the then next Session of Parliament, two Acts relating to the Care and Treatment of Insane Persons in England;" and an Act passed in the Session of Parliament holden in the fifth year of the reign of her said present Majesty, intituled "An Act to continue for three years, and from thence to the end of the then next Session of Parliament, two Acts relating to the Care and Treatment of Insane Persons in England;" and an Act passed in the Session of Parliament holden in the fifth and sixth years of the reign of her said present Majesty, intituled "An Act to amend, and continue for three years, and from thence to the end of the next Session of Parliament, the Laws relating to Houses licensed by the Metropolitan Commissioners and Justices of the Peace for the Reception of Insane Persons, and for the Inspection of County Asylums and Public Hospitals for the Reception of Insane Persons," shall be and the same are hereby repealed, save and except so far as they or any of them repeal any other Act: Provided always, that until the appointment for any Jurisdiction of Visitors and their Clerk under the provisions of this Act the Visitors and Clerk appointed for such Jurisdiction under the said repealed Acts or any of them shall respectively have and perform the powers, authorities, and duties which they would have respectively had or performed if appointed under this Act: Provided also, that all licences heretofore granted shall remain in force for the periods for which they were respectively granted, unless revoked as hereinafter provided; and that all orders, matters, and things which have been granted, made, done, or directed to be done in pursuance of the said repealed Acts or any of them shall be and remain as good, valid, and effectual to all intents and purposes as if the said repealed Acts had not been repealed, except so far as such orders, matters, or things are expressly made void or affected by this Act; and that all fees, charges, and expenses which have become payable under the said repealed Acts or any of them shall be payable in the same manner and from the same funds as would have been applicable thereto in case such Acts had not been repealed.

5 Vict. c. 4.

5 & 6 Vict. c. 87.

Proviso that present Visitors and Clerk shall act under this Act till new ones are appointed and that Licences heretofore granted shall remain in force, unless, &c.

Commissioners in Lunacy under 5 & 6 Vict. c. 84, to be

2. And be it enacted, That the persons already appointed and hereafter to be appointed under an Act passed in the Session of Parliament holden in the fifth and sixth years of the reign of her present Majesty, intituled "An Act to alter

and amend the Practice and Course of Proceeding under
Commissions in the Nature of Writs De lunatico inquirendo,"
whereby the Lord Chancellor is empowered to appoint two
persons, to be called "The Commissioners in Lunacy," shall
henceforth be and be called "The Masters in Lunacy," and
shall take the same rank and precedence as the Masters in
Ordinary of the High Court of Chancery. *henceforth called "The Masters in Lunacy."*

3. And be it enacted, That the Right Honourable Lord
Ashley, the Right Honourable Lord Seymour, the Right
Honourable Robert Vernon Smith, Robert Gordon of Lewis-
ton in the County of Dorset, Esquire, Francis Barlow of
Montagu Square, Esquire, Thomas Turner of Curzon Street,
Esquire, Henry Herbert Southey of Harley Street, Esquire,
John Robert Hume, of Curzon Street aforesaid, Esquire,
Bryan Waller Procter of Gray's Inn, Esquire, James William
Mylne of Lincoln's Inn, Esquire, and John Hancock Hall of
the Middle Temple, Esquire (which said Thomas Turner,
Henry Herbert Southey, and John Robert Hume, and no
other of the said persons, are physicians, and which said Bryan
Waller Procter, James William Mylne, and John Hancock
Hall, and no other of the said persons, are practising barristers
at law of ten years' standing at the bar and upwards), and
their respective successors, to be appointed as hereinafter provided, shall be Commissioners for the purposes of this Act, to
be called "The Commissioners in Lunacy;" and that such
Commissioners for the time being shall respectively hold their
offices during good behaviour, and shall not, so long as they
shall remain such Commissioners, and receive any salary under
this Act, accept, hold, or carry on any other office or situation,
or any profession or employment, from which any gain or profit
shall be derived; and that there shall be paid to each of the
six Commissioners for the time being who shall be physicians,
surgeons, or barristers of five years' standing and upwards,* out
of the moneys or funds hereinafter mentioned, over and above
their respective travelling and other expenses whilst employed
in visiting any houses, hospitals, asylums, gaols, workhouses,
or other places, in pursuance of this Act, the yearly salary of
one thousand and five hundred pounds, by four equal quarterly
payments, on the twenty-ninth day of September, the twenty-
fifth day of December, the twenty-fifth day of March, and the

Appointment of "The Commissioners in Lunacy."

---

* See 16 & 17 Vict. c. 96, s. 39.

twenty-fourth day of June in every year, the first of each such payments (or a proportionate part thereof, to be computed, in the case of the Commissioners appointed by this Act, from the passing of the Act, and in case of the Commissioners to be appointed as hereinafter provided, from the time of the respective appointments of such Commissioners) to be made to such Commissioners respectively on such of the same days of payment as shall first happen after the passing of this Act, or after the dates of their respective appointments, as the case may be.

In case of death, disqualification, refusal, or inability of Commissioners, others to be appointed.

4. And be it enacted, That as often as any Commissioner appointed by this Act or to be appointed under this present provision shall die, or be removed for ill-behaviour, or be disqualified, or resign, or refuse to act, or become unable by illness or otherwise to perform the duties or exercise the powers of this Act, the Lord Chancellor shall appoint a person to be a Commissioner in the room of the Commissioner who shall die, or be removed, or be disqualified, or resign, or refuse or become unable to act as aforesaid, but so that every person so appointed in the room of a physician shall be a physician or surgeon, and every person so appointed in the room of a barrister of five years' standing at the bar * and upwards shall be a practising barrister of not less than five years' standing at the bar, and every person appointed in the room of any other Commissioner shall be neither a physician nor a surgeon, nor a practising barrister; and until such appointment it shall be lawful for the continuing Commissioners or Commissioner to act as if there were no such vacancy.

Provision for retiring pension to incapacitated Commissioners.

5. And be it enacted, That any superannuation allowance to be granted to any Commissioner appointed or to be appointed under this Act shall be granted only in respect of services performed under this Act, and shall be subject to the provisions of an Act passed in the fourth and fifth years of his late

4 & 5 W. 4. c. 24.

Majesty King William the Fourth, intituled "An Act to alter, amend, and consolidate the Laws for regulating the Pensions, Compensation, and Allowances to be made to Persons in respect of their having held Civil Offices in his Majesty's Service," so far as such provisions relate to officers and clerks who had entered or might enter the public service subsequent to the fourth day of August, One thousand eight hundred and twenty-nine.

* See 16 & 17 Vict. c. 96, s. 39.

6. And be it enacted, That every person hereby or here- Commis-
after appointed a Commissioner under this Act shall, before he sioners to
acts in the execution of his duty as a Commissioner, take an following
oath to the following effect : (that is to say), oath.

" I, *A. B.*, do swear, That I will discreetly, impartially, and
faithfully execute all the trusts and powers committed unto
me by virtue of an Act of Parliament made in the ninth year
of the reign of her Majesty Queen Victoria, intituled [*here
insert the title of the Act*]; and that I will keep secret all such
matters as shall come to my knowledge in the execution of
my office (except when required to divulge the same by legal
authority, or so far as I shall feel myself called upon to do so
for the better execution of the duty imposed on me by the
said Act).
" So help me GOD."

Which oath it shall be lawful for the Lord Chancellor to
administer to every such Commissioner ; and any three of the
Commissioners who shall have previously taken the oath are
hereby authorised to administer such oath to any other Commissioner.

7. And be it enacted, That the Commissioners shall cause Commis-
to be made a Seal of the Commission, and shall cause to be sioners
sealed or stamped therewith all licences, orders, and instru- Common
ments granted or made, or issued, or authorised by the Com- Seal.
missioners, in pursuance of this Act, except such orders or
instruments as are hereinafter required or directed to be given
or signed and sealed by one Commissioner or two Commissioners ; and all such licences, orders, and instruments,
or copies thereof, purporting to be sealed or stamped with the
Seal of the Commission, shall be received as evidence of the
same respectively, and of the same respectively having been
granted, made, issued, or authorised by the Commissioners,
without any further proof thereof ; and no such licence,
order, or instrument, or copy thereof, shall be valid, or have
any force or effect, unless the same shall be so sealed or
stamped as aforesaid.

8. And be it enacted, That the Commissioners or any five Commis-
of them shall, as soon as may be after the passing of this Act, sioners
meet at the usual office or place of business now occupied or permanent
used by the Metropolitan Commissioners in Lunacy, or at such chairman.
other place as the Lord Chancellor shall direct, and elect one

of the same Commissioners (not being a physician or a barrister receiving any salary by virtue of this Act) to be the permanent chairman of the Commission; and in case such permanent chairman, or any other permanent chairman who shall thereafter be elected in pursuance of this provision, shall die, or decline or become incapable to act as chairman, or shall cease to be a Commissioner, then and as often as the same shall happen the Commissioners for the time being, or any five of them, at any meeting to be specially summoned for that purpose, shall elect another person to be the permanent chairman of the Commission in the place of the chairman who shall so die, or decline or become incapable to act, or cease to be a Commissioner as aforesaid; and in case the permanent chairman for the time being shall be absent from any meeting it shall be lawful for the majority of the Commissioners present at any such meeting to elect a chairman for that meeting; and in all cases every question shall be decided by a majority of voters (the chairman, whether permanent or temporary, having a vote), and in the event of an equality of votes the chairman for the time being shall have an additional or casting vote.

Appointment of Secretary. 9. And be it enacted, That Robert Wilfred Skeffington Lutwidge,* of Lincoln's Inn, Esquire, shall be the secretary to the Commissioners; and that the said Robert Wilfred Skeffington Lutwidge, and every secretary to be hereafter appointed, shall be removeable from his office by the Lord Chancellor, on the application of the Commissioners; and that as often as the said Robert Wilfred Skeffington Lutwidge, or any secretary to be appointed under this present provision, shall die, or resign, or be removed from his office, the Commissioners, with the approbation of the Lord Chancellor, shall appoint a person to be secretary in the room of the said Robert Wilfred Skeffington Lutwidge, or other the secretary who shall die, or resign, or be removed as aforesaid; and that the secretary for the time being shall, in the performance of all his duties and in all respects, be subject to the inspection, direction, and control of the Commissioners; and that there shall be paid to the secretary for the time being, out of the moneys and funds hereinafter mentioned, the yearly salary of eight hundred pounds, by four equal quarterly payments, on the twenty-ninth day of Septem-

* Mr. Lutwidge was subsequently appointed as one of the Commissioners in Lunacy; he was killed by a lunatic during the present year, and succeeded by Hon. G. Howard.

ber, the twenty-fifth day of December, the twenty-fifth day of March, and the twenty-fourth day of June in every year, the first of such payments (or a proportionate part thereof, to be computed, in the case of the said Robert Wilfred Skeffington Lutwidge, from the passing of this Act, and in case of every other secretary from the time of his appointment) to be made to the said Robert Wilfred Skeffington Lutwidge on such of the same days of payment as shall first happen after the passing of this Act, and to every other secretary for the time being on such of the same days of payment as shall first happen after his appointment.

10. And be it enacted, That any superannuation allowance to be granted to any secretary appointed or to be appointed under this Act shall be granted only in respect of services performed under this Act, and shall be subject to the provisions of an Act passed in the fourth and fifth years of his late Majesty King William the Fourth, intituled " An Act to alter, amend, and consolidate the Laws for regulating the Pensions, Compensation, and Allowances to be made to Persons in respect of their having held Civil Offices in His Majesty's Service," so far as such provisions relate to officers and clerks who had entered or might enter the public service subsequent to the fourth day of August, One thousand eight hundred and twenty-nine.

Provision for retiring pension to Secretary.

4 & 5 W. 4. c. 24.

11. And be it enacted, That it shall be lawful for the Commissioners to appoint, during pleasure, any two persons as clerks to the Commissioners, and to allow to such two clerks any such yearly or other salaries (not exceeding in the whole the yearly sum of two hundred pounds for such two clerks) as the Commissioners shall think proper; and further, that it shall be lawful for the Commissioners, at any time hereafter, in case they shall find it expedient so to do, for the due performance of the business of the Commission, with the consent of the Lord High Treasurer, or of the Commissioners of her Majesty's Treasury, or of any three or more of them, to appoint one or two other clerks (in addition to the two clerks firstly hereinbefore mentioned), and to allow to such one or two additional clerk or clerks any such yearly or other salaries as the Commissioners shall think fit (not exceeding in the whole the yearly sum of two hundred pounds); and such salaries shall be paid out of the moneys or funds hereinafter mentioned.

Power for the Commissioners to appoint two clerks.

12. And be it enacted, That every person appointed to be

x

Secretary and clerks to take an oath.

secretary or clerk as aforesaid shall, before he shall act as such secretary or clerk, take the following oath, to be administered by any one of the Commissioners :—

"I, *A. B.*, do swear, That I will faithfully execute all such trusts and duties as shall be committed to my charge as secretary to the Commissioners in Lunacy [*or* as clerk to the Commissioners in Lunacy, *as the case may be*]; and that I will keep secret all such matters as shall come to my knowledge in the execution of my office (except when required to divulge the same by legal authority).

"So help me GOD."

Clerk of the Metropolitan Commissioners to deliver all documents to the Commissioners under this Act.

13. And be it enacted, That immediately after the passing of this Act the clerk to the Metropolitan Commissioners in Lunacy appointed under the said Act of the second and third years of the reign of his late Majesty King William the Fourth, or under any of the other Acts hereby repealed, shall forthwith deliver up every book, paper, and document, and all goods, property, and effects which may be in his possession by virtue of his said office, or in consequence thereof, or connected with the business thereof, to the Commissioners in Lunacy hereby appointed; and every book, paper, and document, and all goods, property, and effects respectively, which shall be so delivered unto or shall hereafter come into the possession of the Commissioners in Lunacy by virtue of their office, shall thereupon be vested in and shall be deemed to be the property of the Commissioners in Lunacy for the time being.

Jurisdiction within which Commissioners are to grant licences, and termed their immediate jurisdiction, defined.

14. And be it enacted, That it shall be lawful for the Commissioners (if and when they shall think fit) to grant a licence to any person to keep a house for the reception of lunatics, or of any sex or class of lunatics, within the places following; (that is to say) the cities of London and Westminster, the county of Middlesex, the borough of Southwark, and the several parishes and places hereinafter mentioned; (that is to say,) Brixton, Battersea, Barnes, Saint Mary Magdalen Bermondsey, Christ Church Clapham, Saint Giles Camberwell, Dulwich, Saint Paul Deptford, Gravenay, Kew Green, Kennington, Saint Mary Lambeth, Mortlake, Merton, Mitcham, Saint Mary Newington, Norwood, Putney, Peckham, Saint Mary Rotherhithe, Roehampton, Streatham, Stockwell, Tooting, Wimbledon, Wandsworth, and Walworth, in the county of Surrey; Blackheath, Charlton, Deptford, Greenwich,

Lewisham, Lee, Southend, and Woolwich, in the county of Kent; and East Ham, Layton, Laytonstone, Low Layton, Plaistow, West Ham, and Walthamstow, in the county of Essex; and also within every other place (if any) within the distance of seven miles from any part of the said cities of London or Westminster, or of the said borough of Southwark; all which cities, county, borough, parishes, and places aforesaid shall be and are hereafter referred to as the immediate jurisdiction of the Commissioners.

15. And be it enacted, That the Commissioners or some five of them shall meet at the usual office or place of business which shall for the time being be occupied or used by the said Commissioners, or at such other place as the Lord Chancellor may direct, on the first Wednesday in the months of February, May, July, and November in every year, in order to receive applications from persons requiring houses to be licensed for the reception of lunatics within the immediate jurisdiction of the Commissioners, and (if they shall think fit) to license the same; and in case on any such occasion five Commissioners shall not be present the meeting shall take place on the next succeeding Wednesday, and so on weekly until five Commissioners shall be assembled; and the Commissioners assembled at every such meeting shall have power to adjourn such meeting from time to time and to such place as they shall see fit: Provided always, nevertheless, that it shall be lawful for any five of the Commissioners at any other time, at any meeting duly summoned under the provisions in that behalf hereinafter contained, to receive applications from persons requiring houses to be licensed as aforesaid, and, if they shall think fit, to license the same.

Commissioners to hold quarterly and special meetings for granting licences.

16. And be it enacted, That when and so often as any Commissioner shall by writing under his hand require the secretary to convene a meeting of the Commissioners for a purpose or purposes specified in such writing, or for the general despatch of business, such secretary is hereby required to convene such meeting by summons to the other Commissioners, or such of them as shall be then in England and shall have an address known to the secretary, and to give them, as far as circumstances will admit, not less than twenty-four hours' notice of the place, day, and hour, where and on and at which such meeting is intended to be held, and also to state in the summons the purpose or purposes of such meeting,

Provision for summoning special meetings.

as specified by the Commissioner requiring the same to be convened; and then and in every such case it shall be lawful for any three of the Commissioners to assemble themselves to consider, and (if they shall think fit) to execute the purpose or purposes of such meeting: Provided always, nevertheless, that nothing shall be done at any such meeting, at which less than five Commissioners shall be present, which by this Act is required to be done by five Commissioners:* Provided also, that every such meeting shall, as far as circumstances will admit, be held at the usual office or place of business of the Commissioners.

The Justices of the Peace in general or quarter sessions in all other parts of England to license houses for the reception of lunatics, and to appoint visitors.

17. And be it enacted, That in all places not being within the immediate jurisdiction of the Commissioners the justices for the county or borough assembled in general or quarter sessions shall have the same authority within their respective counties or boroughs to license houses for the reception of lunatics as the Commissioners within their immediate jurisdiction; and that the said justices shall, at the Michaelmas general or quarter sessions in every year, appoint three or more justices, and also one physician, surgeon, or apothecary, or more, to act as visitors of every or any house or houses licensed for the reception of lunatics within the said counties or boroughs respectively; and such visitors shall at their first meeting take the oath required by this Act to be taken by the Commissioners, *mutatis mutandis,* such oath to be administered by a justice.

For appointment of a visitor in the place of one dying, being unable, disqualified, &c.

18. And be it enacted, That in case at any time of the death, inability, disqualification, resignation, or refusal to act of any person so appointed a visitor as aforesaid, it shall be lawful for the justices of the county or borough, at any general or quarter sessions, to appoint a visitor in the room of the person who shall die, or be unable, or be disqualified, or resign, or refuse to act as aforesaid.

Lists of visitors to be published by the Clerk of the Peace in a newspaper, and to be sent to the Commissioners.

19. And be it enacted, That a list of the names, places of abode, occupations, or professions of all visitors appointed as hereinbefore is directed shall, within fourteen days from the date of their respective appointments, be published by the Clerk of the Peace of the county or borough for which they shall be respectively appointed, in some newspaper commonly circulated within the same county or borough, and shall, within three days from the date of their respective appointments, be

* See 16 & 17 Vict. c. 96, s. 36.

sent by the Clerk of the Peace to the Commissioners; and every Clerk of the Peace making default in either of the respects aforesaid shall for every such default forfeit a sum not exceeding two pounds.

Penalty for default.

20. And be it enacted, That every such visitor as aforesaid, being a physician, surgeon, or apothecary, shall be paid out of the moneys or funds hereinafter mentioned for every day during which he shall be employed in executing the duties of this Act such sum as the justices of the county or borough shall in general or quarter sessions direct.

Every visitor, being a physician, surgeon, or apothecary, to be remunerated.

21. And be it enacted, That the Clerk of the Peace, or some other person to be appointed by the justices for the county or borough in general or quarter sessions, shall act as clerk to the visitors so appointed as aforesaid, and such clerk shall summon the visitors to meet at such time and place, for the purpose of executing the duties of this Act, as the said justices in general or quarter sessions shall appoint; and every such appointment, summons, and meeting shall be made and held as privately as may be, and in such manner that no proprietor, superintendent, or person interested in or employed about or connected with any house to be visited shall have notice of such intended visitation; and such clerk to the visitors shall, at their first meeting, take the oath required by this Act to be taken by the Secretary of the Commissioners, *mutatis mutandis*, such oath to be administered by one of the visitors, being a justice; and the name, place of abode, occupation, and profession of the clerk to the visitors (whether the same shall be the Clerk of the Peace or any other person) shall within fourteen days after the appointment be published by the Clerk of the Peace for the county or borough in some newspaper commonly circulated therein, and within three days from the date of the appointment be communicated by the said Clerk of the Peace to the Commissioners; and every Clerk of the Peace making default in either of the respects aforesaid shall for every such default forfeit a sum not exceeding two pounds; and every such clerk to the visitors shall be allowed such salary or remuneration for his services (to be paid out of the moneys or funds hereinafter mentioned) as the justices for the county or borough shall in general or quarter sessions direct.

Clerk of the Peace, or some other person, to be appointed to be clerk to visitors.

Oath of clerk. See § 6.

Remuneration of clerk to visitors.

22. And be it enacted, That if the clerk of any visitors shall at any time desire to employ an assistant in the execution

Provision for assistants to the clerk of the visitors.

of the duties of his office, such clerk shall certify such desire and the name of such assistant to one of the visitors, being a justice; and if such visitor shall approve thereof he shall administer the following oath to such assistant:—

Oath of assistant.

" I, *A. B.*, do solemnly swear, That I will faithfully keep secret all such matters and things as shall come to my knowledge in consequence of my employment as assistant to the clerk of the visitors appointed for the county [*or* borough] of   by virtue of an Act of Parliament passed in the ninth year of the reign of her Majesty Queen Victoria, intituled [*here insert the title of the Act*], unless required to divulge the same by legal authority.   " So help me GOD."

And such clerk may thereafter, at his own cost, employ such assistant.

Persons interested in any licensed house, or being medical attendant on any patient therein, disqualified to act as Commissioner, Visitor, Secretary, Clerk, or Assistant.

23. And be it enacted, That no person shall be or act as a Commissioner, or visitor, or secretary, or clerk to the Commissioners, or clerk or assistant clerk to any visitors, or act in granting any licence, who shall then be, or shall within one year then next preceding have been, directly or indirectly interested in any house licensed for the reception of lunatics, or the profits of such reception; and no physician or surgeon (being a Commissioner), and no physician, surgeon, or apothecary (being a visitor), shall sign any certificate for the admission of any patient into any licensed house or hospital,* or shall professionally attend upon any patient in any licensed house or hospital, unless he be directed to visit such patient by the person upon whose order such patient has been received into such licensed house or hospital, or by the Lord Chancellor, or her Majesty's Principal Secretary of State for the time being for the Home Department, or by a committee appointed by the Lord Chancellor; and if any such Commissioner, or visitor, or secretary, or clerk to the Commissioners, or clerk or assistant clerk to any visitors, shall after his appointment be or become so interested in any house licensed for the reception of lunatics, or the profits of such reception, such Commissioner, visitor, secretary, or clerk, or assistant clerk, as the case may be, shall immediately thereupon be disqualified from acting and shall cease to act in such capacity; and if any person, being disqualified as aforesaid, shall take the office of Com-

* Vide 25 & 26 Vict. c. 111, s. 24.

missioner, visitor, secretary, clerk, or assistant clerk, or being a Commissioner, visitor, secretary, clerk, or assistant clerk, shall become disqualified as aforesaid, and shall afterwards continue to act in such capacity, such person shall be guilty of a misdemeanour; and if any physician or surgeon (being a Commissioner), or any physician, surgeon, or apothecary (being a visitor), shall sign any certificate for the admission of any patient into any licensed house or hospital, or shall professionally attend any patient in any licensed house or hospital (except as aforesaid), such physician, surgeon, or apothecary (as the case may be) shall for each offence against this provision forfeit the sum of ten pounds.

Disqualified persons acting a misdemeanour.

Physicians, &c., contravening, penalty 10l.

24. And be it enacted, That every person * who shall desire to have a house licensed for the reception of lunatics shall give a notice, if such house be situate within the immediate jurisdiction of the Commissioners, to the Commissioners; and if elsewhere, to the Clerk of the Peace for the county or borough in which such house is situate, fourteen clear days at the least prior to some quarterly or other meeting of the Commissioners, or to some general or quarter sessions for such county or borough, as the case may be; and such notice shall contain the true Christian and surname, place of abode, and occupation of the person to whom the licence is desired to be granted, and a true and full description of his estate or interest in such house; and in case the person to whom the licence is desired to be granted does not propose to reside himself in the licensed house, the true Christian and surname and occupation of the superintendent who is to reside therein; and such notice, when given for any house which shall not have been previously licensed, shall be accompanied by a plan † of such house, to be drawn upon a scale of not less than one-eighth of an inch to a foot, with a description of the situation thereof, and the length, breadth, and height of and a reference by a figure or letter to, every room and apartment therein, and a statement of the quantity of land, not covered by any building, annexed to such house, and appropriated to the exclusive use, exercise, and recreation of the patients proposed to be received therein, and also a statement of the number of patients proposed to be received into such house, and whether the licence so ap-

Fourteen days' previous notice of intended application for and plan of licensed house to be given to the Commissioners or Clerk of the Peace.

---

* Vide 16 & 17 Vict. c. 96, ss. 1, 2.

† Vide 16 & 17 Vict. c. 96, s. 1, and 25 & 26 Vict. c. 111. s. 14.

plied for is for the reception of male or female patients, or of both; and if for the reception of both, of the number of each sex proposed to be received into such house, and of the means by which the one sex may be kept distinct and apart from the other; and such notice, plan, and statement, when sent to the Clerk of the Peace, shall be laid by him before the justices of the county or borough at such time as they shall take into their consideration the application for such licence : * Provided always, that it shall be lawful for any person to whom a licence shall be granted to remove the superintendent named in the notice, and at any time or times to appoint another superintendent, upon giving a notice containing the true Christian and surname and occupation of the new superintendent to the Commissioners or the visitors of the house, as the case may require : Provided always, that all plans heretofore delivered shall be deemed sufficient for the purposes of this Act, if the Commissioners or justices, as the case may be, shall so think fit.

Notice of all additions and alterations to be given to the Commissioners or Clerk of the Peace.

* 26. And be it enacted, That no addition or alteration shall be made to, in, or about any licensed house, or the appurtenances, unless previous notice in writing of such proposed addition or alteration, accompanied with a plan of such addition or alteration, to be drawn upon the scale aforesaid, and to be accompanied by such description as aforesaid,† shall have been given by the person to whom the licence shall have been granted to the Commissioners or to the Clerk of the Peace, as the case may be, and the consent in writing of the Commissioners, or of two of the visitors, as the case may be, shall have been previously given.

Untrue statement a misdemeanour.

27. And be it enacted, That if any person shall wilfully give an untrue or incorrect notice, plan, statement, or description of any of the things hereinbefore required to be included in any notice, plan, or statement, he shall be guilty of a misdemeanour.

A copy of every licence granted by Justices to be sent to the Commissioners.

28. And be it enacted, That in every case in which a licence for the reception of lunatics shall after the passing of this Act be granted by any justices, the Clerk of the Peace for the county or borough shall, within fourteen days after such licence shall have been granted, send a copy thereof to the

---

* Sec. 25 is repealed by 16 & 17 Vict. c. 96, s. 1.
† Vide 25 & 26 Vict. c. 111, s. 15.

Commissioners; and any Clerk of the Peace omitting to send such copy within such time shall for every such omission forfeit a sum not exceeding two pounds.

29. And be it enacted, That in every case in which any person shall apply for the renewal of a licence already granted or hereafter to be granted, such person, if applying to the Commissioners, shall with such application transmit to the Commissioners, and if applying to any justices * shall with such application transmit to the Clerk of the Peace for the county or borough, and also at the same time to the Commissioners, a statement signed by the person so applying, containing the names and number of the patients of each or either sex then detained in such house, and distinguishing whether such patients respectively are private or pauper patients; and any person who shall hereafter obtain the renewal of a licence without making such return or returns shall for every such offence forfeit the sum of ten pounds; and any person who shall make any such return untruly shall be guilty of a misdemeanour. *Every person applying for the renewal of a licence to furnish a statement of the number and class of patients then detained.*

30. And be it enacted, That every licence shall, as nearly as conveniently may be, be according to the form in the Schedule (A.) annexed to this Act,† and shall be stamped with a ten shilling stamp, and shall be under the seal of the Commissioners, if granted by them, and if by any justices under the hands and seals of three or more such justices in general or quarter sessions assembled, and shall be granted for such period, not exceeding thirteen calendar months, as the Commissioners or justices, as the case may be, shall think fit. *Licences to be made out in a given form, &c., and to be for not more than thirteen months.*

31. And be it enacted, That no licence shall be granted or visitor or clerk appointed by the justices for any borough without the consent in writing of the Recorder of such borough to such grant or appointment. *No licence, &c., in any borough without consent of Recorder.*

32. And be it enacted, That for every licence to be hereafter granted there shall be paid to the Secretary of the Commissioners, or to the Clerk of the Peace, according as the licence shall be granted by the Commissioners or justices (exclusive of the sum to be paid for the stamp) the sum of ten shillings and no more for every patient not being a pauper, and the sum of two shillings and sixpence and no more for every patient *Charge for licences to be granted in pursuance of this Act.*

* Vide 25 & 26 Vict. c. 111, s. 36.

† Vide Schedule (A) annexed to Act 25 & 26 Vict. c. 111, and s. 14 of that Act.

being a pauper, proposed to be received into such house, and if the total amount of such sums of ten shillings and two shillings and sixpence shall not amount to fifteen pounds, then so much more as shall make up the sum of fifteen pounds; and no such licence shall be delivered until the sum payable for

Power to reduce the charge for the licence in certain cases. the same shall be paid : Provided always, that if the period for which a licence shall be granted be less than thirteen calendar months it shall be lawful for the Commissioners or the justices, as the case may be, to reduce the payment to be made on such licence to any sum not less than five pounds.

Application of moneys received for licences by the secretary of the Commissioners. 33. And be it enacted, That all moneys received for licences granted by the Commissioners, and for searches made in pursuance of the provision for that purpose hereinafter contained, shall be retained by the Secretary of the Commissioners, and be applied by him in or towards the payment of the salaries and travelling and other expenses of the Commissioners and of their secretary and clerks, and in or towards the payment or discharge of all or any costs, charges, and expenses incurred by or under the authority of the Commissioners in the execution of or under or by virtue of this Act.

Secretary of the Commissioners to make out an annual account, to be laid before the Lords Commissioners of the Treasury, of all receipts and payments by him under this Act. 34. And be it enacted, That the Secretary of the Commissioners shall make out an account of all moneys received and paid by him as aforesaid, and of all moneys otherwise received and paid by him, and of all charges and expenses incurred under or by virtue of or in the execution of this Act; and such account shall be made up to the first day of August in each year, and shall be signed by five at least of the Commissioners; and such account shall specify the several heads of charge and expenditure, and shall be transmitted to the Lord High Treasurer, or to the Commissioners of her Majesty's Treasury, who shall thereupon audit such account, and, if he or they shall deem it expedient, direct the balance (if any) remaining in the hands of the said secretary to be paid into the Exchequer to the account of the Consolidated Fund; and such accounts shall be laid before Parliament on or before the twenty-fifth day of March in each year, if Parliament be then sitting, or if Parliament be not then sitting, then within one month after the then next sitting of Parliament.

Balance of payments over receipts may be paid out of the Consolidated Fund. 35. And be it enacted, That it shall be lawful for the Lord High Treasurer, or the Commissioners of her Majesty's Treasury, or any three or more of them, and they are hereby directed and empowered, from time to time (on an application to them, agreed to at some quarterly or other meeting of the Commissioners, attended by five at least of the Commissioners, and certified under their hands) to cause to be issued and paid out of the Consolidated Fund to the Secretary of the Commissioners such a sum of money as the Commissioners shall in such application have certified to be requisite to pay and discharge so much of the salaries, costs, charges, and expenses hereinbefore directed to be paid out of the moneys received by the said secretary for licences and otherwise as aforesaid as such moneys shall be inadequate to pay, and the said secretary shall thereupon apply such money in or towards the payment or discharge of such salaries, costs, charges, and expenses respectively; and that it shall be lawful for the Lord High Treasurer or the Commissioners of her Majesty's Treasury, or any three or more of them, from time to time to advance by way of imprest to the said secretary such sum or sums of money as to such Lord High Treasurer or Commissioners of her Majesty's Treasury may appear requisite and reasonable, for or towards the payment or discharge of all or any such salaries, costs, charges, or expenses as aforesaid, such sum or sums to be accounted for by the said secretary in his then next account.

36. And be it enacted, That all moneys to be received for licences granted by any justices shall be applied by the Clerk of the Peace for the county or borough in or towards the payment of the salary or remuneration of the clerk to the visitors for such county or borough, and in or towards the remuneration of such of the same visitors as are hereinbefore directed to be remunerated, and in or towards the payment or discharge of all costs, charges, and expenses incurred by or under the authority of the same justices or visitors in the execution of or under or by virtue of this Act. *Application of moneys received for licences by Clerks of the Peace.*

37. And be it enacted, That the Clerk of the Peace for every county or borough shall keep an account of all moneys received and paid by him as aforesaid, and of all moneys otherwise received or paid by him under or by virtue of or in the execution of this Act; and such account shall respectively be made up to the first day of August in each year, and shall be signed by two at least of the visitors for the county or borough; and every such account shall be laid by the Clerk of the Peace before the justices at the Michaelmas general or quarter sessions, who shall thereupon direct the balance (if any) remaining in the hands of the Clerk of the Peace to be paid into the *Clerks of the Peace to make out annual accounts, to be laid before the justices in session, of all receipts and payments made under this Act.*

hands of the treasurer for such county or borough, in aid and as part of the county or borough rate.

Balance of payments over receipts may be paid out of the funds of the county or borough.

38. And be it enacted, That it shall be lawful for the justices for any county or borough in general or quarter sessions assembled, if they shall think fit, to order to be paid to the Clerk of the Peace of such county or borough, out of the rates or funds thereof, such sum or sums of money as they shall, on examination, deem to be necessary to pay and discharge so much of the salary, remuneration, costs, charges, and expenses hereinbefore directed to be paid out of the moneys received by such Clerk of the Peace for licences and otherwise as aforesaid as such moneys shall be inadequate to pay; and also that it shall be lawful for the justices in general or quarter sessions assembled, if they shall think fit, from time to time to order to be advanced out of the rates or funds of such county or borough, to the Clerk of the Peace, such sum or sums of money as to such justices may appear requisite and reasonable, for or towards the payment or discharge of any such salary, remuneration, costs, charges, or expenses as last aforesaid; and every such sum of money as aforesaid shall be paid and advanced out of the rates or funds of such county or borough by the treasurer thereof, and shall be allowed in his accounts, on the authority of the aforesaid order by the justices for the payment or advance thereof.

Provision in case of the incapacity or death of the person licensed.

39. And be it enacted, That if any person to whom a licence shall have been granted under this Act or under any of the Acts hereinbefore repealed shall by sickness or other sufficient reason become incapable of keeping the licensed house, or shall die before the expiration of the licence, it shall be lawful for the Commissioners or for any three justices for the county or borough, as the case may be, if they shall respectively think fit, by writing endorsed on such licence, under the seal of the Commissioners or under the hands of such three justices, to transfer the said licence, with all the privileges and obligations annexed thereto, for the term then unexpired, to such person as shall at the time of such incapacity or death be the superintendent of such house, or have the care of the patients therein, or to such other person as the Commissioners or such justices respectively shall approve, and in the meantime such licence shall remain in force and have the same effect as if granted to the superintendent of the house; and in case a licence has been or shall be granted to two or more persons

and before the expiration thereof any or either of such persons shall die, leaving the other or others surviving, such licence shall remain in force and have the same effect as if granted to such survivors or survivor.*

40. And be it enacted, That if any licensed house shall be pulled down or occupied under the provisions of any Act of Parliament, or shall by fire, tempest, or other accident be rendered unfit for the accommodation of lunatics, or if the person keeping such house shall desire to transfer the patients to another house, it shall be lawful for the Commissioners (if the new house shall be within their immediate jurisdiction), at any quarterly or other meeting, or for any two or more of the visiting justices for the county or borough within which the new house is situate, as the case may be, upon the payment to the Secretary of the Commissioners or the Clerk of the Peace, as the case may be, of not less than one pound for the licence (exclusive of the sum to be paid for the stamp), to grant to the person whose house has been so pulled down, occupied, or so rendered unfit, or who shall desire to transfer his patients as aforesaid, a licence to keep such other house for the reception of lunatics, for such time as the Commissioners or the said justices, as the case may be shall think fit: Provided always, that the same notice of such intended change of house, and the same plans and statements and descriptions of and as to such intended new house, shall be given as are required when application is first made for a licence for any house,† and shall be accompanied by a statement in writing of the cause of such change of house; and that, except in cases in which the change of house is occasioned by fire or tempest, seven clear days' previous notice of the intended removal shall be sent, by the person to whom the licence for keeping the original house shall have been granted, to the person who signed the order for the reception of each patient, not being a pauper, or the person by whom the last payment on account of such patient shall have been made, and to the relieving officer or overseer of the union or parish to which each patient being a pauper is chargeable, or the person by whom the last payment on account of such patient shall have been made.

Provision in case of a licensed house being taken for public purposes, or accidentally rendered unfit, or of the keeper wishing to transfer his patients to a new house.

41. And be it enacted, That if a majority of the justices of

Power of revocation of licences granted by justices.

* Vide 16 & 17 Vict. c. 96, ss. 1, 2.
† Vide 16 & 17 Vict. c. 96, s. 1.

any county or borough in general or quarter sessions assembled shall recommend to the Lord Chancellor that any licence granted by the justices for such county or borough, either before or after the passing of this Act, shall be revoked, it shall be lawful for the Lord Chancellor to revoke the same by an instrument under his hand and seal, such revocation to take effect at a period to be named in such instrument, not exceeding two calendar months from the time a copy or notice thereof shall have been published in the " London Gazette ; " and a copy or notice of such instrument of revocation shall be published in the " London Gazette," and shall before such publication be transmitted to the person to whom such licence shall have been granted, or to the resident superintendent of the licensed house, or be left at the licensed house : Provided always, that in case of any such revocation being recommended to the Lord Chancellor, notice thereof in writing shall, seven clear days previously to the transmission of such recommendation to the Lord Chancellor, be given to the person the revocation of whose licence shall be recommended, or to the resident superintendent of the licensed house, or shall be left at the licensed house.

Power of revocation and of prohibition of renewal of licences granted by the Commissioners or by justices.

42. And be it enacted, That if the Commissioners shall recommend to the Lord Chancellor that any licence granted either by the Commissioners or by any justices, either before or after the passing of this Act, shall be revoked or shall not be renewed, it shall be lawful for the Lord Chancellor by an instrument under his hand and seal to revoke or prohibit the renewal of such licence ; and in the case of a revocation the same shall take effect at a period to be named in such instrument, not exceeding two calendar months from the time a copy or notice thereof shall have been published in the " London Gazette ; " and a copy or notice of such instrument of revocation shall be published in the " London Gazette," and shall before such publication be transmitted to the person to whom such licence shall have been granted, or to the resident superintendent of the licensed house, or shall be left at the licensed house : Provided always, that in case of any such revocation or prohibition to renew being recommended to the Lord Chancellor, notice thereof in writing shall, seven clear days previously to the transmission of such recommendation to the Lord Chancellor, be given to the person the revocation or prohibition of renewal of whose licence shall be recommended, or to the resident super-

intendent of the licensed house, or shall be left at the licensed house.

43. And be it enacted, That the regulations * as to lunatics of every hospital in which lunatics are or shall be received shall be printed, and complete copies thereof shall be sent to the Commissioners, and also kept hung up in the visitors' room of such hospital; and that every such hospital shall have a physician, surgeon, or apothecary resident therein, as the superintendent and medical attendant thereof; † and such superintendent shall, immediately after the passing of this Act (or immediately after the establishment of such hospital, as the case may be), apply to the Commissioners to have such hospital registered, and thereupon such hospital shall be registered in a book to be kept for that purpose by the Commissioners; and in case the superintendent of any such hospital shall at any time omit to have copies of such regulations sent or hung up as aforesaid, or to apply to have such hospital registered as aforesaid, he shall for every such omission forfeit a sum not exceeding twenty pounds. *(Hospitals receiving lunatics to have their regulations printed, and a resident medical attendant, and to be registered.)*

44. And be it enacted, That after the passing of this Act it shall not be lawful for any person to receive two or more lunatics into any house, unless such house shall be an asylum or an hospital registered under this Act, or a house for the time being duly licensed under this Act, or one of the Acts hereinbefore repealed; and any person who shall receive two or more lunatics into any house other than a house for the time being duly licensed as aforesaid, or an asylum or an hospital duly registered under this Act, shall be guilty of a misdemeanour. *(No house to be kept for the reception of two or more lunatics without a licence.)*

‡ 50. And be it enacted, That every proprietor or superintendent who shall receive any patient into any licensed house or any hospital shall, within two days after reception of such patient, make an entry with respect to such patient in a book to be kept for that purpose to be called "The Book of Admissions," according to the form and containing the particulars required in Schedule (E) annexed to this Act, so far as he can ascertain the same, except as to the form of the mental disorder, and except also as to the discharge or death of the *(Every person receiving a person as a lunatic into any house or hospital to make an entry thereof in a certain form.)*

* Vide 16 & 17 Vict. c. 96, s. 30.

† Vide 16 & 17 Vict. c. 96, s. 36.

‡ Ss. 45, 46, 47, 48, 49 are all repealed by 16 & 17 Vict. c. 96, s. 3.

patient, which shall be made when the same shall happen; and every person who shall so receive any such patient, and shall not within two days thereafter make such entry as aforesaid (except as aforesaid), shall forfeit a sum not exceeding two pounds; and every person who shall knowingly and willingly in any such entry untruly set forth any of the particulars shall be guilty of a misdemeanour.

Form of patient's disorder to be entered in "The Book of Admissions" by the medical attendant.

51. And be it enacted, That the form of the mental disorder of every patient received into any licensed house or any hospital shall, within seven days after his reception, be entered in the said Book of Admissions by the medical attendant of such house or hospital; and every such medical attendant who shall omit to make any such entry within the time aforesaid shall for every such offence forfeit a sum not exceeding two pounds.

Every person receiving a patient into any house or hospital to transmit a notice thereof to the Commissioners, and if within the jurisdiction of any visitors, then also to the clerk of such visitors.

52. And be it enacted, That the proprietor or resident superintendent of every licensed house (whether licensed by the Commissioners or by any justices), and the superintendent of every hospital, shall after two clear days, and before the expiration of seven clear days * from the day on which any patient shall have been received into such house or hospital, transmit a copy of the order and medical certificates or certificate on which such person shall have been received, and also a notice and statement according to the form in Schedule (F) annexed to this Act, to the Commissioners; and the proprietor or resident superintendent of every house licensed within the jurisdiction of any visitors shall also within the same period transmit another copy of such order and certificates or certificate, and a duplicate of such notice and statement, to the clerk of the visitors; and every proprietor or superintendent of any such house or hospital who shall neglect to transmit such copy, notice, or statement to the Commissioners, or (where the same is required) to the clerk of the visitors, shall be guilty of a misdemeanour.

Notices to be given in case of the escape of any patient, and of his being brought back.

53. And be it enacted, That whenever any patient shall escape from any licensed house or any registered hospital the proprietor or superintendent of such house or hospital shall, within two clear days next after such escape, transmit a written notice thereof to the Commissioners; and if such house be

* Vide 25 & 26 Vict. c. 111, s. 28. By this it is seen that the medical certificates must now be forwarded within twenty-four hours from patient's admission.

within the jurisdiction of any visitors, then also to the clerk of such visitors; and such notice shall state the Christian and surname of the patient who has so escaped, and his then state of mind, and also the circumstances connected with such escape; and if such patient shall be brought back to such house or hospital,* such proprietor or resident superintendent shall, within two clear days next after such person shall be so brought back, transmit a written notice thereof to the Commissioners; and also, if such house be within the jurisdiction of any visitors, to the clerk of such visitors; and such notice shall state when such person was so brought back, and the circumstances connected therewith, and whether with or without a fresh order and certificates or certificate; and every proprietor or resident superintendent omitting to transmit such notice, whether of escape or of return, shall for every such omission forfeit a sum not exceeding ten pounds.

54. And be it enacted, That whenever any patient shall be removed or discharged from any licensed house or any hospital, or shall die therein, the proprietor or superintendent of such house or hospital shall, within two clear days next after such removal, discharge, or death, make an entry thereof in a book to be kept for that purpose according to the form and stating the particulars in Schedule (G 1) annexed to this Act, and shall also within the same two days transmit a written notice† thereof, and also of the cause of his death, to the Commissioners, and also, if such house shall be within the jurisdiction of any visitors, to the clerk of such visitors, according to the form and containing the particulars in Schedule (G 2) annexed to this Act; and every proprietor or superintendent of any such house or hospital who shall neglect to make such entry or transmit such notice or notices, or shall therein set forth any thing untruly, shall be guilty of a misdemeanour.

Entry to be made, and notice given, in case of the death, discharge, or removal of any patient.

55. And be it enacted, That in case of the death of any patient in any licensed house or any hospital, a statement of the cause of the death of such patient, with the name of any person present at the death, shall be drawn up and signed by the medical attendant of such house or hospital,‡ and a copy thereof, duly certified by the proprietor or superintendent of such house or hospital, shall by him be transmitted to the Commissioners, and also to the person signing the order for

In case of the death of a patient, a statement of the cause of death to be transmitted to the Commissioners, and, if within the jurisdiction of any visitors, to the clerk of the visitors also.

* Vide 25 & 26 Vict. c. 111, s. 39.
† Vide 16 & 17 Vict. c. 96, s. 19.   ‡ Ibid.

Y

such patient's confinement, and to the registrar of deaths for the district, and if such house be within the jurisdiction of any visitors, then also to the clerk of such visitors, within forty-eight hours after the death of such patient; and every medical attendant, proprietor, or superintendent who shall neglect or omit to draw up, sign, certify, or transmit such statement as aforesaid shall for every such neglect or omission forfeit and pay a sum not exceeding fifty pounds.

Abuse or ill-treatment or neglect of a patient to be treated as a misdemeanour.

56. And be it enacted, That if any superintendent, officer, nurse, attendant, servant, or other person employed in any licensed house or registered hospital shall in any way abuse or ill-treat any patient confined therein, or shall wilfully neglect any such patient, he shall be deemed guilty of a misdemeanour;* and that in the event of the release of any person from confinement in any asylum or private house who shall consider himself to have been unjustly confined, a copy of the certificates and order upon which he has been confined shall at his request be furnished to him or to his attorney by the clerk to the Commissioners, without any fee or reward for the same; and it shall be lawful for the Home Secretary, on the report of the Commissioners or visitors of any asylums, to direct her Majesty's Attorney-General to prosecute on the part of the Crown any person who shall have been concerned in the unlawful taking or confinement of any of her Majesty's subjects as an insane patient, and likewise any person who shall have been concerned in the neglect or ill-treatment of any patient or person so confined.

Houses having 100 patients to have a resident medical attendant, and houses having less to be visited by a medical attendant.

57. And be it enacted, That in every house licensed for one hundred patients or more there shall be a physician, surgeon, or apothecary resident as the superintendent or medical attendant thereof: and that every house licensed for less than one hundred and more than fifty patients (in case such house shall not be kept by or have a resident physician, surgeon, or apothecary †) shall be visited daily by a physician, surgeon, or apothecary; and that every house licensed for less than fifty patients (in case such house shall not be kept by or have a resident physician, surgeon, or apothecary) shall be visited twice in every week by a physician, surgeon, or apothe-

* Vide 16 & 17 Vict. c. 96. ss. 9, 26.

† Vide 25 & 26 Vict. c. 111, s. 47. The medical attendant *must* be registered under the Medical Act.

cary: Provided always, that it shall be lawful for the visitors of any licensed house to direct that such house, and for the Commissioners to direct that any licensed house, shall be visited by a physician, surgeon, or apothecary at any other time or times, not being oftener than once in every day.

58. Provided always, and be it enacted, That when any house is licensed to receive less than eleven lunatics it shall be lawful for any two of the Commissioners or any two of the visitors of such house, if they shall respectively so think fit, by any writing under their hands, to permit that such house shall be visited by a physician, surgeon, or apothecary at such intervals more distant than twice in every week as such Commissioners or visitors shall appoint, but not at a greater interval than once in every two weeks. *The Commissioners and visitors, in houses licensed for less than 11 persons, may lessen the number of medical visits.*

59. And be it enacted, That every physician, surgeon, or apothecary, where there shall be only one, keeping or residing in or visiting any licensed house or any hospital, and where there shall be two or more physicians, surgeons, or apothecaries keeping or residing in or visiting any licensed house or any hospital, then one at least of such physicians, surgeons, or apothecaries shall once in every week (or, in the case of any house at which visits at more distant intervals than once a week are permitted, on every visit) enter and sign in a book to be kept at such house or hospital for that purpose, to be called "The Medical Visitation Book," a report, showing the date thereof, and also the number, sex, and state of health of all the patients then in such house or hospital, the Christian and surname of every patient who shall have been under restraint or in seclusion, or under medical treatment, since the date of the last preceding report, the condition of the house or hospital, and every death, injury, and act of violence which shall have happened to or affected any patient since the then last preceding report, according to the form in Schedule* (H) annexed to this Act; and every such physician, surgeon, or apothecary who shall omit to enter or sign such report as aforesaid shall for every such omission forfeit and pay the sum of twenty pounds; and every such physician, surgeon, or apothecary who shall in any such report as aforesaid enter any thing untruly shall be guilty of a misdemeanour. *A book to be kept, to be called "The Medical Visitation Book," in which a weekly entry is to be made, showing the condition of the house and of the patients.*

60. And be it enacted, That there shall be kept in every licensed house and in every hospital a book to be called "The *A medical case book to be kept.*

* This form is altered. Vide 16 & 17 Vict. c. 96, s. 25.

Y 2

Case Book," in which the physician, surgeon, or apothecary
keeping or residing in or visiting such house or hospital shall
from time to time make entries of the mental state and bodily
condition of each patient, together with a correct description
of the medicine and other remedies prescribed for the treatment of his disorder; and that it shall be lawful for the Commissioners from time to time, by any order under their common
seal, to direct the form in which such case book shall be kept
by such physician, surgeon, or apothecary; and immediately
after a copy of such order shall have been transmitted by the
Secretary of the Commissioners to such physician, surgeon, or
apothecary, such physician, surgeon, or apothecary shall thereupon keep such case book in the form which shall be directed
by such order; and that it shall be lawful for the Commissioners (whenever they shall see fit) to require, by an order in
writing under their common seal, such physician, surgeon, or
apothecary to transmit to the Commissioners a correct copy
of the entries or entry in any case book kept under the provisions of this Act, relative to the case of any lunatic who is
or may have been confined in any such licensed house or hospital; and every such physician, surgeon, or apothecary who
shall neglect to keep the said case book, or to keep the same
according to the form directed by the Commissioners, or to
transmit a copy of the said entry or entries, pursuant to such
order or orders as aforesaid, shall for every such neglect forfeit
any sum not exceeding ten pounds.

All licensed houses and hospitals to be visited by the Com-missioners.

61. And be it enacted, That every * licensed house shall,
without any previous notice, be visited by two at least of the
Commissioners (one of whom shall be a physician or surgeon,
and the other a barrister) four times at the least in every year,
if such house shall be within the immediate jurisdiction of the
Commissioners, and if not, twice at least in every year; and
every † hospital in which lunatics shall be received shall, without any previous notice, be visited by two at least of the said
Commissioners (one of whom shall be a physician or surgeon,
and the other a barrister) once at least in every year; and
every such visit shall be made on such day or days, and at
such hours of the day, and for such length of time, as the
visiting Commissioners shall think fit, and also at such other

---

* Vide 25 & 26 Vict. c. 111, s. 29.

† Vide 25 & 26 Vict. c. 111, s. 30.

times (if any) as the said Commissioners in Lunacy shall direct; and such visiting Commissioners, when visiting such house or hospital, may and shall inspect every part of such house or hospital, and every outhouse, place, and building communicating with such house or hospital, or detached therefrom, but not separated by ground belonging to any other person, and every part of the ground or appurtenances held, used, or occupied therewith, and see every patient then confined in such house or hospital, and inquire whether any patient is under restraint, and why, and inspect the order and certificates or certificate for the reception of every patient who shall have been received into such house or hospital since the last visit of the Commissioners, and in the case of any house licensed by justices shall consider the observations made in the Visitors' Book for such house by the visitors appointed by the justices, and enter in the Visitors' Book of such house or hospital a minute of the then condition of the house or hospital, and of the patients therein, and the number of patients under restraint, with the reasons thereof, as stated, and such irregularity (if any) as may exist in any such order or certificates aforesaid, and also whether the previous suggestions (if any) of the visiting Commissioners or visitors have or have not been attended to, and any observations which they may deem proper as to any of the matters aforesaid or otherwise, and also, if such visit be the first after the granting a licence to the house, shall examine such licence, and, if the same be in conformity with the provisions of this Act, sign the same, but if it be informal, enter in such Visitors' Book in what respect such licence is informal : Provided also, that it shall be lawful for the Lord Chancellor, on a representation by the Commissioners setting forth the expediency of such alteration, by any writing under his hand, to direct that any house licensed by justices shall (during such period as he shall therein specify, or until such his direction shall be revoked) be visited by the Commissioners once only in the year, and also to direct that any house licensed by the Commissioners, and not receiving any pauper patients therein, shall (during such period as he shall therein specify, or until such his direction shall be revoked) be visited by the Commissioners twice only in the year.

62. And be it enacted, That every licensed house within the jurisdiction of any visitors appointed by justices shall be visited by two at least of the said visitors (one of whom shall

Licensed houses not within the immediate

jurisdiction of the Commissioners to be inspected four times a year at least by the visitors.

be a physician, surgeon, or apothecary) four times at the least in every year, on such days, and at such hours in the day, and for such length of time as the said visitors shall think fit, and also at such other times (if any) as the justices by whom such house shall have been licensed shall direct; and such visitors when visiting any such house may and shall inspect every part of such house, and every house, outhouse, place, and building communicating therewith, or detached therefrom, but not separated by ground belonging to any other person, and every part of the ground or appurtenances held, used, or occupied therewith, and see every patient then confined therein, and inquire whether any patient is under restraint, and why, and inspect the order and certificates or certificate for the reception of every patient who shall have been received into such house since the last visit of the visitors, and enter in the Visitors' Book a minute of the then condition of the house, of the patients therein, and the number of patients under restraint, with the reasons thereof as stated, and such irregularity (if any) as may exist in any such order or certificates as aforesaid, and also whether the previous suggestions (if any) of the visitors or visiting Commissioners have or have not been attended to, and any observations which they may deem proper as to any of the matters aforesaid or otherwise.

The proprietors or superintendent of every house and hospital to show every part and every patient to the visiting Commissioners and visitors.

63. And be it enacted, That the proprietor or superintendent of every licensed house or hospital shall show to the Commissioners and visitors * respectively visiting the same every part thereof respectively, and every person detained therein as a lunatic; and every proprietor or superintendent of any licensed house or any hospital who shall conceal or attempt to conceal, or shall refuse or wilfully neglect to show, any part of such house or hospital, or any house, outhouse, place, or building communicating therewith, or detached therefrom, but not separated as aforesaid, or any part of the ground or appurtenances held, used, or occupied therewith, or any person detained or being therein, from any visiting Commissioners or visitors, or from any person authorised under any power or provision of this Act to visit and inspect such house or hospital, or the patients confined therein, or any of them, shall be guilty of a misdemeanour.

64. And be it enacted, That the visiting Commissioners

* Vide 25 & 26 Vict. c. 111, ss. 29, 30.

and visitors respectively, upon their several visitations to every licensed house and to every hospital, shall inquire when divine service is performed, and to what number of the patients, and the effect thereof; and also what occupations or amusements are provided for the patients, and the result thereof; and whether there has been adopted any system of non-coercion, and if so, the result thereof; and also as to the classification of patients; and also as to the condition of the pauper patients (if any) when first received; and also as to the dietary of the pauper patients (if any); and shall also make such other inquiries as to such visiting Commissioners or visitors shall seem expedient; * and every proprietor or superintendent of a licensed house or an hospital who shall not give full and true answers to the best of his knowledge to all questions which the visiting Commissioners and visitors respectively shall ask in reference to the matters aforesaid shall be guilty of a misdemeanour.

Inquiries to be made by the Commissioners and visitors on their several visitations.

65. And be it enacted, That upon every visit of the visiting Commissioners to any licensed house or to any hospital, and upon every visit of the visitors to any licensed house, there shall be laid before such visiting Commissioners or visitors (as the case may be), by the proprietor or superintendent of such licensed house, or of such hospital, a list of all the patients then in such house or hospital (distinguishing pauper patients from other patients, and males from females, and specifying such as are deemed curable), and also the several books by this Act required to be kept by the proprietor or superintendent and by the medical attendant of a licensed house or an hospital, and also all orders and certificates relating to patients admitted since the last visitation of the Commissioners or visitors (as the case may be), and also, in the case of a licensed house, the licence then in force for such house, and also all such other orders, certificates, documents, and papers relating to any of the patients at any time received into such licensed house or hospital as the visiting Commissioners or visitors shall from time to time require to be produced to them; and the said visiting Commissioners or visitors, as the case may be, shall sign the said books as having been produced to them.

Books and documents to be produced to visiting Commissioners and visitors.

66. And be it enacted, That there shall be hung up in some conspicuous part of every licensed house a copy of the

A book to be kept called "The Visitors' Book,"

* Vide 25 & 26 Vict. c. 111, s. 35.

plan given to the Commissioners or justices on applying for the licence of such house ; and that there shall be kept in every licensed house and in every hospital in which lunatics shall be received a Queen's Printer's copy of this * Act, bound up in a book to be called " The Visitors' Book ; " and that the said visiting Commissioners and visitors respectively shall at the time of their respective visitations enter therein the result of the inspections and inquiries hereinbefore directed or authorised to be made by them respectively, with such observations (if any) as they shall think proper ; and that there shall also be kept in every such house and hospital a book to be called " The Patients' Book," and that the said visiting Commissioners and visitors respectively shall at the times of their respective visitations enter therein such observations as they may think fit respecting the state of mind or body of any patient in such house or hospital.

67. And be it enacted, That the proprietor or resident superintendent of every licensed house and of every hospital shall, within three days after every such visit by the visiting Commissioners † as aforesaid, transmit a true and perfect copy of the entries made by them in " The Visitors' Book," " The Patients' Book," and " The Medical Visitation Book," respectively (distinguishing the entries in the several books), to the Commissioners, and shall, within three days after every such visitation by the visitors, transmit a true and perfect copy of the entries made by them as aforesaid (distinguishing as aforesaid) to the Commissioners and also to the clerk of the visitors : and the copies so transmitted to the clerk of the visitors of all such entries relating to any licensed house, and made since the grant or last renewal of the licence thereof, shall be laid before the justices on taking into consideration the renewal of the licence to the house to which such entries shall relate ; ‡ and every such proprietor or superintendent as aforesaid who shall omit to transmit, as hereinbefore directed, a true and perfect copy of every or any such entry as aforesaid shall for every such omission forfeit a sum not exceeding ten pounds.

68. And be it enacted, That the Commissioners visiting any house licensed by justices shall carefully consider and

---

* Vide 16 & 17 Vict. c. 96, s. 37.

† Vide 25 & 26 Vict. c. 111, ss. 29, 30.

‡ Vide 25 & 26 Vict. c. 111, s. 36.

give special attention to the state of mind of any patient therein confined, as to the propriety of whose detention they shall doubt (or as to whose sanity their attention shall be specially called), and shall, if they shall think that the state of mind of such patient is doubtful, and that the propriety of his detention requires further consideration, make and sign a minute thereof in the Patients' Book of such house; and a true and perfect copy of every such minute shall, within two clear days after the same shall have been made, be sent by the proprietor or superintendent of such house to the clerk of the visitors of such house, and such clerk shall forthwith communicate the same to the said visitors, or some two of them (of whom a physician, surgeon, or apothecary shall be one), and such visitors shall thereupon immediately visit such patient, and act as they shall see fit; and every such proprietor or superintendent who shall omit to send a true and perfect copy, as hereinbefore directed, of every or any such last-mentioned minute, and every clerk who shall neglect to communicate the same to two of the visitors as aforesaid, shall be guilty of a misdemeanour.

69. And be it enacted, That the visiting Commissioners shall, after every visitation by them to every licensed house not being within their immediate jurisdiction, and to every hospital, report in writing the general result of their inspection thereof (together with such special circumstances, if any, as they may deem proper to notice) to the Commissioners; and the Secretary of the Commissioners shall thereupon enter the same in a book to be kept for that purpose.

70. And be it enacted, That it shall be lawful for the Commissioners, or any five of them, at any quarterly or special meeting, by any resolution or resolutions under their common seal, or to be entered in a book to be kept for that purpose, and signed by five at least of the Commissioners present at such meeting, from time to time to make such orders and rules as they shall think fit for regulating the duties of the Commissioners, or any of them, or of their secretary, clerks, and servants, or for the due or better performance of the business of the Commission: Provided nevertheless, that the Secretary of the Commissioners shall give to every Commissioner, so far as circumstances will admit, not less than seven days' notice of every such special meeting, and shall in the sum-

mons for such special meeting state the purposes for which the same is intended to be held.

Power in certain cases to visit by night.

71. And be it enacted, That it shall be lawful for any two or more of the Commissioners, or any two visitors, to visit and to inspect any licensed house or hospital at such hour of the night as they shall think fit: Provided nevertheless, that no such visitor shall make any such visitation or inspection except of a licensed house within their jurisdiction.

The person who signed the order for the reception of a private patient may order his discharge or removal.

72. And be it enacted, That if and when any person who signed the order on which any patient (not being a pauper) was received into any licensed house or into any hospital shall by writing under his hand direct that such patient shall be discharged or removed, then and in such case such patient shall forthwith be discharged or removed, as the person who signed the order for his reception shall direct.*

Provision for the discharge of a private patient when the person who signed the order for his reception is incapable.

73. And be it enacted, That if the person who signed the order on which any patient (not being a pauper) was received into any licensed house or into any hospital be incapable by reason of insanity or absence from England, or otherwise, of giving an order for the discharge or removal of such patient, or if such person be dead, then and in any of such cases the husband or wife of such patient, or if there be no such husband or wife, the father of such patient, or if there be no father, the mother of such patient, or if there be no mother, then any one of the nearest of kin for the time being of such patient, or the person who made the last payment on account of such patient, may by any writing under his or her hand give such direction as aforesaid for the discharge or removal of such patient, and thereupon such patient shall be forthwith discharged or removed as the person giving such direction shall direct.†

Mode of removal or discharge of pauper patients.

74. And be it enacted, That the guardians of any parish or union may by a minute of their board, or an officiating clergyman of any parish not under a Board of Guardians, and one of the overseers thereof, or any two justices of the county or borough in which such last-mentioned parish is situate, may by writing under the hands respectively of such clergyman and overseer, or of such justices direct that any pauper patient belonging to such parish or union, and detained in any licensed house or any hospital, shall be discharged or removed there-

* Vide 16 & 17 Vict. c. 96. ss. 19, 20, and 25 & 26 Vict. c. 111, s. 43.   † Ibid.

from, and may direct the mode of such discharge or removal; and if a copy of such minute or such writing be produced to the proprietor or superintendent of such licensed house or such hospital, he shall forthwith discharge or remove such patient, or cause or suffer such patient to be discharged or removed accordingly.*

75. Provided always, nevertheless, and be it enacted, That no patient shall be discharged or removed, under any of the powers hereinbefore contained, from any licensed house or any hospital, if the physician, surgeon, or apothecary by whom the same shall be kept, or who shall be the regular medical attendant thereof, shall by writing under his hand certify that in his opinion such patient is dangerous and unfit to be at large, together with the grounds on which such opinion is founded, unless the Commissioners visiting such house or the visitors of such house shall, after such certificate shall have been produced to them, give their consent in writing that such patient shall be discharged and removed : Provided that nothing herein contained shall prevent any patient from being transferred from any licensed house or any hospital to any other licensed house or any other hospital, or to any asylum, but in such case every such patient shall be placed under the control of an attendant† belonging to the licensed house, hospital, or asylum to or from which he shall be about to be removed for the purpose of such removal, and shall remain under such control until such time as such removal shall be duly effected.

No patient to be removed under any of the preceding powers, if certified to be dangerous, unless the Commissioners or visitors consent, or for the purpose of transfer to some other asylum.

76. And be it enacted, That it shall be lawful for any two or more of the Commissioners to make visits to any patient detained in any house licensed by the Commissioners, on such days and at such hours as they shall think fit; and if after two distinct and separate visits so made (seven days at least to intervene between such visits) it shall appear to such visiting Commissioners that such patient is detained without sufficient cause, it shall be lawful for the Commissioners, if they shall think fit, to make such order as to the Commissioners shall seem meet for the discharge of such patient, and such patient shall be discharged accordingly.

Commissioners may discharge any patient confined in a house licensed by themselves.

77. And be it enacted, That it shall be lawful for any two or more of the Commissioners, of whom one shall be a physi-

Two Commissioners may make

* Vide 16 & 17 Vict. c. 96, s. 19.
† Vide 16 & 17 Vict. c. 96, s. 36.

special visits to discharge any patient confined in a house licensed by justices or in an hospital.

cian and one a barrister, to make special visits to any patient detained in any house licensed by the justices, or in any hospital, on such days and at such hours as they shall think fit; and if after two distinct and separate visits so made it shall appear to such visiting Commissioners that such patient is detained without sufficient cause, they may make such order as to them shall seem meet for the discharge of such patient, and such patient shall be discharged accordingly.

Similar powers for two visitors as to houses within their jurisdiction.

78. And be it enacted, That it shall be lawful for any two or more of the visitors of any licensed house, of whom one shall be a physician, surgeon, or apothecary, to make special visits to any patient detained in such house, on such days and at such hours as they shall think fit; and if after two distinct and separate visits so made it shall appear to such visitors that such patient is detained without sufficient cause, they may make such order as to them shall seem meet for the discharge of such patient, and such patient shall be discharged accordingly.

Every order for the discharge of a patient under the last preceding powers to be signed by the persons exercising them, and to be subject to certain restrictions.

79. Provided always, and be it enacted, That every such order by any Commissioners or visitors for the discharge of a patient from any house licensed by justices, or from any hospital, shall be signed by them, and that each of such special visits shall be by the same Commissioners or visitors; and that it shall not be lawful for such Commissioners or visitors to order the discharge of any patient from any such last-mentioned house or hospital without having previously, if the medical attendant of such house or hospital shall have tendered himself for that purpose, examined him as to his opinion respecting the fitness of such patient to be discharged; and if such Commissioners or visitors shall, after so examining such medical attendant discharge such patient, and such medical attendant shall furnish them with any statement in writing containing his reasons against the discharge of such patient, they shall forthwith transmit such statement to the Commissioners or to the clerk of the visitors, as the case may require, to be kept and registered in a book for that purpose.

The last preceding powers to be exercised under certain other restrictions.

80. Provided also, and be it enacted, That not less than seven days shall intervene between the first and second of such special visits; and that such Commissioners or visitors shall, seven days previously to the second of such special visits, give notice thereof, either by post or by an entry in the Patients' Book, to the proprietor or superintendent of the house

licensed by justices or of the hospital in which the patient intended to be visited is detained; and that such proprietor or superintendent shall forthwith, if possible, transmit by post a copy of such notice, in the case of a patient not being a pauper, to the person by whose authority such patient was received into such house, or by whom the last payment on account of such patient was made, and in the case of a pauper, to the guardians of his parish or union, or if there be no such guardians, to one of the overseers for the time being of his parish, and also in the case of any patient detained in a house licensed by justices, to the clerk of the visitors of such house.

81. Provided always, nevertheless, and be it enacted, That none of the powers of discharge hereinbefore contained shall extend to any person who shall have been found lunatic by inquisition or under any inquiry directed by the Lord Chancellor, in pursuance of the powers in that behalf hereinafter given to him, nor to any lunatic confined under any order or authority of her Majesty's Principal Secretary of State for the Home Department, or under the order of any court of criminal jurisdiction. *Preceding powers not to extend to persons found lunatic by inquisition, or confined under authority of Secretary of State.*

82. And be it enacted, That it shall be lawful for the visitors of any licensed house at any time to determine and regulate the dietary of the pauper patients therein; and that it shall be lawful for the visiting Commissioners at any time to determine and regulate the dietary of the pauper patients in any licensed house or in any hospital; and that if such determination and regulation of any visitors and of the visiting Commissioners shall not agree with each other, then the determination and regulation of the visiting Commissioners shall be followed: Provided always, nevertheless, that every such regulation shall be made to take effect only from such time as not to affect any contract existing on the first day of June last for the maintenance of pauper patients before the first day of June One thousand eight hundred and forty-six, or the expiration of such contract, whichever shall first happen. *Power for visitors and visiting Commissioners to regulate the dietary of pauper patients.*

83. And be it enacted, That if any person shall apply to any visitor in order to be informed whether any particular person is confined in any licensed house within the jurisdiction of such visitor, the said visitor, if he shall think it reasonable to permit such inquiry to be made, shall sign an order to the clerk of the visitors, and the said clerk shall, on receipt of such order, and on payment to him of a sum not exceeding *Power for any visitors to give an order or the clerk of the visitors to search and give information.*

seven shillings for his trouble, make search amongst the
returns made to him in pursuance of this Act whether the
person inquired after is or has been within the then last twelve
calendar months confined in any licensed house within the
jurisdiction of such visitor; and if it shall appear that such
person is or has been so confined, the said clerk shall deliver
to the person so applying a statement in writing, specifying
the situation of the house in which the person so inquired
after appears to be or to have been confined, and of the name of
the proprietor or resident superintendent thereof, and also the
date of the admission of such person into such licensed house,
and (in case of his having been removed or discharged) the
date of his removal or discharge therefrom.

Power for
any Com-
missioner
to give an
order to the
Secretary of
the Com-
missioners
to search
and give
information
whether any
particular
person is or
has been
within
twelve
months con-
fined in any
house or
hospital.
84. And be it enacted, That if any person shall apply to
any Commissioner in order to be informed whether any particular person is confined in any licensed house, or in any
hospital, asylum, or other place by this Act made subject to
the visitation of the Commissioners, such Commissioner, if he
shall think it reasonable to permit such inquiry to be made,
shall sign an order to the Secretary of the Commissioners, and
the secretary shall, on the receipt of such order, and on payment to him of a sum not exceeding seven shillings (to be
applied as hereinbefore provided), make search amongst the
returns made in pursuance of this Act, or of any of the Acts
hereby repealed, whether the person inquired after is or has
been within the last twelve calendar months confined in any
house, hospital, asylum, or place by this Act made subject to
the visitation of the Commissioners; and if it shall appear that
such person is or has been so confined, the secretary shall
deliver to the person so applying a statement in writing,
specifying the situation of the house, hospital, asylum, or
place in which the person so inquired after appears to be or to
have been confined, and also (so far as the said secretary can
ascertain the same from any register or return in his possession)
the name of the proprietor, superintendent, or principal officer
of such house, hospital, asylum, or place, and also the date of
the admission of such person into such licensed house, hospital,
asylum, or other place, and (in case of his having been removed or discharged) the date of his removal or discharge
therefrom.

Any one
Commis-
sioner or
85. And be it enacted, That it shall be lawful for any one
of the Commissioners, as to patients confined in any house,

hospital, or other place (not being a gaol) hereby authorised to be visited by the Commissioners, and also for any one of the visitors of any licensed house, as to patients confined in such house, at any time to give an order in writing under the hand of such one Commissioner or visitor for the admission to any patient of any relation or friend of such patient (or of any medical or other person whom any relation or friend of such patient shall desire to be admitted to him), and such order of admission may be either for a single admission, or for an admission for any limited number of times, or for admission generally at all reasonable times, and either with or without any restriction as to such admission or admissions being in the presence of a keeper or not, or otherwise ; and if the proprietor or superintendent of any such house, hospital, or place shall refuse admission to, or shall prevent or obstruct the admission to any patient of, any relation, friend, or other person who shall produce such order of admission as aforesaid, he shall for every such refusal, prevention, or obstruction forfeit a sum not exceeding twenty pounds. *visitor may give an order for the admission to any patient of any friend or relation, or any person named by a friend or relation.*

86. And be it enacted, That it shall be lawful for the proprietor or superintendent of any licensed house or of any hospital, with the consent in writing of any two of the Commissioners, or in the case of a house licensed by justices, of any two of the visitors of such house, to send or take, under proper control, any patient to any specified place for any definite time for the benefit of his health :* Provided always, nevertheless, that before any such consent as aforesaid shall be given by any Commissioners or visitors the approval in writing of the person who signed the order for the reception of such patient, or by whom the last payment on account of such patient was made, shall be produced to such Commissioners or visitors, unless they shall, on cause being shown, dispense with the same. *Proprietor or superintendent, with consent of two Commissioners or visitors, may take or send a patient to any place for his health.*

87. And be it enacted, That in every case in which any patient shall under any of the powers or provisions of this Act, be removed temporarily from the house or hospital into which the order for his reception was given,† or be transferred from such house or hospital into any new house, and also in every case in which any patient shall escape from any house or hospital, and shall be retaken within fourteen days *In case of the removal of a patient, or of his escape and recapture within fourteen days, the original order for his reception to remain in force.*

* Vide 25 & 26 Vict. c. 111, s. 38.

next after such escape,* the certificate or certificates relating to and the original order for the reception of such patient shall respectively remain in force, in the same manner as the same would have done if such patient had not been so removed or transferred, or had not so escaped and been retaken.

Commissioners to report to the Lord Chancellor periodically.

88. And be it enacted, That the Commissioners shall, at the expiration of every six calendar months, report to the Lord Chancellor the number of visits which they shall have made, the number of patients whom they shall have seen, and the number of miles which they shall have travelled during such months, and shall on the first day of January in each year make a return to the Lord Chancellor of all sums received by them for travelling expenses, or upon any other and what account, and shall also in the month of June † in every year make to the Lord Chancellor a report of the state and condition of the several houses, hospitals, asylums, and other places visited by them under this Act, and of the care of the patients therein, and of such other particulars as they shall think deserving of notice ; and a true copy of such reports, showing the number of visits made, the number of patients seen, and the number of miles travelled, and also a copy of such return of sums received for travelling expenses, or on any other and what account, shall be laid before Parliament within twenty-one days next after the commencement of every Session of Parliament.

Constitution of the private committee.

89. And be it enacted, That the permanent chairman for the time being of the Commissioners, and two other of the Commissioners to be appointed by the Lord Chancellor from time to time as occasion may require (one of whom shall be a physician or surgeon, and the other a barrister), shall be a committee, to be called " the private committee," for the purposes hereinafter mentioned.‡

No person (except a person deriving no profit, or a committee) to take charge of a single lunatic, except upon such order and medical certificates as aforesaid,

90. And be it enacted, That no person (unless he be a person who derives no profit from the charge, or a committee appointed by the Lord Chancellor) shall receive to board or lodge in any house, other than an hospital registered under this Act, or an asylum, or a house licensed under this Act, or under one of the Acts hereinbefore repealed, or take the care

* Vide 25 & 26 Vict. c. 111, s. 39.
† Vide 16 & 17 Vict. c. 96, s. 32.
‡ Repealed by 16 & 17 Vict. c. 96, s. 27.

or charge of any one patient as a lunatic or alleged lunatic, without the like order and medical certificates in respect of such patient as are hereinbefore required on the reception of a patient (not being a pauper) into a licensed* house; and that every person (except a person deriving no profit from the charge, or a committee appointed by the Lord Chancellor) who shall receive to board or lodge in any unlicensed house, not being a registered hospital or an asylum, or take the care or charge of any one patient as a lunatic or alleged lunatic, shall, within seven clear days after so receiving or taking such patient,† transmit to the Secretary of the Commissioners a true and perfect copy of the order and medical certificates on which such patient has been so received, and a statement of the date of such reception, and of the situation of the house into which such patient has been received, and of the Christian and surname and occupation of the occupier thereof, and of the person by whom the care and charge of such patient has been taken;‡ and every such patient shall at least once in every two weeks§ be visited by a physician, surgeon, or apothecary not deriving, and not having a partner, father, son, or brother who derives, any profit from the care or charge of such patient;|| and such physician, surgeon, or apothecary shall enter in a book, to be kept at the house or hospital for that purpose, to be called "The¶ Medical Visitation Book," the date of each of his visits, and a statement of the condition of the patient's health, both mental and bodily, and of the condition of the house in which such patient is, and such book shall be produced to the visiting Commissioner on every visit, and shall be signed by him as having been so produced;** and the person by whom the care or charge of such patient has been taken, or into whose house he has been received as aforesaid, shall transmit to the Secretary of the Commissioners the same notices and statements of

and under certain obligations.

* Vide 16 & 17 Vict. c. 96, s. 8, and 25 & 26 Vict. c. 111, s. 22. By this latter section it will be seen that lunatics found so by inquisition can be received into asylums without medical certificates.

† Vide 25 & 26 Vict. c. 111, s. 28.

‡ Vide 25 & 26 Vict. c. 111, s. 41.

§ Vide 16 & 17 Vict. c. 96, s. 14, and 25 & 26 Vict. c. 111, s. 22, relating to Chancery lunatics.

|| Vide 16 & 17 Vict. c. 96, s. 14.

¶ Vide 25 & 26 Vict. c. 111, s. 42.

** Vide 16 & 17 Vict. c. 96, s. 16.

the death, removal, escape, and recapture of such lunatic, and within the same periods, as are hereinbefore required in the case of the death, removal, escape, and recapture of a patient (not being a pauper) received into a licensed house ; * and that every person who shall receive into an unlicensed house, not being a registered hospital nor an asylum, or take the care or charge of any person therein as a lunatic, without first having such order and medical certificates as aforesaid, or who, having received any such patient, shall not within the several periods aforesaid transmit to the Secretary of the Commissioners such copy, statement, and notices as aforesaid, or shall fail to cause such patient to be so visited by a medical attendant as aforesaid, and every such medical attendant who shall make an untrue entry in the said Medical Visitation Book, shall be guilty of a misdemeanour.

Copy of the order and certificates, &c., with respect to lunatics received into an unlicensed house to be entered in a private register.

91. And be it enacted, That the Secretary to the Commissioners shall preserve every copy transmitted as aforesaid of the order and certificates for the reception of any patient as a lunatic into an unlicensed house, and every statement and notice which may be transmitted to such secretary with respect to any such patient as aforesaid, and shall enter the same (in such form as the private committee shall direct) in a book to be kept for that purpose, to be called " The Private Register," and such private register shall be kept by such secretary in his own custody, and shall be inspected only by the members for the time being of the said private committee,† and by such other persons as the Lord Chancellor shall by writing under his hand appoint.

Members of the private committee to visit unlicensed houses receiving a single patient, and report.

92. And be it enacted, That it shall be lawful for any one member of the said private committee, on the direction of such committee, or of any two members thereof (of whom the one member aforesaid may be one), at all reasonable times to visit every or any unlicensed house in which one patient only is received as a lunatic (unless such patient be so received by a person deriving no profit from the charge, or by a committee appointed by the Lord Chancellor), and to inquire† and report to the said private committee§ on the treatment and state of

* Vide 16 & 17 Vict. c. 96, ss. 17 21, 22. These refer to discharge, change of residence, transfer of patient to care of another person, and temporary absence.

† Vide 16 & 17 Vict. c. 96, s. 27.

‡ Vide 25 & 26 Vict. c. 111, s. 35.

§ Vide 16 & 17 Vict. c. 96, s. 27.

health, both bodily and mental, of such patient; and a copy of every or any such report shall be entered in a private register, to be kept for that purpose, by the Secretary of the Commissioners, and another copy thereof shall, if such private committee think it expedient, be laid before the Lord Chancellor.*

93. And be it enacted, That it shall be lawful for the Lord Chancellor, on the representation of the said private committee, accompanied with a copy of a report made as last aforesaid as to any patient received or detained as a lunatic in an unlicensed house as aforesaid, to make an order that such patient shall be removed from such house, and from the care and charge of the person under whose care and charge such lunatic may be ; and any person detaining such lunatic in such house, or in such care or charge, for the space of three days after a copy of such order shall have been left at such house or served on such person, shall be guilty of a misdemeanour.†

The Lord Chancellor on such report, and the representation of the private committee, may order a lunatic to be removed.

94. And be it enacted, That whenever the Commissioners shall have reason to suppose that the property of any person detained or taken charge of as a lunatic is not duly protected, or that the income thereof is not duly applied for his maintenance, such Commissioners shall make such inquiries relative thereto as they shall think proper, and report thereon to the Lord Chancellor.‡

Commissioners to report if property of lunatics be not duly protected or applied.

95. And be it enacted, That when any person shall have been received or taken charge of as a lunatic upon an order and certificates, or an order and certificate, in pursuance of the provisions of this Act, or of any Act hereinbefore repealed, and shall either have been detained as a lunatic for the twelve months then last past, or shall have been the subject of a report by the Commissioners in pursuance of the provision lastly hereinbefore contained, it shall be lawful for the Lord Chancellor to direct that one of the said Masters in Lunacy shall, and thereupon one of the said Masters shall, personally examine such person, and shall take such evidence and call for such information as to such Master shall seem necessary to satisfy him whether such person is a lunatic, and shall report thereon to the Lord Chancellor, and such report shall be filed with the

The Lord Chancellor to direct the Master in Lunacy to report as to the lunacy of any person detained as a lunatic, and to appoint guardians of his person and estate, and direct the application of his income.

* Vide 16 & 17 Vict. c. 96, s. 15.

† Vide 16 & 17 Vict. c. 96, s. 18.

‡ Vide 16 & 17 Vict. c. 96, s. 23, and 25 & 26 Vict. c. 111, s. 35.

Secretary of Lunatics; and it shall be lawful for the Lord Chancellor from time to time to make orders for the appointment of a guardian, or otherwise for the protection, care, and management of the person of any person who shall by any such report as last aforesaid be found to be a lunatic, and such guardian shall have the same powers and authorities as a committee of the person of a lunatic found such by inquisition now has, and also to make orders for the appointment of a receiver, or otherwise for the protection, care, and management of the estate of such lunatic, and such receiver shall have the same powers and authorities as a receiver of the estate of a lunatic found such by inquisition now has, and also to make orders for the application of the income of such lunatic, or a sufficient part thereof, for his maintenance and support, and in payment of the costs, charges, and expenses attending the protection, care, and management of the person and estate of such lunatic, and also as to the investment or other application for the purpose of accumulation of the overplus, if any, of such income, for the use of such lunatic, as to the Lord Chancellor shall from time to time in each case seem fit: Provided always, that such protection, care, and management shall continue only during such time as such lunatic shall continue to be detained as a lunatic upon an order and certificates or certificate as aforesaid, and for such further time, not exceeding six months, as the Lord Chancellor may fix: Provided also, that it shall be lawful for the Lord Chancellor in any such case, either before or after directing such inquiry by such Master as aforesaid, and whether such Master shall have made a report as aforesaid or not, to direct a commission in the nature of a writ *de lunatico inquirendo* to issue, to inquire of the lunacy of such person.

Masters in Lunacy to have all necessary powers of inquiry, and to make inquiries referred to them.

96. And be it enacted, That such Masters shall have power, in the prosecution of all inquiries and matters which may be referred to them as aforesaid, or otherwise under this Act, to summon persons before them, and to administer oaths, and take evidence, either *vivâ voce* or on affidavit, and to require the production of books, papers, accounts, and documents; and that the Lord Chancellor may by any order (either general or particular) refer to the said Masters any inquiries under the provisions of this Act relating to the person and estate of any lunatic as to whom a report shall be made by a Master as aforesaid, in like manner as inquiries relating to the

persons and estates of lunatics found such by inquisition are now referred to them.

97. And be it enacted, That it shall be lawful for the Lord Chancellor from time to time to make such orders as shall to him seem fit for regulating the form and mode of proceeding before the Lord Chancellor and before the said Masters, and of any other proceedings pursuant to the provisions of this Act, for the due protection, care, and management of the persons and estates of lunatics as to whom such reports shall be made by the said Masters as aforesaid, and also for fixing, altering, and discontinuing the fees to be received and taken in respect of such proceedings, as to the Lord Chancellor shall from time to time seem fit: Provided nevertheless, that all fees to be so received and taken shall be paid into the Bank of England, and placed to the credit of the Accountant-General of the Court of Chancery, to the account intituled "The Suitors' Fee Fund Account," in like manner as and together with the fees payable under the Act passed in the fifth and sixth years of her present Majesty, intituled "An Act to alter and amend the Practice and Course of Proceeding under Commissions in the Nature of Writs *De Lunatico Inquirendo*," and be applied in like manner as such last-mentioned fees.

Lord Chancellor to make orders and regulations, and fix fees.

5 & 6 Vict. c. 84.

98. And be it enacted, That the travelling and other expenses of the said Masters and their clerks shall be paid to them, by virtue of any order or orders of the Court of Chancery, out of the said fund, intituled "The Suitors' Fee Fund Account," in the same manner as their expenses under the said last-mentioned Act.

Masters' expenses how to be paid.

99. And be it enacted, That every proprietor and superintendent of a licensed house or registered hospital, and every other person hereby or by any of the Acts hereinbefore repealed authorised to receive or take charge of a lunatic upon an order, and who shall receive or has received a proper order, in pursuance of this Act or any of the said repealed Acts, accompanied with the required medical certificates or certificate, for the reception, or taking charge of any person as a lunatic, and the assistants and servants of such proprietor, superintendent, or other person, shall have power and authority to take charge of, receive, and detain such patient until he shall die, or be removed or discharged by due authority; and in case of the escape at any time or times of such patient, to

Proprietors, superintendents, and other authorised persons, may plead the order and certificates for receiving any lunatic in bar of all proceedings at law.

retake him at any time within fourteen days after such escape, and again to detain him as aforesaid ; * and in every writ, indictment, information, action, and other proceeding which shall be preferred or brought against any such proprietor, superintendent, or other person authorised as aforesaid, or against any assistant or servant of any such proprietor, superintendent, or authorised person, for taking, confining, detaining, or retaking any person as a lunatic, the party complained of may plead such order and certificates or certificate in defence to any such writ, indictment, information, action, or other proceeding as aforesaid ; and such order and certificates or certificate shall, as respects such party, be a justification for taking, confining, detaining, or retaking such lunatic or alleged lunatic.

Commissioners and visitors may summon witnesses to give evidence, with a penalty for non-compliance.

100. And be it enacted, That it shall be lawful for the Commissioners, or any two of them, and also for the visitors of any licensed house, or any two of such visitors, from time to time, as they shall see occasion, to require, by summons† under the common seal of the Commission, if by the Commissioners, and if by two only of the Commissioners, or by two visitors, then under the hands and seals of such two Commissioners or two visitors, as the case may be (according to the form in Schedule (I) annexed to this Act, or as near thereto as the case will permit), any person to appear before them to testify on oath the truth touching any matters respecting which such Commissioners and visitors respectively are by this Act authorised to inquire (which oath such Commissioners or visitors are hereby empowered to administer) ; and every person who shall not appear before such Commissioners or visitors pursuant to such summons, or shall not assign some reasonable excuse for not so appearing, or shall appear and refuse to be sworn or examined, shall, on being convicted thereof before one of her Majesty's justices for the county or borough within which the place at which such person shall have been by such summons required to appear and give evidence is situate, shall for every such neglect or refusal forfeit a sum not exceeding fifty pounds.

Provision for the payment of witnesses' expenses.

101. And be it enacted, That it shall be lawful for any Commissioners or visitors who shall summon any person to

* Vide 25 & 26 Vict. c. 111, s. 39.
† Vide 25 & 26 Vict. c. 111, s. 46.

appear and give evidence as aforesaid to direct the Secretary of
the Commissioners or the clerk of such visitors, as the case
may be, to pay to such person all reasonable expenses of his
appearance and attendance in pursuance of such summons, the
same to be considered as expenses incurred by such Commissioners and visitors respectively in the execution of this Act,
and to be taken into account and paid accordingly.

102. And be it enacted, That every complaint or information of or for any offence against this Act, where any pecuniary penalty is hereby imposed (except when hereby otherwise provided for), may be made before one justice; and when
any person shall be charged upon oath before a justice for any
such offence against this Act, such justice may summon the
person charged to appear at a time and place to be named in
such summons; and if he shall not appear accordingly, and
upon proof of the due service of the summons (either personally or by leaving the same at his last or usual place of
abode) any two justices may either proceed to hear and determine the case, or may issue their warrant for apprehending
such person and bringing him before any two justices; and
any two justices shall and may, upon the appearing of such
person pursuant to such summons, or upon such person being
apprehended with such warrant, or upon the non-appearance
of such person, hear the matter of every such complaint or
information, and make any such determination thereon as such
justices shall think proper; and upon conviction of any person
such justices may, if they shall think fit, reduce the amount
of the penalty by this Act imposed for such offence to any
sum not less than one-fourth of the amount thereof, and shall
and may issue a warrant under their hands and seals for
levying such penalty or reduced penalty, and all costs and
charges of such summons, warrant, and hearing, and all inci-
dental costs and charges, by distress and sale of the goods and
chattels of the person so convicted; and it shall be lawful for
any such two justices to order any person so convicted to be
detained and kept in the custody of any constable or other
peace officer until return can be conveniently made to such
warrant of distress, unless the said offender shall give security
to the satisfaction of such justices, by way of recognisance or
otherwise, for his appearance before such justices on such day
as shall be appointed for the return of such warrant of distress, such day not being more than seven days from the time

Upon com-
plaint made
of any
offence
against this
Act, justices
to require
the attend-
ance of the
person
charged, and
adjudicate
thereon.

Recovery of
penalties.

of taking any such security; but if upon the return of such warrant of distress it shall appear that no sufficient distress can be had whereupon to levy the said penalty, and such costs and charges as aforesaid, and the same shall not be forthwith paid; or in case it shall appear to the satisfaction of such justices, either by the confession of the offender or otherwise, that the offender hath not sufficient goods and chattels whereupon the said penalty, costs, and charges may be levied, such justices shall and may, by warrant under their hands and seals, **Committal of offenders.** commit such offender to the common gaol or house of correction for any term not exceeding three calendar months, unless such penalty and all such costs and charges as aforesaid shall be sooner paid; and all such penalties, when recovered, shall be paid, when the complaint or information shall be laid **Application of penalties.** or brought by or by the direction of the Commissioners, to the Secretary of the Commissioners, to be by him applied and accounted for as hereinbefore directed with respect to moneys received for licences granted by the Commissioners; and when the complaint or information shall be laid or brought by the direction of any visitors, to the clerk of the peace for the county or borough, to be by him applied and accounted for as hereinbefore directed with respect to moneys received for licences granted by the justices of such county or borough; and the overplus (if any) arising from such distress and sale, after payment of the penalty and all costs and charges as aforesaid, shall be paid, upon demand, to the owner of the goods and chattels so distrained.

Form of conviction before justices. 103. And be it enacted, That the justices before whom any person shall be convicted of any offence against this Act for which a pecuniary penalty is imposed may cause the conviction to be drawn up in the following form, or in any other form to the same effect, as the case may require; and that no conviction under this Act shall be void through want of form :—

BE it remembered, That on the   day of
in the year of our Lord   at
in the County [*or* Borough] of   *A. B.* was convicted
before us   of Her Majesty's Justices of the
Peace for the said County [*or* Borough], for that he the said
            did   and we the said
adjudge the said
for his Offence to pay the Sum of

104. Provided always, and be it enacted, That any person who shall think himself aggrieved by any order or determination of any justices under this Act may, within four calendar months after such order made or given, appeal to the justices at general or quarter sessions, the person appealing having first given at least fourteen clear days' notice in writing of such appeal, and the nature and matter thereof, to the person appealed against, and forthwith after such notice entering into a recognisance before some justice, with two sufficient sureties, conditioned to try such appeal, and to abide the order and award of the said Court thereupon; and the said justices at general or quarter sessions, upon the proof of such notice and recognisance having been given and entered into, shall in a summary way hear and determine such appeal, or, if they think proper, adjourn the hearing thereof until the next general or quarter sessions, and, if they see cause, may mitigate any penalty to not less than one fourth of the amount imposed by this Act, and may order any money to be returned which shall have been levied in pursuance of such order or determination, and shall and may also award such further satisfaction to be made to the party injured, or such costs to either of the parties, as they shall judge reasonable and proper; and all such determinations of the said justices at general or quarter sessions shall be final, binding, and conclusive upon all parties to all intents and purposes whatsoever.

Appeal to Quarter Sessions.

105. And be it enacted, That if any action or suit shall be brought against any person for any thing done in pursuance of this Act or of any of the Acts hereby repealed, the same shall be commenced within twelve calendar months next after the release of the party bringing the action, and shall be laid or brought in the county or borough where the cause of action shall have arisen, and not elsewhere; and the defendant in every such action or suit may, at his election, plead specially or as to the general issue not guilty, and give this Act and the special matter in evidence at any trial to be had thereupon, and that the same was done in pursuance and by the authority of this Act; and if the same shall appear to be so done, or that such action or suit shall be brought in any other county or borough than as aforesaid, or shall not have been commenced within the time before limited for bringing the same, then the jury shall find a verdict for the defendant; and upon a verdict being so found, or if the plantiff shall be nonsuited, or discon-

Actions to be commenced within twelve calendar months.

Evidence in support of plea.

tinue his action or suit after the defendant shall have appeared, or if upon demurrer judgment shall be given against the plaintiff, then the defendant shall recover double costs, and have such remedy for recovering the same as any defendant hath or may have in any other cases by law.

Offenders to be prosecuted, and penalties sued for by the Secretary of the Commissioners and the clerk of any visitors, and by no person without the authority of the Commissioners or visitors.

106. And be it enacted, That it shall be lawful for the Secretary of the Commissioners, on their order, to prosecute any person for any offence against the provisions of this Act, and to sue for and recover any penalty to which any person is made liable by this Act; and all penalties sued for and recovered by such secretary shall be paid to him, and be by him applied and accounted for as hereinbefore directed with respect to moneys received for licences granted by the Commissioners.; and that it shall be lawful for the clerk of any visitors, on their order, to prosecute any person for any offence against the provisions of this Act committed within the jurisdiction of such visitors, and to sue for and recover any penalty to which any person within the jurisdiction of such visitors is made liable by this Act; and all penalties sued for and recovered by any such clerk shall be paid to him, and be by him paid to the Clerk of the Peace for such county or borough, and be by such Clerk of the Peace applied and accounted for as hereinbefore directed with respect to moneys received for licences by such Clerk of the Peace; and it shall not be lawful for any one to prosecute any person for any offence against the provisions of this Act, or to sue for any penalty to which any person is made liable by this Act, except by order of the Commissioners or of visitors having jurisdiction in the place where the cause of prosecution has arisen or the penalty been incurred, or with the consent of her Majesty's Attorney-General or Solicitor-General for England for the time being.

Offenders against the provisions of any of the repealed Acts may be prosecuted under this Act.

107. And be it enacted, That notwithstanding the repeal of the several Acts hereinbefore repealed, every offence heretofore committed against any of the provisions of any of the same Acts may be prosecuted, and every penalty heretofore incurred by any person for any offence against the provisions of any of the same Acts may be sued for and recovered, by the Secretary of the Commissioners, in the same manner and with all the same powers and rights as if such offence had been committed, or such penalty incurred for an offence against the provisions of this Act; and every penalty so recovered shall

be applied in the same manner as a penalty recovered for an offence against the provisions of this Act.

108. And be it enacted, That when any person shall be proceeded against, under the provisions of this Act, for omitting to transmit or send any copy, list, notice, statement, or other document hereinbefore required to be transmitted or sent by such person, and such person shall prove by the testimony of one witness upon oath that the copy, list, notice, statement, or document in respect of which such proceeding is taken was put into the post in due time, or (in case of documents required to be transmitted or sent to the Commissioners or a Clerk of the Peace) left at the office of the Commissioners or of the Clerk of the Peace, and shall have been properly addressed, such proof shall be a bar to all further proceeding in respect of such omission.

No person to be punishable for omitting to send any copy, &c., if proved to have been put in the post, or left at the proper office.

109. And be it enacted, That the costs, charges, and expenses incurred by or under the authority or order of the Commissioners in proceedings under this Act, shall be paid by the Secretary of the Commissioners, and included by him in the account of receipts and payments hereinbefore directed to be kept by him; and that the costs, charges, and expenses incurred by or under the order of any visitors in proceedings under this Act shall be paid by the Clerk of the Peace of their county or borough, and included by him in the account of receipts and payments hereinbefore directed to be kept by him.

Costs incurred by the Commissioners to be paid by their Secretary, and costs incurred by visitors by the Clerk of the Peace.

110. And be it enacted, That two or more of the Commissioners, one at least of whom shall be a physician or surgeon, and one at least a barrister, shall and may, once or oftener in each year, on such day or days, and at such hours of the day, and for such length of time as they shall think fit, visit every asylum for lunatics, and every gaol* in which there shall be or alleged to be any lunatic, and shall inquire whether the provisions of the law have been carried out as to the construction of each asylum visited, and as to its visitation and management, and also as to the regularity of the admissions and discharges of patients therein and therefrom; and whether divine service is performed therein; and whether any system of coercion is in practice therein, and the result thereof; and as to the classification or non-classification of patients therein, and the

Commissioners to visit asylums and gaols.

* Vide 25 & 26 Vict. c. 111, s. 30.

number of attendants on each class; and as to the occupations and amusements of the patients, and the effects thereof ; and as to the condition, as well mental as bodily, of the pauper patients when first received ; and also as to the dietary of the pauper patients ; and shall also make such other inquiries as to every or any such asylum, and all such inquiries as to the lunatics in any gaol, as to such visiting Commissioners shall seem meet.

Provision for the visitation of lunatics under the care of committees, and also of State and criminal lunatics, and other lunatics not comprised in the preceding provisions.
* 112. And be it enacted, That it shall be lawful for the Lord Chancellor, in the case of any lunatic under the care of a committee appointed by the Lord Chancellor, and for the Lord Chancellor, or her Majesty's principal Secretary of State for the Home Department, in the case of any lunatic under the care of any person receiving or taking the charge of such one lunatic only, and deriving no profit from the charge, and in the case of any person confined as a State lunatic, or as a lunatic under the order of any criminal court of justice, and in the case of every other person detained or taken charge of as a lunatic, or represented to be a lunatic, or to be under any re · straint as a lunatic, at any time, by an order in writing under the hand of the Lord Chancellor or the said Secretary of State, as the case may be, directed to the Commissioners or any of them, or to any other person, to require the persons or person to whom such order shall be directed, or any of them, to visit and examine such lunatic or supposed lunatic, and to make a report to the Lord Chancellor, or to her Majesty's principal Secretary of State for the Home Department, of such matters as in such order shall be directed to be inquired into.†

Power for the Lord Chancellor and Secretary of State for the Home Department to authorise a special visitation of any place where a lunatic is represented to be confined.
113. And be it enacted, That it shall be lawful for the Lord Chancellor or her Majesty's principal Secretary of State for the Home Department to employ any Commissioner appointed under this Act, or other person, to inspect or inquire into the state of any asylum, hospital, gaol, house, or place wherein any lunatic, or person represented to be lunatic, shall be confined, or alleged to be confined, and to report to him the result of such inspection and inquiry ; ‡ and every such person so employed and not being a Commissioner, may be paid such sum of money for his attendance and trouble as to the Lord Chancellor or her Majesty's principal Secretary of State for

---

* Sec. 111 is repealed by 16 & 17 Vict. c. 96, s. 28.

† Vide 16 & 17 Vict. c. 96, ss. 33, 34.

‡ Vide 25 & 26 Vict. c. 111, s. 31.

the Home Department shall seem reasonable; and every such person so employed, whether a Commissioner or not, shall be allowed his reasonable travelling or other expenses while so employed; and such sum of money for attendance and trouble, and such expenses, shall be charged on and shall be paid out of the Contingency Fund of the Home Office.

114. And be it enacted, That in this Act and the schedules thereto the words and expressions following shall have the several meanings hereby assigned to them, unless there shall be something in the subject or context repugnant to such construction, that is to say: Interpretation clause.

> "Borough" shall mean every borough, town, and city corporate having a separate quarter sessions, recorder, and clerk of the peace.

> "County" shall mean every county, riding, division of a county, county of a city, county of a town, liberty, and other place having a separate commission of the peace, and not being a "borough" within the meaning aforesaid.

> "The Lord Chancellor" shall mean the Lord High Chancellor, the Lord Keeper or Commissioners of the Great Seal of Great Britain, and other the person or persons for the time being entrusted, by virtue of the Queen's sign manual, with the care and commitment of the custody of the persons and estates of persons found idiot, lunatic, or of unsound mind.

> "Barrister" shall mean a barrister and a serjeant-at-law; and a serjeant-at-law who shall have been called to the bar five years or more before his appointment to be a Commissioner shall be considered as a barrister of five years' standing.

> "Lunatic" shall mean every insane person, and every person being an idiot or lunatic or of unsound mind.

> "Parish" shall mean any parish, township, hamlet, vill, tithing, extra-parochial place, or place maintaining its own poor.

> "Officiating Clergyman of a [or the] Parish" shall mean a clergyman regularly officiating and acting as the

minister or one of the ministers of a parish, chapelry, or ecclesiastical district.*

" Borough Rate " shall mean a borough rate, and any funds assessed upon or raised in or belonging to any borough in the nature of a borough rate, and applicable to the purposes to which borough rates are applicable.

" County Rate " shall mean a county rate, and any funds assessed upon or raised in or belonging to any county in the nature of a county rate, and applicable to the purposes to which county rates are applicable.

" Pauper " shall mean every person maintained wholly or in part at the expense of any parish, union, county, or borough.

" Patient " shall mean every person received or detained as a lunatic, or taken care or charge of as a lunatic.

" Private Patient " shall mean every patient who is not a pauper.

" Proprietor " shall mean every person to whom any licence has been granted under the provisions of any Act hereby repealed, or shall be granted under the provisions of this Act, and every person keeping, owning, having any interest, or exercising any duties or powers of a proprietor in any licensed house.

" Clerk of the Peace " shall mean every clerk of the peace and person acting as such, and every deputy duly appointed.

" Medical Attendant " shall mean every physician, surgeon, and apothecary † who shall keep any licensed house, or shall in his medical capacity attend any licensed house, or any asylum, hospital, or other place where any lunatic shall be confined.

" Justice " shall mean a justice of the peace.

" Asylum " shall mean any lunatic asylum already erected and established under an Act passed in the forty-eighth year of the reign of his late Majesty King George the 48 G. 3, c. 96. Third, intituled " An Act for the better Care and Main-

---

* Vide 16 & 17 Vict. c. 96, s. 36.
† Vide 25 & 26 Vict. c. 111, s. 47.

tenance of Lunatics, being Paupers or Criminals in England," or erected and established, or hereafter to be erected and established, under or which have been made subject or liable to any of the provisions of an Act passed in the ninth year of the reign of his late Majesty King George the Fourth, intituled " An Act to amend the 9 G. 4, c. 40. Laws for the Erection and Regulation of County Lunatic Asylums, and more effectually to provide for the Care and Maintenance of Pauper and Criminal Lunatics in England," or hereafter to be erected and established under the provisions of any Act for the erection or regulation of county or borough lunatic asylums.

" Hospital " shall mean any hospital or part of an hospital or other house or institution (not being an asylum) wherein lunatics are received, and supported wholly or partly by voluntary contributions, or by any charitable bequest or gift, or by applying the excess of payments of some patients for or towards the support, provision, or benefit of other patients.

" Licensed House " shall mean a house licensed under the provisions of this Act, or of some Act hereby repealed, for the reception of lunatics.

" Oath " shall mean an oath, and every affirmation or other declaration or solemnity lawfully substituted for an "oath" in the case of Quakers or other persons exempted by law from the necessity of taking an oath.

Words importing the singular number shall include the plural number, and words importing the plural number shall include the singular number, and words importing the masculine gender shall include females.

115. And be it enacted, That for the purposes of this Act every borough and county shall include every place situate within the limits of such borough or county, and not having a separate commission of the peace ; and for the purposes of this Act every place situate within the limits of any borough or county, and not having a separate commission of the peace, shall be within the jurisdiction of the justices of such borough or county ; and that the justices of every borough shall, for the purposes of this Act, assemble in special sessions at such times as the quarter sessions for such borough shall be holden ;

Boroughs and counties to comprise all places therein not having separate Commission of the Peace.

and that all acts hereinbefore required to be done by the justices of counties in general or quarter sessions assembled may be done by the justices of boroughs at such special sessions.

Act not to extend to Bethlehem Hospital.

116. And be it enacted, That nothing in this Act contained shall extend to the royal hospital of Bethlehem, or any building adjacent thereto and used therewith : Provided always, that it shall be lawful for any Commissioner or other person whom the Lord Chancellor or any one of her Majesty's principal Secretaries of State shall at any time, by an order in writing under the hand of the said Lord Chancellor or Secretary of State, direct, to visit and examine the royal hospital of Bethlehem, and every or any building adjacent thereto as aforesaid, and every or any person confined therein.*

Act to be confined to England and Wales.

117. And be it enacted, That this Act shall extend only to England and Wales.

Alteration of Act.

118. And be it enacted, That this Act may be amended or repealed by any Act to be passed in this present session of Parliament.

---

* Repealed by 16 & 17 Vict. c. 96, s. 25.

Schedules referred to by the foregoing Act.

SCHEDULE (A) * SECTION 30.†

Form of Licence.

KNOW all men, that we, the Commissioners in Lunacy [*or* we
the undersigned Justices of the Peace, acting in and for
in general [*or* quarter *or* special] sessions assembled],
do hereby certify, that *A.B.* of   in the parish of
in the county of   hath delivered to us [*or* the Clerk of
the Peace] a plan and description of a house and premises proposed to be licensed for the reception of lunatics, situate at
in the county of   [*or, in the case of a renewed licence,*
hath delivered to us [*or* the Clerk of the Peace] a list of the number
of patients now detained in a house and premises licensed on the
          day of   . last, for the reception of lunatics,
situate at   in the county of   ], and we, having
considered and approved the same, do hereby authorise and empower the said *A.B.*,   (he intending [*or* not intending]
to reside therein) to use and employ the said house and premises
for the reception of   male [*or*   female, *or*
          male and   female] lunatics, of whom not
more than   shall be private patients, for the space of
          calendar months from this date.

Sealed with our common seal [*or* given under our hands and
seals], this   day of   in the year of our Lord
18

Witness,

Y.Z., Secretary to the Commissioners of Lunacy,

[*or* Clerk of the Peace.]

---

* Vide Schedule (A) annexed to 25 & 26 Vict. c. 111
† Schedules B, C, and D repealed by 16 & 17 Vict. c. 96, s. 3.

SCHEDULE (E)

REGISTRY OF

Date of last previous Admission (if any)	No. in Order of Admission	Date of Admission	Christian and Surname at Length	Sex and Class				Age	Condition as to Marriage			Condition of Life, and previous Occupation	Previous Place of Abode	County, Union, or Parish to which chargeable
				Private		Pauper			Married	Single	Widowed			
				M.	F.	M.	F.							
	1	1846: Jan. 3	William Johnson	–	–	1	–	23	–	1	–	Carpenter	–	– –
	2													
	3													
	4	1848: June 9	William Johnson	–	–	1	–	25	–	1	–	– –	–	– –
	5													
	6													
	7	1852: May 6	William Johnson	–	–	1	–	29	1	–	–	– –	–	– –
	8													

SECTION 50.

ADMISSIONS.

PATIENTS.

By whose Authority sent	Dates of Medical Certificates, and by whom signed	Bodily Condition	Name of Disorder (if any)	Form of Mental Disorder	Supposed Cause of Insanity	Epileptics	Congenital Idiots	Duration of existing Attacks			Number of previous Attacks	Age on First Attack	Date of Discharge or Death	Discharged			Died	Observations
								Years	Months	Weeks				Recovered	Relieved	Not improved		
–	–	–	–	–	Melancholia	–	–	–	–	4	–	2	17	1846: Sept. 1	1				
–	–	–	–	–	–	–	–	–	7	–	–	3	–	1848: Dec. 2	1				
–	–	–	–	–	–	–	–	–	3	–	–	4	–	1853: June 8					

SCHEDULE (F) Section 52.

Notice of Admission.

I HEREBY give you notice, that *A.B.* was received into this house [*or* hospital] as a private [*or* pauper] patient on the day of　　　　and I hereby transmit a copy of the Order and Medical Certificates [*or* Certificate] on which he was received.

Subjoined is a statement with respect to the mental and bodily condition of the above-named patient.

(Signed)

Superintendent [*or* Proprietor] of

Dated this　　　　　　　day of　　　　　　One thousand eight hundred and

STATEMENT.

I HAVE this day seen and personally examined the patient named in the above Notice, and hereby certify that with respect to mental state he [*or* she]　　　　　and that with respect to bodily health and condition he [*or* she]

(Signed)

Medical Proprietor [*or* Superintendent, *or* Attendant].

Dated this　　　　　　day of　　　　　　One thousand eight hundred and

SCHEDULE (G 1) SECTION 54.

REGISTER OF DISCHARGES AND DEATHS.

Date of Discharge or Death	Date of last Admission	No. in Register of Patients	Christian and Surname at Length	Sex and Class				Discharged								Assigned cause of Death.	Age at Death		Observations
				Private		Pauper		Recovered		Relieved		Not improved		Died					
				M.	F.	M.	F.	M.	F.	M.	F.	M.	F.	M.	F.		M.	F.	
1846: Sept. 1	1846: Jan. 3	1	William Johnson	-	-	1	-	1											
1848: Dec. 2	1848: June 9	4	William Johnson	-	-	1	-	1											
1853: June 8	1852: May 6	7	William Johnson	-	-	1	-	-	-	-	-	-	-	1	-	Phthisis	27		

SCHEDULE (G 2) SECTION 54.

*Form of Notice of Discharge or Death.**

I HEREBY give you notice, that   a private [*or* pauper] patient, received into this house [*or* hospital] on the   day of   was discharged therefrom recovered [*or* relieved, *or* not improved,] by the authority of   [*or* died therein], on the   day of

(Signed)

Superintendent [*or* Proprietor] of

house [*or* hospital] at

Dated this   day of   One thousand eight hundred and

In case of death, add " and I further certify, that *A.B.* was present at the death of the said   ; and that the apparent cause of death of the said   [ascertained by post-mortem examination (*if so*)] was   "

---

* This must be sent to Commissioners within two clear days from time of discharge.

SCHEDULE (H) SECTION 54.

FORM OF MEDICAL JOURNAL AND WEEKLY REPORT.

Date	Number of Patients				Names of Patients under Restraint (and by what Means) or in Seclusion		Names of Patients under Medical Treatment		Report on State of Health of Patients and Condition of House or Hospital	Deaths, Injuries, and Violences to Patients
	Private		Pauper							
	M.	F.	M.	F.	Males	Females	Males	Females		

SCHEDULE (I) Section 100.

Form of Summons.

WE, the Commissioners in Lunacy [*or* we whose names are hereunto set and seals affixed, being Two of the Commissioners in Lunacy, *or* Visitors] appointed under or by virtue of an Act passed in the   year of the reign of her present Majesty, intituled [*here insert the Title of the Act*], do hereby summon and require you personally to appear before us at   in the parish of   in the county of   on next the   day of ·   at the hour of in the   noon of the same day, and then and there to be examined, and to testify the truth touching certain matters relating to the execution of the said Act.

Sealed with the Common Seal of " The Commissioners in Lunacy " [*or* given under our hands and seals], this   day of in the year of our Lord One thousand eight hundred and

II.

ANNO DECIMO SEXTO & DECIMO SEPTIMO VIC-
TORIÆ REGINÆ.

CAP. XCVI.

An Act to amend an Act passed in the ninth Year of her Majesty,
for the Regulation of the Care and Treatment of Lunatics.

August 20th, 1853.

WHEREAS an Act was passed in the ninth year of her Majesty, "for the Regulation of the Care and Treatment of Lunatics:" and whereas it is expedient to amend the said Act as hereinafter mentioned: Be it therefore enacted by the Queen's most excellent Majesty, by and with the advice and consent of the Lords Spiritual and Temporal, and Commons, in this present Parliament assembled, and by the authority of the same, as follows:— *8 & 9 Vict. c. 100.*

1. Section twenty-five of the said recited Act shall be repealed, and any one licence to be granted for the reception of lunatics may, in the discretion of the Commissioners or justices granting such licence, include two or more houses belonging to one proprietor or to two or more joint proprietors, provided that no one of such houses be separated from the other or others of them otherwise than by land in the same occupation, and by a road, or by either of such modes; and all houses, buildings, and lands intended to be included in any licence shall be specified, delineated, and described in the plan required by section twenty-four of the said recited Act.* *Section 25 of recited Act repealed, and provision as to what may be included in one licence.*

2. No person having, after the passing of the said recited Act, received for the first time a licence for the reception of lunatics, or hereafter receiving for the first time such licence, shall receive a licence unless he shall reside on the premises licensed; and no two or more persons having, after the passing of the said recited Act, received for the first time a joint licence *The person or one of the persons receiving a licence to reside on the premises.*

* Vide 8 & 9 Vict. c. 100, s. 24; 25 & 26 Vict. c. 111, s. 14.

for the reception of lunatics, or hereafter receiving for the first time such licence, shall receive such licence unless they or one of them shall reside on the premises licensed.*

Sections 45, 46, 47, 48 and 49 of 8 & 9 Vict. c. 100, repealed.

3. Sections forty-five, forty-six, forty-seven, forty-eight, and forty-nine of the said recited Act shall be repealed; but such repeal shall not prevent or defeat any prosecution for any offence committed before the commencement of this Act, and every such offence shall and may be prosecuted, and every pending prosecution continued, as if this Act had not been passed.

No person not a pauper to be received into a hospital or licensed house without a certain order and certificates.

4. Save as hereinafter otherwise provided,† no person (not being a lunatic), for or in respect of whom any money shall be paid or agreed to be paid, shall be boarded or lodged in any licensed house; and, save where otherwise provided or authorised under this or any other Act, no person (not being a pauper) shall be received as a lunatic into any licensed house or hospital without an order under the hand of some person according to the form in Schedule (A) No. 1 annexed to this Act, together with such statement of particulars as is contained in the same schedule, nor without the medical certificates, according to the form in Schedule (A) No. 2 annexed to this Act, of two persons, each of whom shall be a physician, surgeon, or apothecary, and shall not be in partnership with or an assistant to the other,‡ and each of whom shall separately from the other have personally examined the person to whom the certificate signed by him relates not more than seven clear days previously to the reception of such person into such house or hospital; and such order as aforesaid may be signed before or after the medical certificates or either of them; and every person who shall receive any such person as aforesaid into any such house or hospital as aforesaid (save where otherwise provided or authorised under this or any other Act) without such order and medical certificates as aforesaid, shall be guilty of a misdemeanour.§

Proviso that in certain cases any person may be received on a certificate signed by one medical practitioner only.

5. Provided always, That any person (not a pauper) may, under special circumstances preventing the examination of such person by two medical practitioners as aforesaid, be received as

* Vide 25 & 26 Vict. c. 111, s. 16.
† Vide 25 & 26 Vict. c. 111, s. 18.
‡ Vide 25 & 26 Vict. c. 111, s. 24.
§ Vide 8 & 9 Vict. c. 100, s. 106.

a lunatic into any licensed house or any hospital upon such
order as aforesaid, and with the certificate of one physician,
surgeon, or apothecary alone, provided that the statement
accompanying such order set forth the special circumstances
which prevent the examination of such person by two medical
practitioners; but in every such case two other such certificates
shall, within three clear days after his reception into such
house or hospital, be signed by two other persons, each of
whom shall be a physician, surgeon, or apothecary, not in
partnership with or an assistant to the other, or the physician,
surgeon, or apothecary who signed the certificate on which the
patient was received, and not connected with such house or
hospital, and shall within such time and separately from the
other of them have personally examined the person so received
as a lunatic; and every person who, having received any person
as a lunatic into any house or hospital as aforesaid, upon the
certificate of one medical practitioner alone as aforesaid, shall
keep or permit such person to remain in such house or hospital beyond the said period of three clear days without such
further certificates as aforesaid, shall be guilty of a misdemeanour.

6. Provided also, That it shall be lawful for the proprietor *Any person discharged may, with assent of visitors or Commissioners, be retained in licensed house, and a relative or friend may, with like assent, be received therein.* or superintendent of any licensed house,* with the previous
assent in writing of two of the Commissioners, such assent not
to be given until after such Commissioners have, by personal
examination of the patient, satisfied themselves of his desire
to remain, to entertain and keep in such house as a boarder any
person who may have been discharged as a patient from such
house for such time after such discharge as he may desire to
remain, not exceeding the time specified in such assent, and
also, for the benefit of any patient in such house, and with the
previous assent in writing of two of the Commissioners, to receive and accommodate as a boarder therein, for a time to be
specified in the assent, any relative or friend of such patient,
and any two of the Commissioners may from time to time, by
any writing under their hands, extend or revoke any such
assent as aforesaid; and every such patient so retained after
discharge, and every such relative or friend so accommodated,
shall, if required, be produced to the Commissioners and
visitors respectively at their respective visits.

* Vide 25 & 26 Vict. c. 111, s. 18.

Paupers not to be received without a certain order and certificate.

7. Save where otherwise provided or authorised under any Act, no pauper shall be received into any licensed house or any hospital without an order according to the form in Schedule (B) No. 1, annexed to this Act,* under the hand of one justice, or under the hands of an officiating clergyman, and the relieving officer or one of the overseers of the union or parish from which such pauper shall be sent, together with such statement of particulars as is contained in the same schedule, nor without the medical certificate, according to the form in Schedule (B) No. 2, annexed to this Act, of a physician, surgeon, or apothecary, who shall have personally examined the pauper to whom it relates not more than seven clear days previously to his reception; and every person who shall receive any pauper into any such house or hospital as aforesaid (save where otherwise provided or authorised under any Act) without such order and medical certificate as last aforesaid, shall be guilty of a misdemeanour: Provided always, that this enactment shall not by implication or otherwise give any power or authority to make such order, or extend, alter, or affect any power or authority expressly given by any Act to any justice, officiating clergyman, relieving officer, or overseer to make or join in making any such order, or any provisions giving or relating to such power or authority.

The like order and certificates for reception of a single patient as for reception of a private patient into a licensed house.

8. Where, under section ninety of the said recited Act,† the like order and medical certificates are required on the reception or taking the charge or care of any one person as a lunatic or alleged lunatic as are thereinbefore required on the reception of a patient (not being a pauper) into a licensed house, the like order and medical certificates (in lieu of those required as first aforesaid) shall hereafter be required on the reception or taking the charge or care of any such person as are by this Act required on the reception of a patient (not being a pauper) into a licensed house.

Penalty on officers, &c., illtreating lunatics.

9. If any superintendent, officer, nurse, attendant, servant, or other person employed in any registered hospital or licensed house, or any person having the care or charge of any single patient, or any attendant of any single patient, in any way abuse, or ill-treat, or wilfully neglect any patient in such hospital or house, or such single patient, or if any person detaining,

---

* Vide 25 & 26 Vict. c. 111, ss. 25, 26, 31, 32, 33.
† Vide 8 & 9 Vict. c. 100, s. 90.

or taking or having the care or charge, or concerned or taking part in the custody, care, or treatment, of any lunatic or person alleged to be a lunatic, in any way abuse, ill-treat, or wilfully neglect such lunatic or alleged lunatic, he shall be guilty of a misdemeanour, and shall be subject to indictment for every such offence, or to forfeit for every such offence, on a summary conviction thereof before two justices, any sum not exceeding twenty pounds,

10. Every physician, surgeon, and apothecary signing any certificate under or for the purposes of this Act shall specify therein the facts upon which he has formed his opinion that the person to whom such certificate relates is a lunatic, an idiot, or a person of unsound mind, and distinguish in such certificate facts observed by himself from facts communicated to him by others; and no person shall be received into any registered hospital or licensed house, or as a single patient, under any certificate which purports to be founded only upon facts communicated by others. *Medical certificate to specify facts upon which opinion of insanity has been formed.*

11. If after the reception of any lunatic it appear that the order or the medical certificate, or (if more than one) both or either of the medical certificates, upon which he was received, is or are in any respect incorrect or defective, such order and medical certificate or certificates may be amended by the person signing the same at any time within fourteen days next after the reception of such lunatic ; Provided nevertheless, that no such amendment shall have any force or effect unless the same shall receive the sanction of one or more of the Commissioners.* *Orders and medical certificates may be amended.*

12. No physician, surgeon, or apothecary who, or whose father, brother, son, partner, or assistant, is wholly or partly the proprietor of, or a regular professional attendant in, a licensed house or a hospital, shall sign any certificate for the reception of a patient into such house or hospital; and no physician, surgeon, or apothecary shall himself, or by his servants or agents, receive to board or lodge in any unlicensed house, or take the charge or care of any person upon or under any medical certificate signed by himself or his father, brother, son, partner, or assistant; and no physician, surgeon, or apothecary having (either before or after the passing of this Act) signed any certificate for the reception of any person shall be the regu- *Who not to sign certificates, &c.*

* Vide 25 & 26 Vict. c. 111, s. 27.

lar professional attendant of such person while under care or charge under such certificate; and no physician, surgeon, or apothecary who, or whose father, brother, son, partner, or assistant shall sign the order hereinbefore required for the reception of a patient, shall sign any certificate for the reception of the same patient.

A medical man giving false certificates, &c., and a person not being a medical man giving certificates as such, guilty of a misdemeanour.

13. Any physician, surgeon, or apothecary who shall sign any certificate, or do any other act (not declared to be a misdemeanour) contrary to any of the provisions herein contained, shall for every such offence forfeit any sum not exceeding twenty pounds; and any physician, surgeon, or apothecary who shall falsely state or certify anything in any certificate under this Act, and any person who shall sign any certificate under this Act in which he shall be described as a physician, surgeon, or apothecary, not being a physician, surgeon, or apothecary respectively within the meaning of this Act, shall be guilty of a misdemeanour.

Commissioners may permit medical visitation of any single patient less frequently than once a fortnight, but if patient be in the care of a medical man he is to make an entry once a fortnight as to patient's health.

14. It shall be lawful for the Commissioners, by an order under their common seal, where they see fit so to do, to permit the visitation of any single patient by a physician, surgeon, or apothecary less frequently than once in every two weeks, as required by section ninety of the said recited Act, and to prescribe from time to time how often any single patient shall be visited by such a physician, surgeon, or apothecary as therein mentioned; but where such visitation of any single patient so often as once in every two weeks is so dispensed with, and such patient is in the care or charge of a physician, surgeon, or apothecary, such physician, surgeon, or apothecary shall once at the least in every two weeks make an entry in a book to be kept for that purpose, to be called "The Medical Journal," of the condition of the patient's health, both mental and bodily, together with the date of such entry, and such book shall be produced to the visiting Commissioner on every visit, and shall be signed by him as having been so produced; and every such physician, surgeon, or apothecary who shall make an untrue entry in the said book shall be guilty of a misdemeanour.

Visitors of licensed houses may visit single patients on request of Commissioners.

15. It shall be lawful for one or more of the visitors appointed in or for any county or borough under the said recited Act, upon the request in writing of the Commissioners, or any two of them, under their hands, so to do, to visit any person detained in any unlicensed house in such county or borough as

a single patient, and to inquire into and report to the Commissioners on the treatment and state of health, bodily and mental, of such patient, and to inspect the order and certificates on which such person was received; and the provisions of the said recited Act for and concerning the remuneration or payment of any such visitor, being a physician, surgeon, or apothecary, in respect of the execution of the duties of that Act, and for the payment of the costs, charges, and expenses incurred by any visitor in proceedings under that Act, shall extend and be applicable to and for the remuneration or payment of any visitor, being a physician, surgeon, or apothecary, visiting as aforesaid any single patient, and to and for the payment of the costs, charges, and expenses incurred by any visitor in or about such visit as aforesaid.

16. Every physician, surgeon, and apothecary who visits any single patient, or under whose care or charge any single patient shall be, shall on the tenth day of January, or within seven days from that time, in every year report in writing to the Commissioners the state of health, bodily and mental, of such patient, with such other circumstances as he may deem necessary to be communicated to the Commissioners; and it shall be lawful for the Commissioners, at any other time and from time to time as they see occasion, to call for and require from any such physician, surgeon, or apothecary a report in writing relative to any single patient visited by him or under his care or charge in such form and specifying such particulars as the Commissioners may direct. *Annual report to be made to the Commissioners by every medical man visiting or having charge of a single patient.*

17. The provisions contained in sections seventy-two and seventy-three of the said recited Act for the discharge of patients (not being paupers) from licensed houses shall extend and be applicable to and for the discharge of any single patient: Provided always, that this enactment shall not extend to authorise the discharge of any single patient, if the physician, surgeon, or apothecary who has the care or charge of, or visits such patient, certify in writing under his hand that in his opinion such patient is dangerous and unfit to be at large, together with the grounds on which such opinion is founded, unless one of the Commissioners shall consent in writing to the discharge of such patient. *Provisions concerning discharge of patients from licensed houses by relatives extended to single patients.*

18. It shall be lawful for the Lord Chancellor, upon the report of the Commissioners in Lunacy, to order the discharge of any person received or detained as a single patient, or to give such orders and directions in reference to such patient as *Lord Chancellor, upon Report of Commis-*

sioners, may order discharge, &c., of any single patient.

the Lord Chancellor shall think fit; and any person detaining any such patient for the space of three days after a copy of such order for his discharge shall have been served on him, or left at the house in which such person so ordered to be discharged is detained, shall be guilty of a misdemeanour.

On recovery of a patient notice to be given to friends, and in the case of a pauper to guardians, &c., and in default of discharge or removal to Commissioners and visitors.

19. The superintendent or proprietor of every registered hospital and licensed house, and every person having the care or charge of any single patient, shall forthwith, upon the recovery of any patient in such hospital or house, or of such single patient, transmit notice of such recovery in the case of a patient not a pauper to the person who signed the order for his reception, or by whom the last payment on account of such patient was made, and in the case of a pauper to the guardians of his union or parish, or if there be no such guardians to one of the overseers of the poor of his parish, or if such pauper be chargeable to any county, to the Clerk of the Peace thereof, and in case such patient be not discharged or removed within fourteen days from the giving of such notice, such superintendent, proprietor, or person as aforesaid shall immediately after the expiration of such period transmit notice of the recovery of such patient to the Commissioners, and also, in the case of a licensed house within the jurisdiction of any visitors, to the clerk of such visitors, with the date of the notice firstly in this enactment mentioned, and where notice is so given to the clerk of any visitors, he shall forthwith communicate the same to the visitors, or two of them, one of whom shall

Provision in case of death of patient in any hospital or licensed house.

be a physician, surgeon, or apothecary; and in case of the death of any patient in any hospital or licensed house, a statement setting forth the time and cause of the death, and the duration of the disease of which such patient died, shall be prepared and signed by the medical person or persons who attended the patient during the illness which terminated in death, and such statement shall be entered in the "Case Book," and a copy of such statement, certified by the superintendent or proprietor, shall within two days of the date of the death be transmitted to the coroner for the county or borough, and in case such coroner, after receiving such statement, shall think that any reasonable suspicion attends the cause and circumstances of the death of such patient, he shall summon a jury to inquire into the cause of such death.

Provision authorising transfer of

20. Any person, having authority to order the discharge of any patient (not being a pauper) from any asylum, registered

hospital, or licensed house, or of any single patient, may, with the previous consent in writing of two of the Commissioners, direct by an order in writing under his hand the removal of such patient to any asylum, registered hospital, or licensed house, or to the care or charge of any person mentioned or named in such order; and every such order and consent shall be made and given respectively in duplicate, and one of the duplicates shall be delivered to and left with the superintendent or proprietor of the asylum, hospital, or house, from which or the person from whose care or charge the patient is ordered to be removed, and the other duplicate shall be delivered to and left with the superintendent or proprietor of the asylum, hospital, or house into which, or the person into whose care or charge the patient is ordered to be removed; and such order for removal, together with such consent in writing, shall be a sufficient authority for the removal of such patient, and also for his reception into the asylum, registered hospital, or licensed house into which or by the person into whose care or charge he is ordered to be removed : Provided always, that a copy of the order and certificates upon which such patient was received into the asylum, hospital, or house from which he is removed, or as a single patient, by the person from whose care he is removed, certified under the hand of the superintendent or proprietor of such asylum, hospital, or house, or of such person as last aforesaid, to be a true copy, shall be furnished by him free of expense, and shall be delivered, with one duplicate of the said order of removal and consent, to the superintendent or proprietor of the asylum, hospital, or house to which or to the person to whose care or charge such patient is removed.

private and single patients.

21. Every person from whose care or charge any single patient shall be discharged shall transmit to the Commissioners a written notice of such discharge within the like period, and under the like penalty for default, as by the said recited Act is required and provided in the case of the discharge of a patient from a licensed house.

Notice of discharge of single patients to be sent to the Commissioners.

22. It shall be lawful for any person having the care or charge of a single patient to change his residence, and remove such patient to any new residence of such person, in England, provided that seven clear days before such change of residence he give notice in writing thereof, and of the place of such new residence, to the Commissioners and to the person who signed

Provisions as to change of residence of persons having charge of single patients, and temporary

removal of such patients for benefit of health.

the order for the reception of such patient, or by whom the last payment on account of such patient was made; and it shall be lawful for any person having the care or charge of any single patient, having first obtained the consent of two of the Commissioners, to take or send such patient under proper control, to any specified place or places, for any definite time, for the benefit of his health: Provided always, that before any such consent shall be given, the approval in writing of the person who signed the order for the reception of such patient, or by whom the last payment on account of such patient was made, shall be produced to such Commissioners, unless they shall, on cause being shown, dispense with the same.

On representation of Commissioners Lord Chancellor may require statement of property of lunatic.

23. Where any person has already been received as a lunatic under order and certificates, and shall be detained thereunder, and where any person shall hereafter be in like manner received and detained, and the Commissioners represent to the Lord Chancellor that it is desirable that the extent and nature of his income should be ascertained, and the application thereof, the Lord Chancellor may, if he think fit, through the Registrar in Lunacy, require that the person signing the order, or other the person paying for the care and maintenance of the lunatic or having the management of the property, shall transmit to the Lord Chancellor a statement in writing, to the best of his knowledge, of the particulars of the property and income of the lunatic and of the application of the income.

Form of notice of admission.

24. The notice of admission and statement mentioned or referred to in section fifty-two of the said recited Act shall hereafter be according to the form mentioned in Schedule (C) annexed to this Act, in lieu of the form set forth in Schedule (F) to the said recited Act; and such statement shall be signed by the medical superintendent, proprietor, or attendant of the hospital or licensed house from which the same is sent, and the said notice and statement shall be accompanied by a copy of the several documents mentioned in the said notice.*

Form of Medical Visitation Book.

25. The Medical Visitation Book mentioned in section fifty-nine of the said recited Act, shall henceforth be kept in the form set forth in Schedule (D) annexed to this Act, in lieu of the form set forth in Schedule (H) to the said recited Act; and the said section shall be construed as if the particulars mentioned in the several heads of the said form in the said

---

* Vide 25 & 26 Vict. c. 111, s. 28.

Schedule (D) had by the said section been required to be entered in the said book in lieu of the particulars mentioned in the said section.

26. The superintendent or proprietor of every registered hospital or licensed house shall, within one week after the dismissal for misconduct of any nurse or attendant employed in such hospital or house, transmit to the Commissioners, by the post, information in writing under his hand of such dismissal, and of the cause thereof; and every superintendent or proprietor neglecting to transmit such information to the Commissioners within the period aforesaid, shall, for every such offence, forfeit any sum not exceeding ten pounds.

Notice of dismissal for misconduct of attendants to be sent to Commissioners.

27. Section eighty-nine of the said recited Act, constituting from among the Commissioners a private committee for the purposes in the said Act mentioned, shall be repealed, and all the powers vested in, and all the provisions of the said Act applicable to the said private committee, or one or two members thereof, shall be vested in and be applicable to the Commissioners, or one Commissioner, or two Commissioners (as the case may require), as if, where in the said Act the said private committee, or one member or two members thereof (as the case may be), is or are mentioned, or referred to, the Commissioners, or one Commissioner, or two Commissioners (as the case may require), has been mentioned or referred to, instead thereof.

Powers vested in Private Committee to be vested in the Commissioners.

28. Section one hundred and eleven of the said recited Act shall be repealed, and any one or more of the Commissioners shall and may on such day or days, and at such hours in the day, and for such length of time as he or they shall think fit, visit all such parish and union workhouses in which there shall be or be alleged to be any lunatic, as the Commissioners shall by any resolution or resolutions of the board direct, and shall inquire whether the provisions of the law as to lunatics in such parish or union have been carried out, and also as to the dietary. accommodation, and treatment of the lunatics in such workhouses, and shall report in writing thereon to the Poor Law Board.

Repeal of Section 111 of recited Act, and provision as to visitation of workhouses.

29. It shall be lawful for the Commissioners, where, for any reasons to be entered upon the minutes of the board, any case appears to them specially to call for immediate investigation, to authorise and direct, by an order under their common seal, any competent person or persons to visit and examine and

Commissioners may in any special case employ persons to make the necessary inquiries,

and to report to them thereon. report to them upon the mental and bodily state and condition of any lunatic or alleged lunatic in any asylum, hospital, or licensed house, or of any pauper lunatic in a workhouse or elsewhere, or of any lunatic or alleged lunatic under the care or charge of any person as a single patient, and to inquire into and report upon any matters into which the Commissioners are authorised to inquire; and every such person shall, for the special purposes mentioned in such order, have all the powers of a Commissioner; and the Commissioners may allow to every such person a reasonable sum for his services and expenses, such sum to be paid in manner provided by the said recited Act with regard to expenses incurred by or under the authority of the Commissioners in proceedings thereunder;* but this enactment shall not be taken to exonerate the Commissioners from the performance of any duty by law imposed on them.

Regulations for hospitals to be submitted to Secretary of State. 30. The committee having the management or government of every registered hospital shall, within three months after the passing of this Act in the case of every hospital now registered, and within three months after the registration of every hospital hereafter to be registered under the said recited Act, submit the existing regulations, or regulations to be framed by such committee, to one of her Majesty's principal Secretaries of State, for his approval; and any such committee may, with the like approbation, alter and vary such regulations as they think necessary; and all such regulations so approved shall be printed, abided by, and observed, and a copy thereof shall be sent to the Commissioners, and another copy thereof kept hung up in the visitors' room of the hospital.†

Commissioners may make regulations for the government of licensed houses. 31. It shall be lawful for the Commissioners, with the sanction and approbation of one of her Majesty's principal Secretaries of State, from time to time to make regulations for the government of any house licensed for the reception of lunatics; and such regulations of the Commissioners, or a copy thereof, shall be transmitted by their secretary to the proprietor or resident superintendent of every licensed house to which the same relate, and shall be abided by and observed therein.

Time at 32. The report required by section 88 of the said

* Vide 8 & 9 Vict. c. 100, ss. 33–35.
† Vide 8 & 9 Vict. c. 100, s. 43.

recited Act to be made by the Commissioners to the Lord Chancellor in the month of June in every year of the state and condition of the several houses, hospitals, asylums, and other places visited by them under that Act, and of the care of the patients therein, and of such other particulars as they think deserving of notice, shall be made in or before the month of March in every year, and shall be made up to the end of the preceding year.

which reports of Commissioners to the Lord Chancellor as to state of asylums,&c., are to be made.

33. The provision in section 113 of the said recited Act, for and concerning the payment for attendance and trouble of any person (not being a Commissioner) employed under that enactment, and of the travelling or other expenses of any person so employed, and as to the fund out of which such payment is to be made, shall extend and be applicable to and in the case of any person (not being a Commissioner) required to visit and examine any lunatic or supposed lunatic under section 112 of the said recited Act.

Provision for payment of persons employed to inspect places where lunatics are confined extended to persons visiting under s. 112 of 8 & 9 Vict. c. 100.

34. Any person who wilfully obstructs the Commissioners or any of them, or any other person authorised by an order in writing under the hand of the Lord Chancellor or her Majesty's principal Secretary of State for the Home Department, pursuant to the provisions of section 112 or 113 of the said recited Act, to visit and examine any lunatic or supposed lunatic, or to inspect or inquire into the state of any asylum, hospital, gaol, house, or place wherein any lunatic or person represented to be lunatic is confined or alleged to be confined, in the execution of such order ; and any person who wilfully obstructs any person authorised under this Act by any order of the Commissioners to make any visit and examination or inquiry in the execution of such order shall (without prejudice to any proceedings, and in addition to any punishment to which such person obstructing the execution of such order would otherwise be liable) forfeit for every such offence any sum not exceeding twenty pounds.

Penalty on persons obstructing execution of orders of Lord Chancellor or Secretary of State, made under ss. 112 or 113 of recited Act, or of Commissioners made under this Act.

35. Section 116 of the said recited Act shall be repealed, and the Royal Hospital of Bethlehem shall henceforth be subject to the provisions of the said recited Act and of this Act, in the same manner as if the same had not been exempted from the said recited Act, and shall be forthwith registered as an hospital accordingly, in pursuance of section 43 of the said recited Act.

Section 116 of recited Act repealed, and Bethlehem Hospital to be subject to this Act.

Interpretation of terms.

36. In the construction of the said recited Act and of this Act the words "physician," "surgeon," and "apothecary" shall respectively mean * a physician, surgeon, and apothecary duly authorised or licensed to practise as such by or as a member of some college, university, company, or institution legally constituted, and qualified to grant such authority or licence in some part of the United Kingdom, or having been in practice as an apothecary in England or Wales on or before the first day of August, 1815, and being in actual practice as such physician, surgeon, or apothecary. The expression "officiating clergyman of the parish" shall include the chaplain of the workhouse of the same parish, or of the workhouse of the union to which such parish belongs. The expression "single patient" shall mean any person received or taken charge of as a lunatic under section 90 of the said recited Act, or under such section as amended by this Act; and the expression "attendant" shall mean any person, whether male or female, who shall be employed either wholly or partially in the personal care, control, or management of any lunatic in any registered hospital or licensed house, or of any single patient; and in the construction of this Act the word "Board," as used in relation to the Commissioners in Lunacy, shall mean any three or more of the Commissioners assembled at a meeting convened in pursuance of section 16 of the said recited Act, or holden under any order or rule for the time being in force made under section 70 of the said recited Act for regulating the duties of the Commissioners.

Recited Act and this Act to be construed as one Act, &c.

37. The said recited Act and this Act shall be construed together as one Act, and a Queen's Printer's copy of this Act shall be bound up in the "Visitors' Book" of every hospital and licensed house together with the said recited Act.

Act not to affect provisions relating to criminal lunatics, 39 & 40 G. 3, c. 94; 1 & 2 Vict. c. 14, and 3 & 4 Vict. c. 54, save as herein provided.

38. Nothing in this Act shall affect the provisions of any of the following Acts (that is to say): An Act of the session holden in the thirty-ninth and fortieth years of King George the Third, chapter 94; an Act of the session holden in the first and second years of her Majesty, chapter 14; and an Act of the session holden in the third and fourth years of her Majesty, chapter 54, or any other provisions concerning criminal lunatics, save as hereinafter provided; that is to say, it shall

* Vide 25 & 26 Vict. c. 111, s. 47. By this it is seen that the medical man must be registered according to the Medical Act.

be lawful for one of her Majesty's principal Secretaries of State to issue his warrant to remove or discharge any insane person who shall be in custody under the provisions of the said Act of the third and fourth years of her Majesty, chapter 54, provided it shall be duly certified to such Secretary of State, by two physicians or surgeons, that such insane person was harmless, and might be discharged from restraint as an insane person, without danger to himself or to others, in like manner as if it had been certified to such Secretary of State that such person had become of sound mind, anything in the said Act or any other Act to the contrary thereof in any wise notwithstanding.

39. And whereas by the said recited Act it is provided that every person to be appointed in the room of any Commissioner, being a barrister of five years' standing at the bar and upwards, shall be a practising barrister of not less than five years' standing at the bar : And whereas it is expedient to amend the said provisions as hereinafter mentioned ; the present or any future secretary to the Commissioners, if at the time of his appointment to be such secretary he was or shall have been a practising barrister of not less than five years' standing at the bar, shall be eligible to be appointed a Commissioner in the room of any such Commissioner as aforesaid. *Secretary to the Commissioners, if at the time of his appointment a practising barrister of five years' standing, eligible to be appointed a Commissioner.*

40. This Act shall commence and come into operation on the first day of November, 1853. *Commencement of Act.*

Schedules to the foregoing Act.

SCHEDULE (A) No. 1, SECTIONS 4, 8.

Order for the Reception of a Private Patient.

I, the undersigned, hereby request you to receive *A.B.*, a Lunatic [*or* an idiot, *or* a person of unsound mind,] as a patient into your house [*or* hospital]. Subjoined is a statement respecting the said *A.B.*

         (Signed)   Name.

                            Occupation (if any).

                            Place of abode.

                            Degree of relationship (if any), or other circumstance of connection with the patient.

Dated this   day of   One thousand eight hundred and

To   Proprietor [*or* Superintendent] of [*describing the house or hospital by situation and name, if any*].

STATEMENT.

[*If any particulars in this Statement be not known, the fact to be so stated.*]

Name of patient, with Christian name at length.

Sex and age.

Married, single, or widowed.

Condition of life, and previous occupation (if any).

The religious persuasion, as far as known.

Previous place of abode.

Whether first attack.

Age (if known) on first attack.

When and where previously under care and treatment.

Duration of existing attack.

Supposed cause.

Whether subject to epilepsy.

Whether suicidal.

Whether dangerous to others.

---

* Vide 25 & 26 Vict. c. 111, ss. 23, 25, 26. By the amended Act we see that the order is only available for one month, and the person signing it must have seen the patient within a month.

Whether found lunatic by inquisition, and date of commission or order for inquisition.

Special circumstances (if any) preventing the patient being examined, before admission, separately by two medical practitioners.

(Signed)*   Name.

[*Where the person signing the Statement is not the person who signs the Order, the following particulars concerning the person signing the Statement are to be added ; viz.,*]

Occupation (if any).

Place of abode.

Degree of relationship (if any) or other circumstances of connection with the patient.]

SCHEDULE (A) No. 2, SECTIONS 4, 5, 8, 10, 11, 12, 13.

Form of Medical Certificate.

I, the undersigned [*here set forth the qualification entitling the person certifying to practise as a Physician, Surgeon, or Apothecary, ex. gra.,* being a Fellow of the Royal College of Physicians in London], and being in actual practice as a [Physician, Surgeon, *or* Apothecary, *as the case may be*], hereby certify, That I, on the day of   at   [*here insert the street and number of the house (if any) or other like particulars*], in the county of   , separately from any other Medical Practitioner, personally examined *A.B.* of [*insert residence and profession or occupation, if any*], and that the said *A.B.* is a lunatic [*or* an idiot, *or* a person of unsound mind], and a proper person to be taken charge of and detained under care and treatment, and that I have formed this opinion upon the following grounds ; viz.

1. Facts indicating insanity observed by myself [*here state the facts*].

2. Other facts (if any) indicating insanity communicated to me by others [*here state the information, and from whom*].

(Signed)†

Place of abode.

Dated this   day of   One thousand eight hundred and

---

* Vide 25 & 26 Vict. c. 111, s. 24. This will enumerate those who are prohibited from signing.

† Vide 25 & 26 Vict. c. 111, s. 24.

SCHEDULE (B) No. 1, SECTION 7.

Order for the Reception of a Pauper Patient.

I, *C.D.* [*or, in the case of a Clergyman and Relieving Officer, &c.,* we, *C.D.* and *E.F.*], the undersigned, having called to my (*or* our) assistance a Physician, [*or* Surgeon, *or* Apothecary, *as the case may be,*] and having personally examined *A.B.*, a Pauper, and being satisfied that the said *A.B.* is a Lunatic [*or* an Idiot, *or* a person of unsound mind,] and a proper person to be taken charge of and detained under care and treatment, hereby direct you to receive the said *A.B.* as a patient into your house [*or* hospital]. Subjoined is a Statement respecting the said *A.B.*

          (Signed)   *C.D.*

     A Justice of the Peace for the County, City, or Borough of

     [*or* an *or* the Officiating Clergyman of the Parish of   ].

          (Signed)   *E.F.*

     The Relieving Officer of the Union or Parish of

         [*or* an Overseer of the Parish of   ].

Dated the   day of   One thousand eight hundred and

To   Proprietor [*or* Superintendent.] of [*describing the house or hospital*].

STATEMENT.

[*If any particulars in this Statement be not known, to be so stated.*]

Name of patient, and Christian name at length.
Sex and age.
Married, single, or widowed.
Condition of life, and previous occupation (if any).
The religious persuasion, as far as known.
Previous place of abode.
Whether first attack.
Age (if known) on first attack.
When and where previously under care and treatment.
Duration of existing attack.
Supposed cause.
Whether subject to epilepsy.
Whether suicidal.

Whether dangerous to others

Parish or Union to which the Lunatic is chargeable.

Name and Christian name and place of abode of nearest known relative of the patient, and degree of relationship (if known).*

> I certify that, to the best of my knowledge, the above particulars are correctly stated.
>
> (Signed)
>
> Relieving Officer [*or* Overseer].

SCHEDULE (B) No. 2, SECTIONS 7, 10, 11, 12, 13.

Form of Medical Certificate.†

I, the undersigned [*here set forth the qualification entitling the person certifying to practise as a Physician, Surgeon, or Apothecary, ex. gra.*, being a Fellow of the Royal College of Physicians in London], and being in actual practice as a [Physician, Surgeon, *or* Apothecary, *as the case may be*], hereby certify, that I, on the day of   at   [*here insert the Street and Number of the House (if any) or other like particulars*], in the County of   , personally examined *A.B.* of [*insert Residence and Profession or Occupation (if any)*], and that the said *A.B.* is a Lunatic, [*or* an Idiot, *or* a Person of Unsound Mind], and a proper person to be taken charge of and detained under care and treatment, and that I have formed this opinion upon the following grounds ; viz.—

1. Facts indicating Insanity observed by myself [*here state the facts*].

2. Other Facts (if any) indicating Insanity communicated to me by others [*here state the information, and from whom*].

> (Signed) ‡
>
> Place of Abode.

Dated this   day of   One thousand eight hundred and

---

* Vide 25 & 26 Vict. c. 111, s. 25.

† Vide 25 & 26 Vict. c. 111, ss. 26–27.

‡ Vide 8 & 9 Vict. c 100, s. 23.

SCHEDULE (C) Section 24.

Notice of Admission.

I hereby give you Notice, that *A.B.* was admitted into this House [or Hospital] as a Private [or Pauper] Patient on the day of   and I hereby transmit a Copy of the Order and Medical Certificates [or Certificate] on which he was received. [*If a Private Patient be received upon One Certificate only, the special Circumstances which have prevented the Patient from being examined by Two Medical Practitioners to be here stated, as in the Statement accompanying the Order for Admission*].

Subjoined is a Statement with respect to the mental and bodily Condition of the above-named Patient.

(Signed)

Superintendent [or Proprietor] of

Dated the *   day of   One thousand eight hundred and

Statement.

I have this Day [*some Day not less than Two clear Days after the Admission of the Patient*] seen and examined the Patient mentioned in the above Notice, and hereby certify that with respect to mental State he [or she]   and that with respect to bodily Health and Condition he [or she]

(Signed)

Medical Proprietor [or Superintendent, or Attendant] of

Dated the *   day of   One thousand eight hundred and

---

* Vide 8 & 9 Vict. c. 100, s. 52 ; 25 & 26 Vict. c. 111, s. 28.

This notice must be sent within one clear day, and the statement after the expiration of two and before the expiration of seven.

SCHEDULE (D) SECTION.

Form of Medical Visitation Book.

Date	Number and Class of Patients				Patients who are, or since the last entry have been under restraint, or in seclusion, when and for what period, and reasons, and, in cases of restraint, by what means				Patients under Medical Treatment, and for what (if any) bodily disorder		Deaths, Injuries, and Violence to Patients since the last entry
	Private		Pauper		Restraint		Seclusion				
	M.	F.	M.	F.	Males	Females	Males	Females	Males	Females	

III.

ANNO VICESIMO QUINTO & VICESIMO SEXTO VICTORIÆ REGINÆ.

CAP. CXI.

An Act to amend the Law relating to Lunatics.

August 7, 1862.

WHEREAS it is expedient to amend the law relating to lunatics, other than those found lunatics by inquisition, or lunatics
convicted of crime, or acquitted on the ground of insanity:
Be it enacted by the Queen's most excellent Majesty, by and
with the advice and consent of the Lords Spiritual and Temporal, and Commons, in this present Parliament assembled, and
by the authority of the same, as follows, (that is to say),

Preliminary.

1. In the construction and for the purposes of this Act (if
not inconsistent with the context or subject matter) the follow-

Interpreta-
tion of
terms.
ing terms shall have the respective meanings hereinafter assigned to them, that is to say,

> "Lunacy Act, chapter 100," shall mean an Act passed
> in the session holden in the eighth and ninth years
> of the reign of her present Majesty, chapter 100, and
> intituled, "An Act for the Regulation of the Care and
> Treatment of Lunatics." *

> "Lunacy Act, chapter 96," shall mean an Act passed
> in the session holden in the sixteenth and seventeenth
> years of the reign of her present Majesty, chapter 96,
> intituled "An Act to amend an Act passed in the ninth
> year of her Majesty, for the Regulation of the Care and
> Treatment of Lunatics."

> "Lunacy Act, chapter 97," shall mean an Act passed in
> the session holden in the sixteenth and seventeenth
> years of the reign of her present Majesty, chapter 97,
> intituled "An Act to consolidate and amend the Laws
> for the Provision and Regulation of Lunatic Asylums

* 16 & 17 Vict. c. 96.

for Counties and Boroughs, and for the Maintenance and Care of Pauper Lunatics, in England."

"The Lunacy Acts" shall include the three Acts above mentioned and this Act.

"Asylum" shall have the same meaning as it has in the Lunacy Act, chapter 97.

"Registered Hospital" shall mean any hospital registered for the reception of lunatics.

2. This Act shall be construed as one Act with the Lunacy Acts, chapters 100, 96, and 97, and words defined by the said Acts or any of them shall have the same meaning in this Act. *Construction of Act.*

3. This Act may be cited for all purposes as the "Lunacy Acts Amendment Act, 1862." *Short title.*

Establishment of County Asylums.

4. Whereas by section 31 of the Lunacy Act, chapter 97, it is provided, "that the said visitors shall from time to time make their report to the general or quarter sessions of the county or borough, counties or boroughs, for which they (or such of them as have not been elected by subscribers, as therein mentioned) have been elected, of the several plans, estimates, and contracts which have been agreed upon, and of the sum or sums of money necessary to be raised and levied for defraying the purchase moneys and expenses thereof on the county or borough, or, in the case of such union as therein mentioned, on each or every of the counties or boroughs; which plans, estimates, and contracts shall be subject to the approbation of the court or courts of general or quarter sessions of such county or counties, and of the justices of such borough or boroughs, before the same are completed or carried into execution" (save in the case therein mentioned). *Plans, &c., of visitors, when not approved by the Quarter Sessions, to be submitted to Secretary of State.*

Where a plan, estimate, or contract agreed upon by any committee of visitors on behalf of a union of counties, or of a union of counties and boroughs, is disapproved of by one or more, but not all, of the courts of general or quarter sessions, or other bodies of justices whose approbation is required, in pursuance of the said enactment, each court of general or quarter sessions or body of justices disapproving of the same shall, within four months after such plan, estimate, or contract is reported to them, or where the same has been reported to them before the passing of this Act, then within one month after the holding of the first court of general or quarter sessions of the county, or the first meeting of the justices of the borough after the passing of this Act, as the case may be, set forth their objections, with any observations they may think fit in relation thereto, in a report in writing, and forthwith transmit the same to one of her Majesty's principal Secretaries of State, and the Secretary of State shall cause such inquiries to be made in relation to the matter as he may deem proper, and shall by writing under his hand direct the plan, estimate, or contract in question, with or without any alteration therein, or such other plan, estimate, or contract for the like purpose, as he may think fit, to be proceeded with and carried into execution.

The decision of the Secretary of State, given in pursuance of this section, shall be final, and shall be acted upon without further report or approval.

Estimates to accompany plans. 5. Together with every plan for building, or providing, or enlarging, or improving, any asylum for pauper lunatics, which is to be submitted to the Commissioners in Lunacy, under section 45 of the said Lunacy Act, chapter 97, an estimate of the cost and expense of carrying such plan into execution shall be also submitted to the said Commissioners.

Excess of payment may be paid to a building and repair fund. 6. Where the committee of visitors enter into any agreement for the reception into the county asylum of pauper lunatics belonging to a county or borough which has not contributed to the erecting or providing such asylum, and think fit under the Lunacy Act, chapter 97, section 54, to fix a greater weekly sum than is charged by them in respect of lunatics sent from or settled in some place, parish, or borough, which has contributed to the building or providing such asylum, they may, if they think fit, pay over the excess created by the payment of such greater weekly sum to a building and repair fund, to be applied by them to the altering, repairing, or improving such asylum, and shall annually submit to the general or quarter sessions, a detailed statement of the manner in which such fund has been expended.

Provision as to contract for reception of lunatics. 7. Where any contract has been made by a committee of visitors of any county or borough under the Lunacy Act, chapter 97, section 42, for the reception into any asylum, hospital, or licensed house of the whole or a portion of the pauper lunatics of such county or borough, it shall be lawful for the justices of such county or borough, so long as such contract is

subsisting, to defray out of the county or borough rate so
much of the weekly charge agreed upon for each pauper lunatic received therein as may, in the opinion of such committee
of visitors, represent the sum due for the use of such asylum,
hospital or licensed house, not exceeding, however, one fourth
of the whole of such weekly charge, in exoneration to that
extent of the union to which the maintenance of any such
pauper lunatic may be chargeable.

8. It shall be lawful for the visitors of any asylum and the
guardians of any parish or union within the district for which
the asylum has been provided, if they shall see fit, to make
arrangements, subject to the approval of the Commissioners
and the president of the Poor Law Board, for the reception and
care of a limited number of chronic lunatics in the workhouse
of the parish or union, to be selected by the superintendent of
the asylum, and certified by him to be fit and proper so to be
removed.

Provision for care of chronic lunatics.

9. The committee of visitors of any asylum may provide
accommodation for the burial of pauper lunatics dying in the
asylum by acquiring a new burial ground, or by enlarging any
existing burial ground; they may purchase for the purposes
aforesaid any land, and may grant any land when purchased, or
any land already belonging to them, to any person or body of
persons, to be held on trust for a new burial ground or as part
of an existing burial ground, or they may themselves hold
such land on trust as a new burial ground or as part of an
existing burial ground; they may also contribute any sums of
money to any person or body of persons on condition of such
person or body of persons agreeing to provide accommodation
for the burial of such paupers as aforesaid in any burial
ground; they may also take steps for the consecration of any
new burial ground or enlarged burial ground, or any part
thereof, and in the case of a new burial ground they may provide for the appointment of a chaplain therein; they may enter
into any agreements necessary for carrying into effect the
powers conferred by this section, but the exercise of such
powers shall be subject to the restrictions following:

Lunatics in asylum.

Firstly, That not more than two statute acres shall in the
case of any one asylum be purchased or granted as a
new burial ground, or for an enlargement of an existing
burial ground.

Secondly, That the sanction of the court of general or quarter sessions and of one of Her Majesty's principal Secretaries of State shall be given to any plan that may be proposed by any visitors for carrying into effect this section.

All expenses incurred by any visitors in providing accommodation for the burial of pauper lunatics, in pursuance of this Act, shall be deemed to be moneys, costs, and expenses payable for the purposes of the Lunacy Act, chapter 97, and may be defrayed accordingly.

8 & 9 Vict. c. 18, incorporated.

10. All the provisions of "The Lands Clauses Act, 1845," except the provisions of that Act "with respect to the purchase and taking of any lands otherwise than by agreement," "with respect to the recovery of forfeitures, penalties, and costs," "with respect to lands acquired by the promoters of the undertaking, under the provisions of the Lands Clauses Consolidation Act, 1845, or the Special Act, or any Act incorporated therewith, but which shall not be required for the purposes thereof," "and with respect to the provision to be made for affording access to the Special Act by all parties interested," shall be incorporated with this Act; and for the purposes of this Act the expression "the promoters of the undertaking," wherever used in the said Lands Clauses Consolidation Act, shall mean any such committee of visitors as aforesaid.

Taking on lease additional land for use of asylum.

11. It shall be lawful for any committee of visitors, with the sanction of the court of general or quarter sessions, to hire or take on lease, from year to year or for any term of years, at such rent, and upon such terms, and under such covenants as they think fit, any land or buildings, either for the employment or occupation of the patients in the asylum, or for the temporary accommodation of any pauper lunatics for whom the accommodation in the asylum may be inadequate.

The restrictions in section 33 of the Lunacy Act, chapter 97, as to the term for which the committee of visitors are thereby authorised to take a lease, or to rent land, shall not apply to land or buildings to be hired or taken under this provision.

The land and buildings so to be hired or taken shall, while used for the purposes of this section, be deemed part of the asylum, and all existing provisions as to the asylum or part of the asylum shall be applicable thereto accordingly.

Superannuation of officers in asylum.

12. The power vested in the visitors of an asylum of granting an annuity by way of superannuation to any person that

has been an officer or servant in such asylum for not less than twenty years, under section 57 of the Lunacy Act, chapter 97, may be exercised by them when any such person has been an officer or servant for not less than fifteen years, in the same manner as if the time of such service had been twenty years; and in calculating the amount of superannuation regard may be had, if the visitors think fit, to the value of the lodgings, rations, or other allowances enjoyed by the person superannuated: Provided, that no annuity by way of superannuation granted by the visitors of any asylum under the provisions of this Act, or of the Lunacy Act, chapter 97, shall be chargeable on or payable out of the rates of any county until such annuity shall have been confirmed by a resolution of the justices of such county in general or quarter sessions assembled.

13. Where the offices of superintendent and matron of any asylum are held by man and wife, and an order has been made under the Lunacy Act, chapter 97, granting an annuity by way of superannuation to the superintendent, it shall be lawful for the committee of visitors of such asylum, if they think fit to do so, and if the matron has been an officer in the asylum for not less than twenty years, to grant to her such annuity by way of superannuation as they in their discretion think proportionate to her merits and time of service, although she may not have become incapable of executing her office from sickness, age, or infirmity; and every annuity granted in pursuance of this section shall be payable out of the rates lawfully applicable to the building or repairing of such asylum: Provided, firstly, that the annual amount by way of superannuation paid to any matron under this section shall not exceed two-thirds of the salary payable at the time of her retirement; secondly, that no such superannuation shall be granted unless notice of the meeting at which the same is to be granted, and of the intention to determine thereat the question of such superannuation, have been given in such manner and so long before the time appointed for such meeting as is provided in the said Act with respect to notices of meetings of committees of visitors, nor unless three visitors concur in and sign the order granting the same; thirdly, if any such matron as aforesaid at any time thereafter is appointed to any public office, or to any office under the Lunacy Act, in respect of which she receives a salary, the payment of the compensation awarded to her under this Act shall be suspended so long as she receives such salary,

Provision for superannuation of matrons.

if the amount thereof is greater than the amount of compensation, or, if not, shall be diminished by the amount of such salary.

Licensed Houses.

Inspection by Commissioners before licence granted by justices.

14. Before the grant by the justices of a licence for the reception of lunatics to a house which has not been previously licensed for that purpose, the notice given by the applicant, and the plan and statements accompanying the same, or copies of such notice, plan, and statements respectively,* shall be transmitted by the applicant to the Commissioners, and the Commissioners shall inspect, or cause to be inspected, the house and land or appurtenances proposed to be included in the licence, and shall ascertain, with reference as well to the situation as to the structure, arrangements, and condition of the premises, whether the same are suitable for the reception of the patients proposed to be received therein, and the Commissioners shall transmit to the clerk of the peace for the county or borough a report in reference to such application; and no licence shall be granted by the justices of the county or borough, in pursuance of such application, until the report of the Commissioners with reference thereto has been received by the said clerk of the peace, and taken into consideration by the justices in general or quarter or special sessions assembled.

Where a licence is granted by the justices of a county or borough in respect of a house not previously licensed, such licence shall, as nearly as conveniently may be, be according to the form in the schedule marked A to this Act, instead of in the form prescribed by the Lunacy Act, chapter 100.

Notice of alterations to be given to the Commissioners.

15. Before the consent of any visitors is given to any addition or alteration being made in or about any licensed house, or the appurtenances, the notice of the proposed addition or alteration, and plan thereof, and accompanying description given to the clerk of the peace, or copies thereof respectively, shall be transmitted by him to the Commissioners, who shall, after making or causing to be made such inquiries or inspection (if any) as they may deem proper, transmit to the said clerk of the peace a report stating their approval or disapproval thereof; and the visitors shall not consent to such addition or alteration until they have received and considered such report.

* Vide 8 & 9 Vict. c. 100, s. 24; 16 & 17 Vict. c. 96, s. 1.

16. Whereas by the 2nd section of the Lunacy Act, chapter 96, it is enacted, " that no person having, after the passing of the Lunacy Act, chapter 100, received for the first time a licence for the reception of lunatics, or thereafter receiving for the first time such licence, shall receive a licence unless he resides on the premises licensed ; and no two or more persons having, after the passing of the last-mentioned Act, received for the first time a joint licence for the reception of lunatics, or thereafter receiving for the first time such joint licence, shall receive such licence unless they or one of them should reside on the premises licensed :" And whereas it is expedient that in the licensed houses to which the said section does not apply, by reason of the proprietor or proprietors thereof having first received a licence prior to the date mentioned in the said section, the following provision shall be made : Be it enacted, That in all cases of licensed houses, where the proprietor or proprietors thereof have first received their licence or licences before the date of the passing of the Lunacy Act, chapter 100, the physician, surgeon, or apothecary required by Act of Parliament to reside in or visit such house shall be approved, in the case of a house licensed by the Commissioners, by the Commissioners ; and in the case of a house licensed by justices, by the justices ; and any proprietor of a licensed house to which this section applies who permits any physician, surgeon, or apothecary who has not been approved by the Commissioners, or by the justices, as the case may be, to reside in or visit at such house in such capacity as aforesaid for a period exceeding one calendar month, shall incur a penalty not exceeding five pounds for every day beyond such month during which such physician, surgeon, or apothecary so resides or visits. The above-mentioned period of one month shall be reckoned in the case of a physician, surgeon, or apothecary so resident or visiting at the time of the passing of this Act from the date of the passing thereof, and in the case of any fresh appointment of any such physician, surgeon, or apothecary as aforesaid from the date of such appointment.

Provision as to non-resident proprietors.

17. If any person empowered by licence issued under the Lunacy Act, chapter 100, to employ his house and premises for the reception of lunatics receives into his house any patients beyond the number specified in his licence, or fails to comply with the regulations of his licence in respect of the sex of the patients to be received, or the class of patients,

Penalty on infringing terms of licence.

whether private or not, to be received, he shall, in respect of each patient received in contravention of his licence, incur a penalty not exceeding fifty pounds.

Extension of powers to take boarders in houses.

18. It shall be lawful for the proprietor or superintendent of any licensed house, with the previous assent in writing of two or more of the Commissioners, or in the case of a house licensed by justices of two or more of the visitors, to entertain and keep in such house as a boarder for such time as may be specified in the assent any person who may have been within five years immediately preceding the giving of such assent a patient in any asylum, hospital, or licensed house, or under care as a single patient.*

Admission and Visitation of Patients.

Provision for sending pauper lunatics to asylums.

19. Whereas by the 67th section of the Lunacy Act, chapter 97, it is amongst other things enacted as follows: " That every relieving officer of any parish within a union or under a board of guardians, and every overseer of a parish of which there is no relieving officer, who shall have knowledge either by such notice or otherwise that any pauper resident in such parish is or is deemed to be a lunatic and a proper person to be sent to an asylum, shall within three days after obtaining such knowledge give notice thereof to some justice of the county or borough within which such parish is situate:" Now be it enacted, That the said section shall be construed as if the words " and a proper person to be sent to an asylum " had been omitted in the said recited enactment.

Lunatics proper to be sent to asylums.

20. No person shall be detained in any workhouse, being a lunatic or alleged lunatic, beyond the period of fourteen days, unless in the opinion, given in writing, of the medical officer of the union or parish to which the workhouse belongs such person is a proper person to be kept in a workhouse, nor unless the accommodation in the workhouse is sufficient for his reception, and any person detained in a workhouse in contravention of this section shall be deemed to be a proper person to be sent to an asylum within the meaning of section 67 of the Lunacy Act, chapter 97; and in the event of any person being detained in a workhouse in contravention of this section, the medical officer shall for all the purposes of the Lunacy Act, chapter 97, be deemed to have knowledge that a pauper resident with-

* Vide 16 & 17 Vict. c. 96, ss. 4, 6.

in his district is a lunatic, and a proper person to be sent to an asylum, and it shall be his duty to act accordingly, and further to sign such certificate as is contained in Schedule F to the said Act, No. 3, with a view to more certainly securing the reception into an asylum of such pauper lunatic as aforesaid.

21. The list of lunatic paupers required by section 66 of the Lunacy Act, chapter 97, to be made out by the medical officer, shall be in the form in the Schedule marked B hereto, and not in the form required by the said section, and shall, as respects such of the lunatics therein mentioned as may be in any workhouse, state whether, in the opinion of the medical officer, the workhouse is or not sufficient for the accommodation of the lunatics detained therein, and whether or not the lunatics detained therein are proper persons to be kept in a workhouse. *Amendment of form of list as respects pauper lunatics in workhouses.*

22. When a person has been found lunatic by inquisition, an order, signed by the committee appointed by the Lord Chancellor, and having annexed thereto an office copy of the order appointing such committee, shall be a sufficient authority for the reception of such person into any asylum,* hospital, licensed house, or other house, without any further order or any such medical certificates as are required by section 90 of the Lunacy Act, chapter 100, and sections 4 and 8 of the Lunacy Act, chapter 96, and the provisions of the section 90 of the Lunacy Act, chapter 100, as to the visitation of every single patient once in every two weeks by a physician, surgeon, or apothecary, shall not apply to any person found lunatic by inquisition as aforesaid. *Order for reception and medical visitation of persons found lunatic by inquisition.*

23. No order for the reception of a private patient into any asylum or registered hospital, licensed or other house, made in pursuance of the Lunacy Acts, chapters 96 and 97, or either of them, shall authorise the reception of such patient after the expiration of one calendar month from its date, nor unless the person subscribing such order has himself seen the patient within one month prior to its date, nor unless a statement of the time and place when such person last saw the patient is added to such order. *Persons signing orders for admission to have seen patient within one month.*

24. The following persons shall be prohibited from signing any certificate or order for the reception of any private patient into any licensed or other house:† *Certain persons prohibited from signing orders for admission.*

* Vide 8 & 9 Vict. c. 100, s. 90 ; 16 & 17 Vict. c. 96, ss. 4, 8.

† Vide 16 & 17 Vict. c. 96, Sched. A.

First, Any person receiving any percentage on or otherwise interested in the payments to be made by or on account of any patient received into a licensed or other house:

Second, Any medical attendant as defined by the Lunacy Act, chapter 100.*

Relative of pauper to be named in order of admission.

25. Where an order is made, in pursuance of the Lunacy Acts or any of them, for the reception of any private or pauper lunatic into any asylum, registered hospital, † or licensed house, there shall be inserted in every such order, wherever it be possible, the name and address of one or more of the relations of the lunatic; and in the event of his death it shall be the duty of the clerk of such asylum, the superintendent of such hospital, and the proprietor or superintendent of such licensed house, to send by post notice of his death in a prepaid letter addressed to such relation or one of such relations.

Same order and certificates to justify detention as pauper of private patient.

26. The order and certificate required by law for the detention of a patient as a pauper shall extend to authorise his detention, although it may afterwards appear that he is entitled to be classified as a private patient; and the order and certificates required by law for the detention of a patient as a private patient shall authorise his detention, although it may afterwards appear that he ought to be classified as a pauper patient.†

Provision as to defective certificates.

27. Where any medical certificate upon which a patient has been received into any asylum, registered hospital, licensed or other house, or either of such certificates, is deemed by the Commissioners incorrect or defective, and the same are or is not duly amended to their satisfaction within fourteen days after the reception by the superintendent or proprietor of such asylum, registered hospital, or licensed or other house of a direction or writing from the Commissioners requiring amendment of the same, the Commissioners or any two of them may, if they see fit, make an order for the patient's discharge.

Transmission of documents to Commissioners on admission of patient.

28. The documents required by the Lunacy Act, chapter 100, sections 52 and 90, and the Lunacy Act, chapter 97, section 89, to be sent to the Commissioners in Lunacy, after two clear days, and before the expiration of seven clear days from the day on which any private patient has been received into any licensed house, registered hospital, or asylum, shall, with the exception of the statement now required to be subjoined to the

* Vide 8 & 9 Vict. c. 100. s. 114.
† Vide 16 & 17 Vict. c. 96, Sched. A, B.

notice of admission into any asylum, hospital, or licensed house, be transmitted to the said Commissioners within one clear day from the day on which any patient has been received into any such house, hospital, or asylum as aforesaid, and the said sections shall, so far as relates to the said documents, other than the said statement, be construed as if the words "one clear day" were substituted therein for the words "after two clear days, and before the expiration of seven clear days;" nevertheless the said excepted statement shall be transmitted as heretofore, save that it shall be separate from the said notice, and shall refer to the order of admission by the date thereof, instead of referring to it as the above notice, and the words referring to the said statement as being subjoined shall be omitted in the said notice.

29. Every licensed house may be visited at any time, and, if situate within their immediate jurisdiction,* shall be visited twice at least in every year by any one or more of the Commissioners, in addition to the visits now required to be made by two at least of the Commissioners; † and if not within the immediate jurisdiction of the Commissioners, may be visited at any time, and shall be visited twice at least in every year by one or more of the visitors, in addition to the visits now required to be made by two at least of the visitors.‡ *Visits by Commissioners.*

Every Commissioner visiting alone shall have the same powers as two Commissioners would have under section 61 of the Lunacy Act, chapter 100; and all the provisions of the said Act contained in sections 63, 64, 65, 66, and 67 shall apply to a Commissioner or visitor visiting alone, as the case may be, in the same manner as they would apply under the said Act to two or more Commissioners or two or more visitors visiting together.

30. Any one or more of the Commissioners may at any time visit every asylum and hospital for lunatics, and every gaol in which there may be, or alleged to be, any lunatic, in addition to the visits now required or empowered to be made by two at least of the Commissioners, and every Commissioner so visiting alone shall have the same powers as two or more Commissioners would perform and have, in the case of an asylum or gaol, in pursuance of the 110th section of the Lunacy Act, chapter *Single Commissioner to visit asylums and gaols.*

* Vide 8 & 9 Vict. c. 100, s. 14.
† Vide 8 & 9 Vict. c. 100, s. 61.
‡ Vide 8 & 9 Vict. c. 100, s. 62.

100, and in the case of a hospital in pursuance of section 61 of the Lunacy Act, chapter 100.

Power to remove lunatic from workhouse to asylum.

31. Where upon the visitation of any workhouse by any two or more of the Commissioners in Lunacy it appears to them that any lunatic or alleged lunatic therein is not a proper person to be kept in a workhouse, they may by an order under their hands direct such lunatic to be received into an asylum, and any order so made shall have the same effect, and be obeyed by the same persons, and subject them to the same penalties in case of disobedience, as an order made by a justice for the reception of a lunatic into an asylum under the 67th section of the Lunacy Act, chapter 97 : Provided always, that it shall be lawful for the guardians of the union or parish to which any workhouse belongs to appeal against such order at any time within one calendar month from the making thereof to her Majesty's principal Secretary of State for the Home Department, who shall thereupon exercise the power given to him by section 113 of the Lunacy Act, chapter 100, save that he shall not appoint thereunder the Commissioners who made the order appealed against, or either of them ; and the order in the matter of the Secretary of State, made upon the report of the special visitation, shall be binding on all parties concerned.

Removal of single pauper patients to asylums.

32. Any two or more of the Commissioners in Lunacy may visit any pauper lunatic or alleged lunatic not in an asylum, hospital, licensed house, or workhouse, and may, if they think fit so to do, call to their assistance a physician, surgeon, or apothecary and examine such pauper ; and if such physician, surgeon, or apothecary sign a certificate with respect to such pauper, according to the form in Schedule F, No. 3, annexed to the Lunacy Act, chapter 97, and the Commissioners are satisfied that such pauper is a lunatic, and a proper person to be taken charge of and detained under care and treatment, they may, by an order under their hands, direct such lunatic or alleged lunatic to be received into an asylum, and any order so made shall have the same effect, and be obeyed by the same persons, and subject them to the same penalties in case of disobedience, as an order made by a justice for the reception of a lunatic into an asylum under the 67th section of the Lunacy Act, chapter 97.

Effect of order for removal.

33. The order made by any two or more of the Commissioners in Lunacy in pursuance of this Act may authorise the admission of a lunatic not only into any asylum of the county or borough in which the parish or place from which the lunatic

is sent is situate, but also into any other asylum for the reception of pauper lunatics of such county or borough; and also into any asylum for any other county or borough, or any hospital registered or house licensed for the reception of lunatics, under the same circumstances and subject to the same conditions under which an order of the justice or justices may authorise such admission, in pursuance of section 72 of the Lunacy Act, chapter 97.

34. The superintendent of every asylum shall, once at the least in each half year, transmit to the guardians of every union, and of every parish under a board of guardians, and the overseers of every parish not in a union nor under a board of guardians, a statement of the condition of every pauper lunatic chargeable to such union or parish.

Statement of condition of pauper lunatics to be transmitted to guardians.

35. The inquiries authorised to be made under section 64 of the Lunacy Act, chapter 100, or under section 92 of the same Act, and the provisions amending the same, may include inquiries as to the moneys paid to the superintendent or proprietor on account of any lunatic under the care of such superintendent or proprietor.

Amendment of Sect. 64, of 8 & 9 Vict. c. 100.

36. The proprietor * of every licensed house within the jurisdiction of visitors appointed by justices shall, within three days after a visit by the visiting Commissioners or Commissioner, transmit a true and perfect copy of the entries made by them or him in the Visitors' Book, the Patients' Book, and the Medical Visitation Book, respectively, distinguishing the entries in the several books, to the clerk of the visitors as well as to the Commissioners,† and the copies so transmitted to the clerk of the visitors of all such entries in the Visitors' Book relating to any such licensed house, and made since the grant or last renewal of the licence thereof, shall be laid before the justices on taking into consideration the renewal of the licence to the house to which such entries relate ; and every such proprietor as aforesaid who shall omit to transmit as hereinbefore mentioned a true and perfect copy of every or any such entry as aforesaid, shall for every such omission forfeit a sum not exceeding ten pounds.

Copies of entries of Commissioners and visitors.

37. The visiting committee of every union, and of every parish under a board of guardians, and the overseers of every

Visiting Committee to enter observations in a book respecting dietary,

* Vide 8 & 9 Vict. c. 100, s. 114.

† Vide 25 & 26 Vict. c. 111, s. 29.

accommodation, &c., of lunatics in workhouses.

parish not in a union nor under a board of guardians, shall once at the least in each quarter of a year enter in a book to be provided and kept by the master of the workhouse such observations as they may think fit to make respecting the dietary, accommodation, and treatment of the lunatics or alleged lunatics for the time being in the workhouse of their union or parish, and the book containing the observations made in pursuance of this section by the visiting guardians or overseers shall be laid by the master before the Commissioner or Commissioners on his or their next visit.

Miscellaneous Clauses.

Patients may be permitted to be absent on trial from hospitals and private houses.

38. Section 86 of the Lunacy Act, chapter 100, and section 17 of the Act eighteenth and nineteenth Victoria, chapter 105, shall extend to authorise the proprietor or superintendent of any licensed house or hospital, with such consent, and to be given on such approval as thereby required, to permit any patient to be absent from such hospital or house upon trial for such period as may be thought fit.

Two of the Commissioners, as regards any hospital or any licensed house, and two of the committee of governors of any hospital, and two of the visitors of any licensed house, as regards any licensed house within the jurisdiction of visitors, may of their own authority permit any pauper patient therein to be absent from such hospital or house upon trial for such period as they may think fit, and may make or order to be made an allowance to such pauper, not exceeding what would be the charge for him in such hospital or house, which allowance shall be charged for him, and be payable as if he were actually in such hospital or house, but shall be paid over to him, or for his benefit, as the said Commissioners or visitors may direct.

In case any person so allowed to be absent on trial for any period do not return at the expiration thereof, and a medical certificate as to his state of mind, certifying that his detention as a lunatic is no longer necessary, be not sent to the proprietor or superintendent of such licensed house or hospital, he may at any time within fourteen days after the expiration of the same period be retaken as in the case of an escape.*

* Vide 8 & 9 Vict. c. 100, ss. 53 & 99.

39. If any officer or servant in any hospital or licensed house through wilful neglect or connivance permits any patient to escape from such hospital or licensed house, or secretes or abets or connives at the escape of any patient from such hospital or licensed house, he shall for every such offence incur a penalty not exceeding twenty pounds.

Penalty on officer conniving at the escape of lunatics.

40. Every letter written by a private patient in any asylum, hospital, or licensed house, or by any single patient, and addressed to the Commissioners in Lunacy or committee, or in the case of houses within the jurisdiction of visitors to the visitors or any of them, shall, unless special regulations to the contrary have been given by such Commissioners or visitors, be forwarded unopened.

Correspondence of private patients.

Every letter written by a private patient in any asylum, hospital, or licensed house, or by any single patient, and addressed to any person other than the Commissioners or committee or visitors or one of them, shall be forwarded to the person to whom it is addressed, unless the superintendent in the case of an asylum or hospital, the proprietor in the case of a licensed house, and the person having the charge of a single patient in the case of a single patient, prohibit the forwarding of such letter, by endorsement to that effect under his hand on the letter, in which case he shall lay all letters so endorsed before the visiting Commissioners, committee, or visitors, as the case may be, on their next visit.

Any superintendent, proprietor, or person in charge of a single patient failing to comply with the provisions of this section as to laying any letter before the Commissioners or committee or visitors that is not forwarded to the address of the person to whom it is directed, or being privy to the detention by any other person of any letter detained in contravention of this section, shall incur a penalty not exceeding twenty pounds in respect of each offence ; and any person detaining any letter in contravention of this section shall incur, in respect of each letter so detained, a penalty not exceeding twenty pounds.

41. Every person having the care or charge of a single patient shall, in addition to the notice required to be given by the 90th section of the Lunacy Act, chapter 100, before the expiration of seven clear days from the day on which he has taken the patient under his care or charge, transmit to the Commissioners a statement of the condition of the patient, according to the form in Schedule F annexed to the said last-

Statement as to condition of single patients.

mentioned Act, such statement to be signed by the physician, surgeon, or apothecary visiting the patient in pursuance of the 90th section of the Lunacy Act, chapter 100.

If any person having the care or charge of a single patient fails to transmit such statement as aforesaid within such time as is required by this section, he shall be guilty of a misdemeanour.

Commissioners empowered to prescribe forms, &c., of Medical Visitation Book.

42. In the case of single patients, the Commissioners may, from time to time, make regulations as to the form of and the particulars to be entered in the "Medical Visitation Book," required to be kept by the 90th section of the Lunacy Act, chapter 100, and if the person having the care or charge of a single patient fails to comply with the regulations so made, he shall in respect of each offence incur a penalty not exceeding five pounds.

Discharge of a private patient.

43. If there be no person capable or qualified, under section 72 or section 73 of the said Lunacy Act, chapter 100, to direct the discharge or removal of any such patient as therein mentioned from any registered hospital or licensed house, the Commissioners may order the discharge or removal of such patient, as they may think fit.

Report to Coroner of death of single patient.

44. The superintendent of every asylum, and every person having the care or charge of a single patient, shall, in the event of the death of any patient, transmit to the coroner of the county or borough the same statement as is required by law to be transmitted in the case of the death of any patient in any hospital or licensed house, and if such coroner, after receiving such statement, thinks that any reasonable suspicion attends the cause and circumstances of the death of such patient, he shall summon a jury to inquire into the circumstances of such death.

Any superintendent or person in charge who makes default in complying with the requisitions of this section, shall be guilty of a misdemeanour.

Chargeability of pauper lunatics whose settlements cannot be ascertained where found in certain boroughs.

45. Section 14, of the Act of the Session holden in the eighteenth and nineteenth years of her Majesty, chapter 105, shall be repealed, and in lieu thereof be it enacted, Where any pauper lunatic is not settled in the parish by which or at the instance of some officer or officiating clergyman of which he is sent to an asylum, registered hospital, or licensed house, and it cannot be ascertained in what parish such pauper lunatic is settled, and such lunatic is found in a borough which has a sepa-

rate court of sessions of the peace, and is not liable, under the Act of the Session, holden in the fifth and sixth years of King William IV., chapter 76, section 117, to the payment of a proportion of the sums expended out of the county rate, or is found in any borough which under the Act of the Session, holden in the twelfth and thirteenth years of her Majesty, chapter 82, is exempted from liability to contribute to the payment of the expenses incurred for maintaining pauper lunatics chargeable to the county in which such borough is situate, such lunatic shall be adjudged to be chargeable to the borough in which he is found; and it shall not be lawful for any justices to adjudge such lunatic to be chargeable to any county, nor to make any order upon the treasurer of any county for the payment of any expenses whatsoever incurred or to be incurred in respect of such lunatic.

All the provisions in the Lunacy Act, chapter 97, as to the mode of determining that a pauper lunatic is chargeable to a county, and as to the orders to be made for payment of expenses and other moneys in respect of such lunatic, and for the repayment thereof to the treasurer of a county, shall extend to the case of a borough to which a lunatic is made chargeable under this section as if the said provisions were re-enacted in this Act, and such borough were therein mentioned or referred to instead of a county.

46. Any two or more Commissioners or visitors, in exercise of the powers given to them by the one hundredth section of the Lunacy Act, chapter 100, may, if they think fit, examine on oath any person appearing before them as a witness, notwithstanding a summons may not have been served on him in pursuance of the said section.

Amendment of 8 & 9 Vict. c. 100, s. 100, as to power of administering oaths.

47. The term physician, surgeon, or apothecary, wherever used in the Lunacy Acts, shall mean a person registered under "The Medical Act," passed in the session holden in the twenty-first and twenty-second years of the reign of her present Majesty, chapter 90.

Definition of physician, surgeon, or apothecary.

48. So much of section 132 of the Lunacy Act, chapter 97, as enacts that in that Act, unless there be something in the subject or context repugnant to such construction, the word "county" shall mean a county of a city, or county of a town, shall, except with respect to the city of London, be repealed, and all the provisions of the said Act, and of the Acts amending the same, shall be read and construed accordingly.

Part of sect. 132 of 16 & 17 Vict. c. 97 repealed.

SCHEDULE A.*

Form of Licence.

KNOW all Men, That we, the undersigned Justices of the Peace, acting in and for　　　　　　　　in General [*or* Quarter *or* Special] Sessions assembled, do hereby certify that *A.B.* of in the Parish of　　　　　　　　　in the County of hath delivered to the Clerk of the Peace a Plan and Description of a House and Premises proposed to be licensed for the Reception of Lunatics, situate at　　　　　　　　in the County of and which has not been previously licensed for that Purpose, and hath applied to us for a Licence thereof: And whereas the Particulars of the said Application have been transmitted to the Commissioners in Lunacy, and their Report in reference to the said Application has been received, and has been taken into consideration by us; and we, having considered and approved the Application, do hereby authorise and empower the said *A.B.* (he intending *or* not intending to reside therein) to use and employ the said House and Premises for the Reception of　　　　　　Male [*or* Female, *or*　　　　　Male and　　　　　Female] Lunatics, of whom not more than　　　　　shall be Private Patients, for the Space of Calendar Months from this Date.

　　Given under our Hand and Seals, this　　　　　　　　Day of
　　　　　　in the Year of our Lord One thousand eight
hundred and
　　　　　　　　Witness, *Y.Z., Clerk of the Peace.*

SCHEDULE B.

　County of
　Union [*or* Parish of]
　District of

QUARTERLY LIST of LUNATIC PAUPERS within the District of the
　Union of　　　　　　[*or* the Parish of　　　　　], in the County
　or Borough of　　　　　, not in any Asylum, Registered Hospital,
　or Licensed House.

　* Vide 8 & 9 Vict. c. 100, s. 30. And Sched. A of said Act.

Name.	Sex.	Age.	Form of Mental Disorder.	Duration of present Attack of Insanity, and if idiotic, whether or not from birth.	Resident in Workhouse.	Non-Resident in Workhouse, where and with whom resident.	Date of Visit.	In what Condition, and, if ever restrained, why, and by what Means, and how often.

I declare that I have personally examined the several Persons whose Names are specified in the above List on the Days set opposite their Names; and I certify, firstly, with respect to those appearing by the above List to be in the Workhouse, that the Accommodation in the Workhouse is sufficient for their Reception, and that they are all [*or* all except *A.B.* and *C.D.*] proper Patients to be kept in the Workhouse; and, secondly, with respect to those appearing by the above List to be resident elsewhere than in the Workhouse, that they are all [*or* all except *A.B.* and *C.D.*] properly taken care of, and may properly remain out of an Asylum.

I declare that the Persons in the above List are to the best of my knowledge the only Pauper Lunatics in the District of the Union of   [*or* in the Parish of   ] who are not in an Asylum, Registered Hospital, or duly Licensed House.

(Signed)   A.B.,

Medical officer of the   District
of the Union [or Parish] of

  Dated the   day of   One thousand eight hundred and

D D

FORMS OF NOTICES

REFERRED TO IN THE CHAPTER ON PAUPER LUNATICS.

———◆◇◆———

16 & 17 Vict. c. 97, s. 67 ; 25 & 26 Vict. c. 111, s. 19. No. 17.

MEDICAL OFFICER'S NOTICE TO RELIEVING OFFICER OF PAUPER LUNATIC.

To[1]

    Relieving Officer of the[2]   of

I, the undersigned, a Medical Officer of the[3]   Union,
in the Count of
which comprises the said[2]   of
having knowledge that one[4]
a Pauper, resident in the said[2]   of
which is within the District of which I am the Medical Officer, is[5]
[deemed to be] a Lunatic, DO HEREBY GIVE YOU NOTICE of the premises, that you may take the steps which the law requires you to
do in such behalf.

     As witness my Hand this   day of
        in the year of our Lord One thousand eight hundred and

                             Medical Officer.

———————

[1] *Insert name of Relieving Officer.*
[2] *Insert* Parish *or* Township, *as the case may be.*
[3] *Insert name of Union.*
[4] *Insert name of Lunatic.*
[5] *Here the Officer must state* is *or* is deemed to be, *as he thinks most proper under the circumstances of the case.*

16 & 17 Vict. c. 97, s. 67 ; 25 & 26 Vict. c. 111, s. 19. No. 18.

RELIEVING OFFICER'S NOTICE TO JUSTICE OF PAUPER LUNATIC.

To[1]

    one of Her Majesty's Justices of the Peace, acting in and for
        the[2]   of

I, the undersigned, a Relieving Officer of the[3]
Union, in the Count   of
having knowledge that one[4]
a Pauper, resident in the[5]   of
in the said[2]   which[5]   is comprised within
the said Union, and of which I am the Relieving Officer, is[6] [deemed
to be] a Lunatic, DO HEREBY GIVE YOU NOTICE of the premises, in
order that you may take such steps in such behalf as the law requires.

    As witness my Hand this   day of
        in the year of our Lord One thousand eight hundred and

                              Relieving Officer.

---

[1] *Insert name of Justice of the Peace.*   [5] *Insert* Parish *or* Township, *as the*
[2] *County or Borough.*   *case may be.*
[3] *Insert name of the Union.*   [6] *State according to the Notice.*
[4] *Insert name of Lunatic.*

---

16 & 17 Vict. c. 97, s. 67. No. 19. 25 & 26 Vict. c. 111, s. 19.

ORDER OF THE JUSTICE TO BRING PAUPER LUNATIC BEFORE HIM.

To[1]   of
    Relieving Officer of the[2]
    Union, in the[3]   of

I, the undersigned, one of Her Majesty's Justices of the Peace,
acting in and for the[6]   of
having received notice from you of your knowledge that one[7]
                    a Pauper resident in
the[4]   of[5]   which[4]
is comprised within the Union aforesaid, and of which[4]
you are the Relieving Officer, is[8] [deemed to be] a Lunatic, DO by
this Order under my Hand and Seal, require you to bring the said
alleged Lunatic before me, or before some other Justice of the
said   who shall then and

there be present, on   day next, the
being within three days from the time when such notice was given
to me as aforesaid, at   in
the⁶   aforesaid, to be dealt with as the law requires.

      GIVEN under my Hand and Seal, this   day of
      in the year of our Lord One thousand eight hundred and
          at   in the
      aforesaid.

                             (L.S.)

---

¹ *Insert name of the Relieving Officer.*   ⁵ *Name of Parish or Township.*
² *Insert name of Union.*   ⁶ *County or Borough.*
³ *Name of County.*   ⁷ *Name of Pauper Lunatic.*
⁴ *Insert* Parish *or* Township.   ⁸ *State* is *or* is deemed to be.

---

16 & 17 Vict. c. 97, s. 67.   No. 20.   25 & 26 Vict. c. 111, Sec. 19.

REQUEST OF JUSTICE TO MEDICAL PRACTITIONER TO ASSIST HIM IN THE EXAMINATION OF A PAUPER LUNATIC.

      To¹
          of   ²

      Sir,
WHEREAS one³
a Pauper resident in the⁴   of
in the⁵   of   which⁴
is comprised in the ⁶   Union, who is alleged to be a
Lunatic, having been brought before me, one of Her Majesty's
Justices of the Peace acting in and for the said⁵   with
the intent that I should issue an Order in such behalf accordingly,
I DO THEREFORE hereby request you to attend before me this
day⁷   at   in the⁵
of   to examine such alleged Lunatic, and
render me all the assistance in your power in relation to the matter
aforesaid.

               I am,
                     Your obèdient servant,

---

¹ *Insert name of Medical Practitioner.*   ⁴ *Insert* Parish *or* Township.
² *Insert* Physician, Surgeon, *or* Apothecary,   ⁵ *County or Borough.*
    as the case may be.   ⁶ *Name of Union.*
³ *Name of Pauper.*   ⁷ *Or the day of the hearing.*

16 & 17 Vict. c. 97, s. 89. Schedule F. No. 4. (3.)

NOTICE OF ADMISSION OF A PAUPER PATIENT.

I HEREBY GIVE YOU NOTICE, That [1]
was admitted into this Asylum as a Pauper Patient, on the
     day of   18 , and I hereby transmit a Copy of
the Order and Statement and Medical Certificate on which [2] he was
received.

Subjoined is a Statement with respect to the Mental and Bodily
Condition of the above-named Patient.

(Signed)

Clerk of   Asylum.

Dated this   day of
One thousand eight hundred and

To the Commissioners in Lunacy.

STATEMENT.

I have this day [3] seen and examined [1]
the Patient mentioned in the above Notice, and hereby Certify, that
with respect to Mental State [2] he

.

.

and that with respect to Bodily Health and Condition [2] he

.

.

(Signed)

Medical Officer of   Asylum.

Dated this   day of
One thousand eight hundred and

----

[1] *Here insert the Patient's name.*
[2] *Insert* she *where necessary.*
[3] Some day not less than *two* nor more than *seven* clear days after the admission of the Patient.

NOTE.—The 16 & 17 Vict. c. 97 requires the Clerk of the Asylum, after the *second* and before the end of the *seventh* clear day from the day of the admission of the Lunatic into the Asylum, to transmit this document to the Commissioners in Lunacy, subject to a penalty of 20*l.* for his omission.

16 & 17 Vict. c. 97, s. 73.   Sched. (F.) No. 1.

COPY OF THE ORDER FOR THE RECEPTION OF A PAUPER PATIENT.

the undersigned, having called to[2]   Assistance a[3]
and having personally examined
a Pauper,[4] and being satisfied that the said
is a[5]   [6]

and a proper person to be taken charge of
and detained under Care and Treatment, hereby direct you to receive the said   as a
Patient into your Asylum.

Subjoined is a Statement respecting the said

(Signed)

Dated the   day of   One
thousand eight hundred and

To

Superintendent of the Asylum for the
of

---

[1] I, *C. D.*, a justice of the peace for the county, city, or borough of ——; *or in case of two justices, or of a clergyman and relieving officer, or overseer*, We, *C. D.*, and *E. F.*

[2] My *or* our.

[3] Physician, *or* surgeon, *or* apothecary, *as the case may be.*

[4] *Omit the words* a pauper, *when the lunatic is not a pauper.*

[5] Lunatic, *or* an idiot, *or* a person of unsound mind.

[6] *Add, where the lunatic is sent as being wandering at large, the words* wandering at large, *and in the case of a lunatic sent by virtue of the authority given to two justices, add* not under proper care and control, *or* and is cruelly treated *or* neglected by the person having the care or charge of him, *as may appear to the justices to be the case.*

[7] Justices of the peace for the county or borough of ——; *or* an *or* the officiating clergyman of the parish of ——. *To be signed by two justices where required by the Act.*

[8] The relieving officer of the union *or* parish of ——, *or* an overseer of the parish of ——.

[9] *State the special circumstances (if any) in the blank space.*

Where the order directs the lunatic to be received into any asylum other than an

STATEMENT.

*If any Particulars in this Statement be not known, the Fact
to be so stated.*

Name of Patient, and Christian }
  Name, at length   . . }

Sex and Age   .   .   .   .

Married, Single, or Widowed .

Condition of Life, and Previous }
  Occupation (if any) .   . }

The Religious Persuasion, as far }
  as known   .   .   . }

Previous Place of Abode . .

Whether first Attack .   .   .

Age (if known) on first Attack .

When and where previously }
  under Care and Treatment }

Duration of existing Attack.   .

Supposed Cause .   .   .

Whether subject to Epilepsy .

Whether Suicidal .   .   .

Whether Dangerous to others .

Parish or Union to which the }
  Lunatic is chargeable (if a }
  Pauper. or destitute Lunatic) }

Name and Christian Name, and }
  Place of Abode of nearest }
  known relative of the Patient, }
  and degree of Relationship }
  (if known)   .   .   . }

    I Certify that, to the best of my knowledge, the above particulars are correctly stated,

(Signed)

---

*asylum of the county or borough in which the parish or place from which the lunatic
is sent is situate, or into a registered hospital or licensed house, it should state that
the justice or justices, or other persons making the order, is or are satisfied that there
is no asylum of such county or borough, or that the asylum or asylums thereof is or
are full; or (as the case may require) the special circumstances by reason whereof
the lunatic cannot conveniently be taken to an asylum for such first-mentioned county
or borough.*

16 & 17 Vict. c. 97, s. 73. Sched. (F.) No. 3.

COPY OF THE MEDICAL CERTIFICATE.

I, the undersigned, being a[1]

and being in actual Practice as a[2]   hereby Certify,
that I, on the   day of   at[3]
in the County of
[4]
personally examined[5]

and that the said
is a[6]   and a proper Person to be
taken charge of and detained under Care and Treatment, and that
I have formed this opinion upon the following grounds; viz.—

    1. Facts indicating Insanity observed by myself[7]—

    2. Other Facts indicating Insanity communicated to me by
       others[8]

           (Signed)

           Place of Abode

Dated this   day of   One
      thousand eight hundred and

---

[1] *Here set forth the qualification entitling the person certifying to practise as a physician, surgeon, or apothecary, e.g.:*—Fellow of the Royal College of Physicians in London, Licentiate of the Apothecaries' Company, *or as the case may be.*
[2] Physician, surgeon, or apothecary, *as the case may be.*
[3] *Here insert the street and number of house (if any) or other like particulars.*
[4] *In any case where more than one medical certificate is required by this Act, here insert,* separately from any other medical practitioner.
[5] *A. B. of* ——. *Insert residence, and profession or occupation (if any).*
[6] Lunatic, or an idiot, or a person of unsound mind.
[7] *Here state the facts.*
[8] *Here state the information (if any) and from whom.*

16 & 17 Vict. c. 97, s. 79. No. 41.

ORDER FOR DISCHARGE OF LUNATIC FROM ASYLUM BY THE VISITORS THEREOF.

[1] WE, the undersigned, being Justices of the Peace acting in and for the [1] of and two of the Visitors of the Lunatic Asylum situate at [2] in the [1] of DO HEREBY, with the advice in writing of the Medical Officer thereof, ORDER one [3] a Lunatic, now detained in the said Asylum to be discharged therefrom [4]

of

to wit.

GIVEN under our Hands and Seals, this day of in the year of our Lord One thousand eight hundred and at in the aforesaid.

(L. S.)

(L. S.)

----

[1] *County or Borough.*
[2] *Place of Lunatic Asylum.*
[3] *Name of Lunatic.*
[4] *Add* forthwith, *or* on the day of

CERTIFICATE OF MEDICAL OFFICER.

I, the Medical Officer of the Lunatic Asylum at in the [1] of from which it hath been proposed that one a Lunatic, now detained in the said Asylum, should be ordered by two of the Visitors of the said Asylum to be discharged, DO HEREBY CERTIFY to such Justices that such Lunatic in my judgment may be discharged from such Asylum.

As witness my Hand, this day of at

(L. S.)

8 & 9 Vict. c. 100, s. 74. No. 49.

ORDER FOR DISCHARGE OR REMOVAL OF A PAUPER LUNATIC FROM A LICENSED HOUSE.

To[1]   the[2]   of the[3]
    at[4]   in the[5]   of

Sir,—I am directed by the Board of Guardians of the[6]
    in the[5]   of   to transmit to you a Copy
of a Minute of the Board respecting a Pauper Lunatic now confined
in your[3]   and to request that the same may receive due
attention from you.

                I am,
                   Yours truly,

                              Clerk to the said Guardians.*

        Dated this   day of

---

[1] *Insert Name.*
[2] Proprietor *or* Superintendent.
[3] *Licensed House or Registered Hospital.*

[4] *Insert Name of Place.*
[5] County *or* Borough.
[6] *Insert* Union *or* Parish.

* Upon receipt of a Copy of this Minute, the Proprietor or Superintendent shall forthwith discharge or remove such Patient, or cause or suffer such Patient to be removed, unless the Physician, Surgeon, or Apothecary keeping the same, or the regular Medical Attendant thereof, in writing under his hand, certify that in his opinion such Patient is dangerous and unfit to be at large, together with the grounds on which such opinion is founded. 8 & 9 Vict. c. 100, ss. 74, 75.

COPY OF A MINUTE OF THE BOARD OF GUARDIANS OF THE

              Dated the   day of

    Resolved,—That[7]   a Pauper Lunatic belonging
to this[6]   and now detained in the[3]   at[4]
       in the[5]   of   shall be forthwith
[8]   therefrom, and that[9]   be[3]   in the manner
following: that is to say—[10]

                    (signed)

                        Presiding Chairman.

---

[7] *Name of Lunatic.*
[8] Removed *or* discharged.

[9] He *or* she.
[10] *Here set out the mode of discharge or removal.*

16 & 17 Vict. c. 97, s. 68. No. 22.

INFORMATION AS TO A LUNATIC WANDERING AT LARGE.

³⎤ THE INFORMATION of¹   of²

of   ⎱ in the³   of   taken upon
   ⎰ oath before me, the undersigned, one of Her Majesty's
   ⎰ Justices of the Peace acting in and for the³

to wit. ⎦ of   this day and year underwritten, who
informeth me that one⁴   is wandering at large
within the limits of my jurisdiction, that is to say, within the³
of   and is deemed to be a Lunatic.

WHEREFORE the said Informant applies to me to issue my Order, under my Hand and Seal, in such behalf, according to the Statute in such case made and provided.

SWORN before me, this   day of   in the year of our
Lord One thousand eight hundred and   at
in the³   of

----

¹ *Insert name of Informant.*
² *His place of abode.*
³ *Insert* County *or* Borough.
⁴ *Name of Lunatic.*

----

16 & 17 Vict. c. 97, s. 68. No. 23.

ORDER OF JUSTICE TO BRING A WANDERING LUNATIC BEFORE HIM.

³⎤ To¹   of²   in

of   ⎱ the³   of   the⁴
   ⎰ of the⁵   of

to wit. ⎦ WHEREAS one⁶   of   hath this
day appeared before me, the undersigned, one of Her
Majesty's Justices of the Peace acting in and for the³   of
and upon his oath hath informed me that one⁶
is wandering at large within the limits of my jurisdiction,
that is to say, within the³   of   and is deemed to
be a Lunatic.

THIS THEREFORE is to require you forthwith to apprehend the said⁶
and bring⁷   before me, or before some other
Justice having jurisdiction in the said³   if the said

shall be apprehended therein, to be dealt with as the aw may require.

And this shall be your sufficient warrant.

Given under my Hand and Seal, this   day of   in the year of our Lord One thousand eight hundred and   at   in the

(L. S

---

[1] *Insert name of Person to whom Order is addressed.*
[2] *Place of his abode.*
[3] County *or* Borough.
[4] Constable, Relieving Officer, *or* Overseer of the Poor.
[5] Parish *or* Township.
[6] *Insert from the Information.*
[7] *Insert* him *or* her *as the case may require.*

---

16 & 17 Vict. c. 97, s. 68. No. 24.

REQUEST OF JUSTICE TO MEDICAL PRACTITIONER TO ASSIST HIM IN THE EXAMINATION OF A WANDERING LUNATIC.

To[1]   of   [2]

Sir,—WHEREAS Information having been made before me, on oath, that one[3]   wandering at large within the limits of my jurisdiction, is deemed to be a Lunatic, I have, by an Order under my Hand and Seal, ordered him to be brought before me, at   in the   or before some other Justices having jurisdiction in the said[4]   to be dealt with as the law may require: I DO THEREFORE hereby request you to attend before me, or such other Justices, at the time and place aforesaid, to examine such alleged Lunatic, and to render me or them every assistance in your power in relation to the matter aforesaid.

I am,

Your obedient servant,

---

[1] *Insert name of Medical Practitioner.*
[2] *Insert* Physician, Surgeon, *or* Apothecary, *as the case may be.*
[3] *Name of Lunatic.*
[4] *Insert* County *or* Borough.

16 & 17 Vict. c. 97, s. 68.   No. 25.

INFORMATION AS TO A LUNATIC NOT UNDER PROPER CARE AND CONTROL, OR CRUELLY TREATED OR NEGLECTED.

⁴⎫   The Information of¹   of

of ⎰ [the²   of the³   of   ], in

⎱the⁴   of   given upon oath before me,

     the undersigned, one of Her Majesty's Justices of the

to wit. ⎭ Peace acting in and for the said⁴   the day and

year underwritten, who informeth me that one⁵

of the said³   in the⁴   aforesaid, and within the

limits of my jurisdiction, not a Pauper, and not a Person wandering at large, is deemed to be a Lunatic, and is⁶

Wherefore the said Informant applies to me to inquire into the matters aforesaid, and deal with the same as the case shall appear to me to require.

Sworn before me, this   day of   in the year of our Lord One thousand eight hundred and   at in the

---

¹ *Insert name of the Informant.*
² *Insert* Constable, Relieving Officer, *or* Overseer, *as the case may be; or if any other person give information, erase the words within the brackets.*
³ *Insert* Parish *or* Township.
⁴ County *or* Borough.
⁵ *Name of Lunatic.*
⁶ *Insert, as the case may be,* not under proper care and control; *or* cruelly treated by his (*or* her) relative, *or* by the person having the care *or* charge of him *or* her; *or* neglected by his (*or* her) relative, *or* by the person having the care *or* charge of him (*or* her).

---

16 & 17 Vict. c. 97, s. 68.   No. 27.

ORDER OF JUSTICE TO BRING LUNATIC, NOT A PAUPER, BUT ALLEGED TO BE NEGLECTED OR ILL-TREATED BEFORE TWO JUSTICES.

³⎫   To¹

of ⎰ of²   in the³

⎱ of   the⁴

⁴ ⎰ of the⁵   of

to wit. ⎭ in the³   of

Whereas Information having been given before me, the undersigned, one of Her Majesty's Justices of the Peace acting in and for the[2]   of   on oath

that one[6]   of

the[7]   of   in

the[3]   of   and with-

in the limits of my jurisdiction, not a Pauper, and not a person

wandering at large, was deemed to be a Lunatic, and was[8]

.

.   I did by an Order under my Hand

and Seal, bearing date[9]

.   order one[9]

being a[9]   to visit and examine the said[6]

.   and make inquiry into the matters

aforesaid, and report to me his opinion thereon. AND WHEREAS the

said[9]   hath visited and examined the said[6]

.   and made inquiry into

such matters, and hath reported to me in writing his opinion there-

on. AND WHEREAS upon such report it appears to me that the

matters of such Information are true.

Now THEREFORE I do hereby order you to take the said[6]

                        and bring[10]   before two Justices,

at   in the[3]   aforesaid, on the

day of   there to be dealt with as the law shall require.

GIVEN under my Hand, this   day of

in the year of our Lord One thousand eight hundred

and   at

in the

(L.S.)

---

[1] *Name of person to whom the Order is to be addressed.*

[2] *Place of his abode.*

[3] County *or* Borough.

[4] Constable, Relieving Officer, *or* Overseer of the Poor.

[5] Parish *or* Township.

[6] *Name of Lunatic.*

[7] *Place of his abode.*

[8] *Insert, as the case may be,* not under proper care and control ; *or* cruelly treated by his (*or* her) relative, *or* the person having the care *or* control of him (*or* her) ; *or* neglected by his (*or* her) relative, *or* by the person having the care *or* control of him (*or* her).

[9] *Insert* Physician, Surgeon, *or* Apothecary, *from the Order.*

[10] *Insert* him *or* her.

16 & 17 Vict. c. 97, s. 68. No. 26.

ORDER OF A JUSTICE TO A MEDICAL PRACTITIONER TO VISIT A LUNATIC ALLEGED TO BE ILL-TREATED OR NEGLECTED.

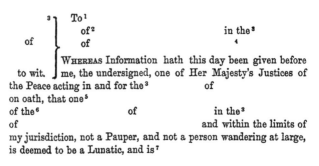

To [1]

of [2]   in the [3]

of   of   4

to wit.   WHEREAS Information hath this day been given before me, the undersigned, one of Her Majesty's Justices of the Peace acting in and for the [3]   of on oath, that one [5]
of the [6]   of   in the [3]
of   and within the limits of my jurisdiction, not a Pauper, and not a person wandering at large, is deemed to be a Lunatic, and is [7]

Now THEREFORE I do hereby Order you to visit and examine such Person and make inquiry into the matters aforesaid, and to report in writing to me your opinion thereupon with all due speed, and for your so doing this shall be your sufficient authority.

GIVEN under my Hand and Seal, this   day of in the year of our Lord One thousand eight hundred and   at in the   of

                         (L.S.)

---

[1] *Name of* Physician, Surgeon, *or* Apothecary.
[2] *Place of his residence.*
[3] County *or* Borough.
[4] *Insert here* Physician, Surgeon, *or* Apothecary, *as the case may be.*
[5] *Name of Lunatic.*
[6] Parish *or* Township.
    Insert, as the case may be, not under proper care and control; *or* cruelly treated by his (*or* her) relative, *or* by the person having the care *or* charge of him (*or* her); *or* neglected by his (*or* her) relative, *or* by the person having the care *or* charge of him (*or* her).

16 & 17 Vict. c. 97, s. 68. No. 28.

REQUEST OF TWO JUSTICES TO MEDICAL PRACTI-TIONERS TO ASSIST THEM IN THE EXAMINATION OF A LUNATIC ALLEGED TO BE ILL-TREATED OR NEGLECTED.

To [1]
of [2]

Sir,

WHEREAS [4]   one of Her Majesty's Justices of the Peace acting in and for the [5] of   having, after information on oath before him that one [6]
          of [7]   deemed to be a Lunatic, was [8]

and after due enquiry into the matters of such information, ordered the said [6]   to be brought before us, the undersigned, Justices of the Peace for the said [5]   on   at
                    in the said [5]   there to be dealt with as the law shall require.

WE DO THEREFORE hereby request you to attend before us, at the time aforesaid, to examine such alleged Lunatic, and to render us all the assistance in your power in relation to the matter aforesaid.

We are,
          Your obedient servants,

---

[1] *Insert name of Medical Practitioner.*
[2] *His abode.*
[3] Physician, Surgeon, *or* Apothecary.
[4] *Insert name of Justice*; *if one of those signing this Request, insert,* I, the undersigned, A. B.
[5] County *or* Borough.
[6] *Name of Lunatic.*
[7] *Place of his abode.*
[8] *Insert, as the case may be,* not under proper care and control; *or* cruelly treated by his (*or* her) relative, *or* by the person having the care *or* control of him (*or* her); *or* neglected by his (*or* her) relative, *or* by the person having the care *or* control of him (*or* her).

E E

16 & 17 Vict. c. 97, s. 77. No. 40.

ORDER FOR REMOVAL OF PAUPER LUNATIC TO AN ASYLUM BY THE VISITORS THEREOF.

[4] To [1]
of
of   the [2]   of the [3]

to wit.   WE, the undersigned, being Justices of the Peace acting in and for the [4]   of
and two of the visitors of the Lunatic Asylum, situate at [5]
                    in the [4]   of
                    and belonging [6]   to the
said [4]   DO HEREBY ORDER YOU, with all due speed, to remove one [7]
a Pauper Lunatic chargeable to the   aforesaid, and now confined in the [8]   of
to the said Asylum at [5]

     GIVEN under our Hands and Seals, this   day
        of   in the year of our Lord One thousand
     eight hundred and   at
          in the   aforesaid.

                              (L.S.)

                              (L.S.)

---

[1] *Name of Officer.*   [5] *Place of Lunatic Asylum.*
[2] Overseer, Relieving Officer, *or other Officer.*   [6] *Add* wholly *or* in part.
[3] Union, Parish, *or* County.   [7] *Name of Lunatic.*
[4] County, *or* Borough.   [8] Asylum, Registered Hospital, *or* Licensed House.

CERTIFICATE OF MEDICAL OFFICER.

I, the Medical Officer of the Lunatic Asylum at
         in the [4]   of
from which one
a Pauper Lunatic, now in the said Asylum, hath been ordered by two of the visitors of the Pauper Lunatic Asylum at
         in the [4]   of
to be removed thereto, DO HEREBY CERTIFY that such Lunatic is in a fit condition of bodily health to be removed, in pursuance of such Order.

     As witness my Hand, this   day of
       18   at

                              (L.S.)

INDEX.

———◇◇———

A

ABSENCE,
 leave of, granted to private patients from asylums, 53, 335, 396
 of pauper patients, 99

ACTIONS,
 for illegal detention of a single patient, 88, 89
 for reception of a lunatic without medical certificate, 161
 against the person who signed the order, 163–165
 against a non-registered practitioner for signing a certificate, 168, 169
 brought against proprietor, what may be pleaded in, 341, 342
 limitation of, 345
 for wilfully obstructing orders of Commissioners, Lord Chancellor, or Secretary of State, 373

ACTS,
 Lunacy Act, 8, 9 Vict. c. 100 (1845), 299–360
  ,, ,, 16, 17 Vict. c. 96 (1853), 361–378
 Amendment Act, 25, 26 Vict. c. 111 (1862), 382–401
 copy of (1845) to be bound up in Visitors' Book, 327–374
 section in Vagrant (1744), 7

ADMISSION,
 of private patients into asylums, 41, 56–81
 instructions by Commissioners, relative to, 252–256
 order for, 56–59, 252, 254, 376
 notice of, sent to Commissioners, 44, 356
 form of, 370
 of Chancery patients into asylums, 139, 391
 of single patients into unlicensed houses, 82–89, 336, 364
  ,, Chancery lunatics into unlicensed houses, 133, 336
 of pauper lunatics into county asylums, 94–97
  ,,   ,, licensed houses, 100, 390, 364

B

I

J

JURISDICTION OF COMMISSIONERS IN LUNACY,
   places within, 30, 306
JURY,
   when one may be demanded by alleged lunatic, 116
   Commission, *de lunatico inquirendo*, without a, 117
   power of Master to summon a, 122
   jury to be had if lunatic is beyond jurisdiction, 120
   examination of alleged lunatic by, 123
JUSTICES OF THE PEACE, *ex-officio* visitors of asylums, 30, 308
   pauper lunatic ordered to be brought before, 95, 98
   notice given to, that a lunatic is resident in parish, 97, 404
   in the examination of the lunatic may be assisted by a medical
      man, 98, 405
   lunatic wandering at large to be brought before, 103, 412
   licensed house beyond the jurisdiction of Commissioners
      granted by, 30, 308
   granting of licences by, 206
   offence against Lunacy Act, person to be brought before, 343
   form of conviction by, 344
   who meant by, 350
   order issued to bring pauper lunatic before the, 404
   assisted by a medical man in examination of wandering lunatic,
      413, 417
   provisions respecting ill-treatment of wandering lunatic, orders
      issued by, 414-417

K

KLEPTOMANIA, 278-280 ·

L

LIABILITIES,
   of proprietors and superintendents of asylums, 160-162
   of person who signed order, 163-165
   of medical men signing certificates, 165-169
LICENCES,
   for houses situated beyond the jurisdiction of Commissioners
      granted by justices of the peace, 30, 308
   of houses within the jurisdiction of the Commissioners, 34, 313
   form of, 34, 353, 400
   Commissioners', remarks on, 34-38
   duration of, 38, 313

F F

ORDER
>   for admission of private patient, 56–59, 252, 254, 320, 362
>   amendment of, 365, 392
>   form of, for private patients, 376
>   form of, for pauper lunatics, 407
>   for single patients into unlicensed house, 83–85, 336, 364
>   persons prohibited from signing the, 56, 365, 391
>   liabilities of persons signing, 163, 362
>   only available for one month from date of signing, 58, 391
>   for admission into St. Luke's Hospital, 145
>   ,,   Bethlehem ditto, 156
>   for admission into county asylums, 95–97, 407
>   for Commission of lunacy, 117, 120
>   power of court to refuse such, 118
>   for delivering up lunatic's documents, 131
>   issued after Commission, 132
>   for supersedeas, 136
>   In SCOTLAND,—
>   granted by sheriff, 172
>   In IRELAND,—
>   for admission, 190, 191

P

PARISH,
>   meaning of, 349

PATIENTS. (*See* LUNATICS—SINGLE PATIENT—PRIVATE PATIENTS.)
>   meaning of term in Act, 350
>   book of, 46

PAUPER PATIENTS, 94–110, 364
>   meaning of term in Act, 94, 350
>   proceedings prior to admission into county asylum of, 94
>   notice sent to relieving officer of parish, 94–97, 390, 403
>   section of Act especially referring to, 94–97
>   summary of chief sections relating to, 97–98
>   examined by minister of parish, 97, 407
>   ordered to be brought before a justice of the peace, 98, 390, 404
>   one medical certificate only required for, 98, 364
>   provision for sending to licensed houses, or workhouses, 98,
>   100, 390, 394
>   leave of absence of, 99, 335
>   discharge of by Visitors, 99, 332, 410
>   reception of by relatives at home, 99
>   death of, 99, 321, 368

W

Y

LONDON: PRINTED BY
SPOTTISWOODE AND CO., NEW-STREET SQUARE
AND PARLIAMENT STREET